DEATH IN THE LOCKER ROOM

ONE DAY A YOUNG KID IN HIGH SCHOOL CAME INTO MY GYM and showed me some pills he said his high school coach gave him to help him get stronger. The coach told him they were amino acids and vitamins, but they turned out to be Dianabol. I then spoke to a policeman, who told me not to even bother and follow up because it's just a misdemeanor. The coach would get in more trouble for a marijuana cigarette. We tell all the kids who come to us not to take anything unless they know what it is.

Cheryl Jones
97-pound World Powerlifting Champion

DEATH IN THE LOCKER ROOM
Steroids & Sports

Bob Goldman

with
Patricia Bush, Ph.D.
Ronald Klatz, D.O.

Title Creation by June Colbert

CENTURY PUBLISHING
LONDON

The use of public photographs in this text in no way implies that those people pictured have ever, are, or ever will, take illegal drugs. The pictures are used only to depict the excitement of sport competition.

The typefaces used in this book are Triumvirate Bold Italic and Paladium Text and Bold Italic. Typesetting and camera-ready art was done by Point West, Inc., Carol Stream, Illinois 60188.

1   2   3   4   5   6   87   86   85   84

Icarus Press, Inc.
P.O. Box 1225
South Bend, Indiana 46624

Copyright © Bob Goldman, Ronald Klatz,
Patricia Bush, 1984

All rights reserved

First published in Great Britain in 1984
by Century Publishing Co. Ltd.
Portland House
12-13 Greek Street, London W1V 5LE
ISBN 0 7126 0954 7

To the late John B. Ziegler, M.D.—
colleague, teacher, and dear friend—
I dedicate this work.
And to my parents, Arnold and Alice,
and my grandmother, Rose.

TABLE OF CONTENTS

FOREWORD

For many years the problem of drug abuse in sports was hidden and behind the scenes, almost a taboo issue. Perhaps people were afraid it would present a negative picture of sport competition and athletic advancement. Only recently has this critical problem been thrust into the public's mind and eye.

Here in the United States, there were concerns about our supremacy and ability to compete in view of the suspicion that Eastern athletes were taking drugs, being monitored, and working closely with their sports scientists and pharmacologists. Some of our athletes felt coerced into drug abuse as their only chance of winning.

During this time period, spanning the last decade, it is commendable that Bob Goldman, a world class athlete-medical scientist, has meticulously collected information pertaining to the health aspects and ethical concerns surrounding this dilemma. This important work brings together in narrative book form the many events that have occurred via the media's perceptions as well as extensive documentation of the world's scientific research literature over a nine-year period.

In 1979, Lord Killanin, then president of the International Olympic Committee, suggested that the most important issue facing the future of the Olympic games would be the problems relating to drug abuse in athletic performance.

William E. Simon, current president of the United State Olympic Committee, courageously has taken a strong position of leadership with the highest of ethical directives to clean up all of sport and preserve the health, integrity, and right of athletes to compete honestly and with their own true natural capabilities. He and executive director of the United States Olympic Committee, F. Don Miller, have worked closely with the U.S. Olympic Council on Sports Medicine to design a strong program of drug testing, education, and medical research.

The significance of this program is that it is destined to be the strongest in the world and is the first national effort of any program to eliminate this threat to athletic health and freedom. In addition to the significant and vital cooperation William E. Simon and F. Don Miller have created with the sports medicine resources in this country, they are now coordinating a conglomerate of the best high tech scientific training and sports medicine research programs to give athletes access to the best possible training systems, to become the finest athletes on earth—without drugs.

This is a multi-disciplinary attack, a potent force in solving the drug problem. We have the people to bring not only the best of sports science to the athlete but those who carry ethics and truth. Science itself is neutral; there is no right or wrong. The law of gravity, for example, is neither good nor bad. What is not neutral are the scientists, the practitioners, who take new concepts and make them good or bad as they present them to the athletes. The comprehensive Olympic Sports Medicine program will make drugs obsolete and a nonissue. By carefully integrating all this research and knowledge and making it useful and accessible to all our athletes, we can take one quantum leap beyond what 1,200 years of Olympic games have witnessed—to cultivate the athletes' innate peak potential.

Under the strong direction of William E. Simon, F. Don Miller, and our sports scientists, in a country of 250 million people with the greatest natural resources in the world, we will have not only the best sports medicine program, but we will have established a strong foundation of wisdom. This book is one of the building blocks. You will see an Olympic team in 1988 that will be the best in the world. All that needs to be created is the proper line of communication between athletes, coaches, science, and the Olympic Committee that will filter down to all levels of competition.

Irving I. Dardik, M.D., F.A.C.S.
Chairman, U.S. Olympic Committee Council on Sports Medicine

PREFACE

"...And it's not likely to go away. Until, that is, the bodies are piled high in the wings to the left and right of the playing fields, sportsmen defrocked of their power, and athletes' reputations as black as the midnight sky...and the phrase "physical culture" evolves in its maturity to about the credibility level of a garbage landfill on a one hundred degree day, with all the disease that festers beneath the rotting refuse."

Denie

JANUARY 1972

The air is thick and musty and the boom of the heavy bass of inner-city disco music reverberates through the large gymnasium, teeming with bodies covered in skin-tight, sleek, nylon wrestling gear. I have a sick feeling in the pit of my stomach, after having not eaten for three days, in order to make weight for the New York Wrestling Championships. Having to lose twenty-one pounds in the last five days, my guts feel as if they had been bound with wire and dropped down an elevator shaft. Daydreaming for a minute and blocking out the sound of grunts and thuds as bodies clash in battle on the mats, I reflect on this past week: The wearing of three layers of sweat suits so I'd sweat more; running and wrestling until I passed out in puddles of sweat-laden garb in a pool of body perspiration; the countless flights of stairs climbed; the tonnage of weight moved in endless repetitions, until muscle fibers screamed for relief as the weights clanged to the floor. What am I doing here? And why do I want to win this tournament so badly? Three weeks ago, in an accident, I separated my wrestling coach's shoulder going over moves together. Was this the drive?—to win, for him?

Like a twig snapping, I am removed from this dazed state by a teammate's tapping on my shoulder. "Your name's been called," he says slowly.

I had won my first three matches decidedly, but not without incident. I can taste the dried blood in my mouth from the elbow that conveniently found its way there. I think two of my fingers are broken, but the white tape is hiding most of the swelling that is peeking out from the uneven cracks. I'm so dehydrated, my lips keep sticking together and my tongue cleaves to the roof of my mouth. My lips cracked, I retort, "So soon?"

I begin to feel the adrenalin, what's left of it, surge in my body as I walk past the judge's table, and in the corner of my eye I catch a glitter of the trophy's reflections, the award we are all fighting for.

What seems like only an instant later, the whistle sounds, as my muscles are again interlocked in battle. I feel my muscles swell as the fatigue is replaced by rage and desire to win. Seconds of combat feel like minutes. My opponent makes the fatal mistake, and I clamp on him like a vice. It is over. As the referee holds up my arm, the room begins to spin and darken, my legs go to soft rubber, and I fall, like a loose sack of potatoes, to the floor. I ache all over, bloodied and sweat-laden—yet it feels so warm and wonderful inside. I won, and that was all I cared about.

I understand only too well the obsession with athletic victory. However, over the past decade, I have come to see the pain and agony of others caught within its grip. Athletic competition is the final avenue where men and women from all nations might join arms and embrace after the battle, where all benefit in some way.

The experience is the finest, with the pinnacle experience of all being the Olympics. But this crystal is flawed. Only the winner is rewarded, and gold medals have become MX missiles on the winner's side, nationalistic pride counted by the quantity of medals won . . . at any cost. Today's hero, tomorrow's has-been, with the athlete caught in the middle.

We are all easy victims to the pride syndrome. I too cheered with glee as our boys beat the Russians in hockey for the gold at Lake Placid in '80. The players became immediate national heroes. The Olympics are no longer athletic but are political power confrontations, with all of us as pawns.

It's big business. For example, the 1984 Olympics issued an official credit card, American Express; an official gasoline, an official video game maker, insurance company, camera, candy bar, car, drink, and beer—to name a few. All for a price.

But what it all comes down to in most peoples' minds is East v.

West, Communism v. the Free World. I had a dream since a young child of going to the Olympics in wrestling. Dan Gable was my idol, and I was filled with American pride as he blew everyone off the mat. Repeated knee injuries kept me from my dream, so world records for the *Guinness Book of World Records* provided my semblance of the dream. But how far will an athlete go to reach his or her dream?

This book is the story of dreams, some shattered into nightmares. I want very much for the Olympics to survive and for our athletes to live normal lives after the trumpets have sounded and the camera flashes have died out. The drug-abuse epidemic threatens to swallow this dream. I hope this book will be the catalyst to make people angry enough to do something about it.

ACKNOWLEDGEMENTS

During the past decade I spent writing this book, I had the pleasure of getting to know and correspond with many fine people. I remember working at the gymnasium part-time after school years back and taking my big weekly check of $33.50 to the bank to exchange for dimes so that I could run to the library to photocopy new articles. I would then stick them inside my jacket and run home to store them in boxes I kept hidden in my basement files. These boxes have since been replaced with an elaborate, scientific series of filing systems I've amassed during the last third of my life.

In many ways, I had to be a detective to hunt down the facts, but without the valuable cooperation of the many I wish to acknowledge here, this book would never have seen print.

June Colbert and Denie have been with me over this past ten years, and I am much indebted to their belief in this project. Ben Weider, president of the International Federation of Body Builders, has dedicated his life to promoting this health sport and has single-handedly established chapters in over 100 countries around the world. He stood by me throughout, despite the criticism of this previously unpopular stand on steroids in sport. That took much courage, considering his other obligations.

My department chairman, Robert E. Kappler, D.O., provided me with the resources and time to complete the final manuscript, and without his foresight, this project would never have been completed.

With great respect and admiration, I must acknowledge certain members of the U.S. Olympic Committee, who have demonstrated the courage and leadership to put a halt to this drug madness. I am indebted to William E. Simon, president of the USOC for his ability to establish order, leadership, and direction for the future; executive director of the USOC, F. Don Miller, for his years of dedication to the betterment and advancement of Olympic sport; Irving I. Dardik, M.D., chairman of the USOC Council on Sports Medicine, for his support, foresight, creativity, and for placing the athlete first; Kenneth Clarke, Ph.D., director, Olympic Training Center; Robert O. Voy, M.D., chief medical officer, sports medicine division, Olympic Training Center; and Jack Kelly, first vice president of the USOC, an Olympian's Olympian.

James A. Nicholas, M.D., and Anthony Maddalo, M.D., of the Institute of Sports Medicine and Athletic Trauma at Lenox Hill, as well as Allan J. Ryan, M.D., editor-in-chief of *The Physician and Sportsmedicine*, provided invaluable assistance in refining some of my earlier work in this field.

I wish to thank the skilled media professionals who shared their insight into this complex dilemma: Neil Amdur, *New York Times*; Bart Barnes, *Washington Post*; Stephen Beitler, Joe Henderson, and Caryn Landau, *Runner's World*; Jack Bell, American Medical Association; Walter Bingham, Stephan Kanfer, and Peter Stoler, *TIME*; Marc Bloom, *The Runner*; Joe Carnicelli and Pat McCormack, UPI; Matt Clark, *Newsweek*; Vince Eversano, *Inside Sports*; Henry Freeman and Tom Weir, *USA Today*; Larry Fox, *New York Daily News*; Phil Gunby, *Journal of the American Medical Association*; Randy Harvey, *Los Angeles Times*; John Husar, *Chicago Tribune*; John Jeansonne, *Newsday*; Roy Karten and Al Sanoff, *US News and World Report*; Barry Kaufman, D.D.S., NBC-TV (Chicago); Robert Kennedy, *Muscle Mag International*; Jerry Kindela and Ric Wayne, *Flex*; Ken Kontor, National Strength and Conditioning Associaion; Mark Kram, *Detroit Free Press*; Mark Mulvoy and Linda Verigan, *Sports Illustrated*; Thyra Resch, ABC-TV; Bill Reynolds, *Muscle & Fitness*; Mark Ritter, *Muscle Training Illustrated*; Yuri Shalamov; Barry Shapiro, *Sport*; Pat Walker, *Body in Motion*; Mike Wolf, Ph.D, *Self*; and John Zinsser, *Reader's Digest*.

I am indebted to the following sports stars for their time and personal interest: Muhammud Ali, Paul Anderson, Franco Columbu, Ric Draysin, Bev Francis, Dan Gable, John Grimek, Mark Johnson, Cheryl Jones, Jack LaLanne, Dan Lurie, Joe Namath, Richard Ornstein, Al Oerter, Bill Pearl, Susan Perkins, Robby Robinson, Arnold Schwarzenegger, Harry Schwartz, William Shatner, Ken Sprague,

Maris Sternberg, Pat Stewart, Chet Yorton, Jennifer Weyland, and Joe Weider, who trained a number of the above stars.

I am deeply appreciative to Doris Barrilleaúx, who provided photographs and philosophy from the woman's angle. Terry Todd, Ph.D., and his wife Jan were a pleasure to work with and have done much to expose the problem of drugs in sport.

I wish to thank those individuals and publishers who were kind enough to lend their support: Pat Columban, McGraw-Hill; Mary Lou Coyle, Prentice-Hall; Joyce I. Connell, Little, Brown; M.A. Dunleavy, Lea & Febiger; Elizabeth S. Escamilla; Jarlath Graham, Crain Books; Steven Groshek and Audrey G. Krigman, M.D., Ciba Pharmaceuticals; Arlene LaMantia, Yearbook Medical Publishers; Rayond Lams, Appleton-Century-Crofts; Jim Lewis of Australia; Richard Nuzzo, *Medical Communications*; D. A. Parrott, *British Medical Journal*, John C. Quinn, *USA Today*; Susan Sisko, *New York Post*; Sharon Sudderth, *American Journal of Sports Medicine*; Urban & Schwarzenberg, West Germany; Mary Lou Welch, American Heart Association; and Joyce Williams, W.B. Saunders Company.

The following university athletic departments assisted with photographs and information: Chicago State, DePaul, Harvard, Notre Dame, UCLA, Illinois, Iowa, Southern California, George Williams College, and Yale.

With great respect, I wish to acknowledge the following researchers, some of whom I know through their fine work and others I know personally: R.N. Alsever, M.D.; Gideon Ariel, Ph.D.; Professors Arnold Beckett and Raymond Brooks, University of London; Donald Catlin, M.D., and Carmine Clemente, Ph.D., UCLA; Tony Daly, M.D.; Douglas Decker, M.S. and Dennis Levenson, M.D., University of Chicago; Manfred Donike, M.D., Biochemistry Institute, West Germany; C.E. Finch, Ph.D., University of Southern California; Lawrence A. Golding, Ph.D.; R.W. Gotlin, M.D.; Dan F. Hanley, M.D.; John Harvey, Jr., M.D.; Jerome M. Hershman, M.D.; Charles Huggins, M.D., and Thomas Jones, M.D., University of Chicago; Charles D. Kochakian, Ph.D., and H.L. Kruskemper, Ph.D., two of the world's experts on anabolic steroid biochemistry; Jerzy Kosowicz, M.D., Warsaw, Poland; David Lamb, Ph.D.; John Lombardo, Cleveland Clinic; Prince Alexandre de Merode, International Olympic Committee chairman; Wylie L. Overly, M.D.; V. Rogozkin, Research Institute of Physical Culture, Leningrad; S. Solberg, University of Tromsø, Norway; Jacques Wallach, M.D.; Paul Ward, Ph.D; William N. Taylor, M.D.; and James E. Wright, Ph.D., who has performed exceptional contemporary work.

I am deeply indebted to my publisher, Icarus Press. Bruce and Laila Fingerhut put their heart, soul, and pocketbook into this project. They are very special people and more than any author could ask for as publishers. They promised to keep the integrity of my work intact—fact is, they added to it.

I would like to thank my colleagues at the Chicago College of Osteopathic Medicine, who were never too busy to answer questions or lend assistance.

By department: *Anatomy* — Edgar F. Allin, M.D., Randy L. Pachnik, D.P.M.; *Biochemistry* — Wells Farnsworth, Ph.D., David F. Mann, Ph.D., Doris Yasnoff Norwell, Ph.D.; *Osteopathic Medicine* — Dean Cohen, D.O., Richard Feely, D.O.; Karen Gajda, D.O.; Debora Heath, Kenneth Nelson, D.O., Michael Settecase, D.O.; *Microbiology* — Aaron Alexander, Ph.D., John Burdick, Ph.D., Marianne Hahn, Ph.D.; *Pathology*—Louis W. Gierke, D.O.; Prahba Gupta, M.D., Donald W. Hendrickson, D.O.; *Pharmacology*—Venkatray Prabhu, Ph.D., Dan Richardson, Ph.D., Kenneth Suarez, Ph.D.; *Physiology*—Martin S. Balin, M.D., Ph.D., Albert Kelso, Ph.D., Robert S. Tarr, Ph.D.; *Nephrology*—Don L. Hollandsworth, D.O., Mayer L. Horensten, D.O., Gary Slick, D.O.; *Internal Medicine*—Thomas W. Allen, D.O., Mark Efrusy, D.O., John Kniaz, D.O., Michael R. Olden, D.O., John Zuzga, D.O., Behnam Zakhireh, M.D., Francis X. Blais, D.O., V. Paul Bertrand, D.O., David P. Chenicoff, D.O., George T. Caleel, D.O., Hadi Hedayati, M.D., Lawrence Haspel, D.O., Robert L. Litchfield, D.O., Ward E. Perrin, D.O., Bruce Redman, D.O., J. Jerry Rodos, D.O.; *Cardiology*—David Braunstein, D.O., C. Richard Smith, D.O., Paul M. Wolfson, D.O.; *Surgery*—Aris Athens, D.O., Richard T. Caleel, D.O., Vincent J. DiRito, D.O., Graham O. Davies, D.D.S., Glen Einspanier, D.O., Anthony M. Grimaldi, D.O., Louis Habryl, D.O., Herb Kollinger, D.O., P. Robert Lomardo, D.O., Albert F. Milford, D.O., James C. Murray, D.O., Raymond W. Schleuter, D.O., John H. Sloan, D.O., Herbert Tirjer, D.O., Richard Warel, D.O.; *Psychiatry*—Wendel W. Carpenter, Ph.D., Charles E. Payne, O.F.M.; *Library Services*—Vicki Bloom, Kathy Depres, Tom Hagler, Jean Pariza, Estell Harris-Nwadiei, Lorenza Sturgis, Sandra A. Worley, M.S.; *Education*—Richard J. Agostinelli, R. P.h., Joel S. Alpert, Ph.D., Harold L. Hakes, Ph.D., J.D., John L. Karrat, D.O., Michael Lynch, D.O., Shirley Lewis, Mark E. McKeigue, D.O., Sandra Retzky, D.O. Harold Rose, D.O., Tineke Schouten; and school president Thaddeus P. Kawalek, Ph.D., whose support was vital. My thanks also to my secretaries, Alison K. Hubbard, M.A., Alfreda Green, and Barbara Williams.

The following people assisted peripherally over the years: Lloyd Blankfein, J.D., Bill Boggs, Robert Bram, David Butler, Adrian Byrd, Perris Calderon, Carl Ciazzo, D.C., Lesli Cohen, Jack Cohen, Wayne and Karen Demilia, Tom DiNatale, Doug Ditzel, D.O., Frank George, D.O., Paul and Mark Goldman, Ed Gersin, Art Hafner, Ph.D., Arnold Johnson, Ph.D., Peter Julian, M.S., Bob Kelly, Myron King, Jack Kirshman, Mitch Kaufman, Linda Klatz, Larry Kuhel, Sam F. Lamensdorf, Jr., Arnold Mandell, M.D., David Melzer, D.O., Sandi Merle, Jean Martineau, Steve MeKuly, Gabe Mirkin, M.D., Mike McGovern, Ph.D., Larry Page, D.O., Frank Paoletti, Sam Patroff, Frank Pellegrini, Ph.D., Jeffrey Plitt, Glen Pollack, Murray and Ben Posner, Phil Rosenthal, Mike and Patty Rothman, Bob Saunders, W. Norman Scott, M.D., Martin Silverberg, Amy Sklar, J.D., Bettina Smith, Lee Stein, Larry and Shelly Strickler, George Snyder, Gary Vogel, Bernard Waldman, David Webster, Carole L. Weidman, J.D., Steve Weinberger, John Wilton, Ruth Zelkha, Ira Hurley, and Bob Gajda.

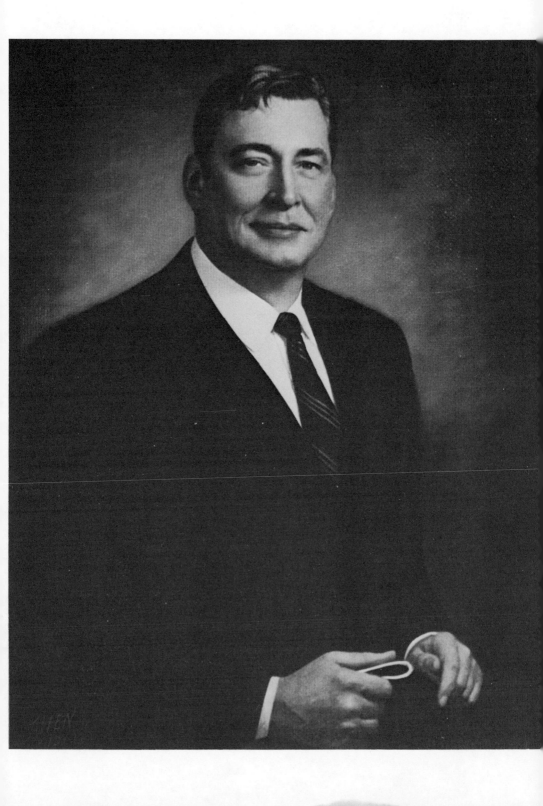

INTRODUCTION

The time is ripe. We need the truth. I would never have imagined that the moral state of the sports world would change so drastically. I was team physician for a number of American national teams and have had the opportunity to train many of the past Olympic champions. The first time I was exposed to anabolic steroid use was during the 1956 World games. The Russians were using straight testosterone. What caught my attention was the young athletes having to get catherized, which is a tube they insert into the urinary tract so they can urinate. This procedure is usually used for old men who have prostate trouble. The Russians were abusing the drugs heavily. Another thing I noticed was that you would see a really good weight lifter or strength athlete one year, and then he would burn out, and you wouldn't see him anymore. At subsequent competitions, I would ask what happened to these athletes, but I never received an answer.

I came back to the United States after we won everything, and I told the heads of the American athletic committees back in the 1950s that the Eastern Bloc countries and Russians were going to use every trick to win, especially in strength sports. They like stamina and strength sports, such as weightlifting, wrestling, and field events, all over Europe as a show of national strength.

When I came back home, I developed the original anabolic steroids with Ciba Pharmaceutical. It was simple to put together. We took testosterone and took out the secondary groups, using prostatic enlargements, which are enlarged endocrine glands. I took the drugs to test the benefits and safety for use by athletes. I gave them very

1

low dosages (5 mg.). A short while later, I found out they were taking far in excess of this behind my back and developing all sorts of medical pathologies. I wanted nothing to do with IQs of this level, so I discontinued this area of my experimentation. The athletes got their hands on the drugs in the 1960s and in just fifteen to twenty-five years have turned it into one big mess.

When I started the practice of medicine, treating the farmers and Indians in Montana, you couldn't get them to take a pill. The only time I could be sure they took their medication was when we finally got in penicillin injections. People had a strong aversion to taking a pill then, but now things have changed. Now everyone is pill happy. It started in the 1950s and by the 1960s had taken a firm hold on the public's life blood. I couldn't understand it. At least then I didn't have trouble giving medication any longer, but now the public is drug crazy.

It is bad enough to have to deal with drug addicts, but now healthy athletes are putting themselves in the same category. It's a disgrace. I imagine at times the athletes are forced into it from peer pressure and the blind desire to win, or even at times given drugs without their knowledge.

Who plays sports for fun anymore? Back in my college football days, we truly enjoyed athletic competition for the sake of friendly combat. The Olympics were a time for people of all nations to join in the interplay of true brotherhood among nations. It was as much a celebration as it was an athletic event. Now it is one cheap political ploy. With the coming future Olympics, it will probably be as fixed as an illegal horserace.

The Russian Olympic doctor I befriended told me that in his country an individual is worth absolutely nothing. They take these young girls and give them hormones to slow their maturity. It would be very interesting if we could get to examine a few of these girls. When a woman matures normally she gets heavier, but I am not talking about fat. Her bones get heavier, and her tendons stronger. Just like a big 250-pound man can curl hundreds of pounds of weights, but he can't climb up a rope like a light man can. They give them the drugs to keep them light and young. There is no way we can get at their medical records, but if we could we might find some beautiful research results that would read something like this: The young gymnasts would probably be sterile, experience a number of abnormalities and, if fertile, probably be incapable of carrying a pregnancy to full term. This is far from the child-bearing potential of undrugged female gymnasts.

I hope this book will answer a lot of questions that have puzzled many people. The time is right. As frightening as many of the facts and theories are, they are correct. I have seen the problems occur in my patients. The public has the right to know, and I feel this book is the vehicle. Not only are the athletes' lives in danger but that of our children and even the unborn. Medications using hormones generations ago are today producing breast cancer in the daughters of the users of these hormones. The word must be spread now. This is an epidemic, a war we must not lose. There are too many lives at stake. This book just might help to bring some morality and sanity back to our athletic world.

John B. Ziegler, M.D.

DRUGS & SPORTS

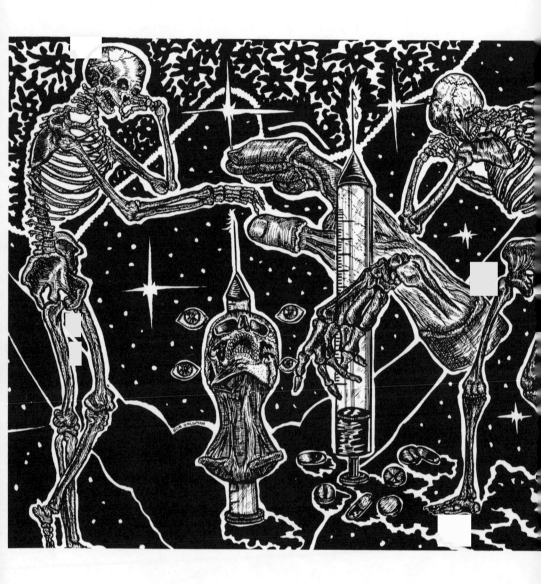

Drawing by Bob Goldman.

1
DEATH OF AN ATHLETE

The association of tumors of the liver with the use of anabolic steroids has been increasingly documented in recent years.
> *Doctors Prat, Gray, Stolley, and Coleman of the Cornell Medical Center, writing in the Journal of the American Medical Association*

THE LAST TIME I SAW JOHN* WAS THE DAY BEFORE HE DIED. I ALMOST burst into tears. I had to pretend I was admiring the view from his hospital room, so I could get control over my face and my voice.

This emaciated body, his swollen belly visibly raising the hospital sheets, this my friend, this idol of teenagers, was a towering six-foot-two-inch giant of a man when last I saw him. Now I could hardly recognize him. When I saw him last, he weighed 220 pounds; he'd lost nearly 100 of those pounds. When I saw him last, he had a thick head of black hair; now he was almost entirely bald, and the formerly heavy black eyebrows that emphasized his expressions were entirely gone. When I saw him last, his sweat-beaded skin moved firmly over his muscles as he worked out; now his skin hung on him wrinkled, dry, flaccid, crepey, ash-green in color, *old, sick*. When I saw him last, his voice boomed across the gym, unmistakable above the sounds of straining men and boys running, grunting, jumping, pounding, cursing, yelling; now he was gasping for air, his voice a hoarse whisper almost unintelligible as he greeted me the way he al-

*Not his real name.

ways had, "Hi Bob; when're you gonna let me show you how to put some muscles on that skinny body of yours?" This time I wasn't up to the snappy comebacks and just said it straight, "Just as soon as you get out of here, old buddy."

John was thirty-five years old and he was DYING. *Dying*, this man who could pick you up and break you in half. *Dying*, this man who had been bodybuilding since he was fifteen; who watched what he ate; who didn't smoke, didn't drink, didn't stay up late. This man who was married, and had two kids of his own and dozens of kids at the gym whom he helped and who worshipped him. This nearly perfect specimen of a human being was dying, and I couldn't understand it.

Now he was asking me about the guys down at the gym and making jokes about the nurses and telling me it was the chemotherapy he'd been given that made him sick and made his hair fall out, that he was sure he'd got *it* licked and not to worry, that he'd show the doctors a thing or two. He'd be back and then look out.

I'd met John when I was in college. I'd been working out, lifting weights and such since I was in high school. I grew up in a very tough neighborhood in Brooklyn, so working out made me strong enough to stay out of trouble while retaining my self-respect. In college I did six sports, but I still wanted to work through my formal routines to stay in shape, so I found a health club near school. And there I met John. John had such presence that he clearly dominated any situation he was in. He was one of those men that, despite a truly modest gentle manner, simply could not help standing out in a crowd. It wasn't from him but from others that I learned that he held a major world title, dozens of lesser titles, and had been a football star. From him I learned that a man can hold a major world title and still be very nice, very popular, very unassuming, and very willing to help struggling young athletes. He was never too busy to help the kids, and they idolized him. He was kind; he was patient; he was truly a good man.

And he took drugs. From the time I met him and for at least three years after that—to the time his illness was diagnosed—John took anabolic steroids, sold to him and others out of a suitcase by a man called Marcel who was known as the athletes' "French connection." It wasn't a secret. John came to the gym every day, and he kept the drugs and paraphernalia in his locker. No one thought too much of it because so many athletes took anabolic steroids. At this gym, not everyone took them, but no one was criticized for doing it. It was tacitly understood that John wanted to keep his championship body from aging and to retain his size and strength. Athletes all over the world were known to be taking anabolic steroids to build weight, strength, and endurance, so they could become champions like John. Granted, John was, in his early thirties, competitively over-the-hill. Still who could criticize him if he wanted to retain his achingly acquired state of physical perfection for as long as possible? Granted, many athletes were suspicious of anabolic steroids and refused to take them. Rumors of impotence and hair growing in strange places and paralysis from misplaced injections and worse circulated, but no one knew for sure, and meanwhile serious articles in sports magazines were cautiously hinting at their benefits, and everyone knew several athletes who were taking them and seemed to be doing all right physically, often better than all right in competition.

And then John got sick. It took awhile before the diagnosis was certain—kidney tumor, rare. By the time the diagnosis was confirmed by all the liver and kidney-function tests, the scans, the SGOTs, the tumor, the cancer, had metastasized through the bloodstream to the lungs and other parts of John's body.

John was given chemotherapy, which delayed his death. The drugs had terrible side effects—nausea, repetitive vomiting, a throat so raw he spat blood, and hair that came out in handfuls (the least of his problems considering the other side effects and the potential outcome of the disease). They gave him conventional antinauseant drugs of the sort people take for motion sickness, but they only dampened his nausea and delayed the inevitable, thus extending the whole unpleasant business. John took just six months to die.

In retrospect I judged it a supreme irony that John told me he had heard that smoking marijuana might prevent the terrible nausea that accompanied his chemotherapy, but that he didn't want to do it because it might get back to the kids, and he didn't want to set a bad example.

At that time I didn't know much about the drugs that were to consume the next nine years of my life. About fifteen years ago, I'd begun hearing about some drugs called steroids that could make a person grow and become stronger very quickly. Because I was a biology major in college, I knew that the chemistry of the body was a delicate, interlocking homeostatic system, and that many of the growth and sexual-maturation hormones that the body produced naturally were steroids. It seemed to me then that one was only asking for trouble by interfering in one of nature's most important arrangements. It was one thing for sick people to take steroids to correct some malfunction of their bodies, but it was quite another for normal healthy super-fit people to take them to try and beat other people in competitive sports.

As time passed, I began to hear about steroids in many places—not just in gyms but as common knowledge among people discussing sports. I began seeing articles about them in sports magazines and to realize steroid use was an international concern. Even young people—those I coached in wrestling at the local high school and at football camp—were talking about them.

And then anabolic steroids showed up closer to home.

I found that one of my friends, whom I had played high school football with, was injecting himself with steroids. There he was at the gym pumping a drug into his body with apparently no concern. He didn't seem to realize that what he was doing might be dangerous. He treated his action as though he were taking a multiple vitamin capsule. What seemed ironic to me was that I knew this was a fellow who wouldn't smoke, wouldn't eat candy, or even stay out very late; he was that concerned about his health.

Six months after this episode, John got sick.

I have two younger brothers. Both of them have always participated in all the sports they could, and they bodybuild and work out in gyms as I do. It was soon after John's death that one of my brothers told me that many of the kids down at the gym, the same one where I used to work out, were taking anabolic steroids. And these kids were fifteen and sixteen years old!

On top of this, I noticed a small article in the newspaper referring to an article in the prestigious *Journal of the American Medical Association*, suggesting that John's death may have been caused by anabolic steroids. I went to the nearest medical library as soon as I could, and I read there that anabolic steroids were capable of causing a rare type of kidney tumor that was nearly always fatal in adults.

That day at the library I managed to find a few more articles on anabolic steroids, and my concerns grew. The scientific literature indicated that anabolic steroids also could inhibit growth in young athletes; cause high blood pressure, sterility, bleeding from the intestinal tract, and hypoglycemia; increase the risk of heart attack; masculinize women; produce unsightly acne; deepen the voice; and change the distribution of body hair.

The potential side effects of anabolic steroids were clearly very dangerous, and some were permanent. Yet I knew from what I'd read, heard, and seen, that many athletes were taking large doses of these drugs over long periods of time without a semblance of medical supervision. And now high school and perhaps younger children were taking them so they could be stronger and bigger faster. I also knew that none of them had an idea of the dangers anabolic steroids presented. They were taking very powerful drugs as though they were some kind of new health food.

I decided I would try to learn all I could about anabolic steroids and drug-taking in sports in general. Then I would try to see that athletes had appropriate information on the dangers and possible benefits of taking drugs so that when they made their decisions—to take or not to take drugs—they would have weighed the cost-benefits and would make informed decisions.

At that time I was much more receptive to the idea that there must be some good in anabolic steroids. After all, so many people, respected athletes, took them. It seemed to me they must do more good than harm at least on average. It was possible that John's death, and that of another man I knew who had died immediately following an anabolic steroid injection at his gym, were rare and unusual.

Now that I've finished my research, I'm no longer open-minded. *I can state unequivocally that drugs, especially anabolic steroids, have no business in sports.* Anabolic steroids bestow few benefits, and none that are worth the terrible risks of taking them. Anabolic steroids should be reserved for very sick, debilitated persons and administered by qualified physicians, who constantly monitor the progress of their patients and watch for the development of side effects.

Seven years of my research were entirely taken up with reading every medical text and journal article that I could find on steroids and hormone chemistry (the science of endocrinology). My goal was to learn all there was to know about the kinds, uses, abuses, chemical structures, side effects, and sources of anabolic steroids. Although I'd had a good deal of organic chemistry, biology, and physiology in college, steroids were almost a new area of science for me. My college texts mentioned steroid chemistry only briefly. Somewhat more was to be found on endogenous hormones relative to normal growth and sexual development and functioning, but I found little on what happens when synthetic hormones are introduced from outside the body.

Only recently have we learned about the dangerous side effects, such as thrombosis and possible liver tumors, that are associated with the long-term use of oral contraceptives.

Before I was finished, I had read nearly 800 scientific articles about steroids, and I had learned that the science of endocrinology is in its infancy. Much research remains to be done before anyone completely understands how steroids, especially anabolic steroids, work. Meanwhile, for anyone to take them without close medical supervision (*not* a team physician) is exceedingly foolish. Such supervision must include blood and liver function tests.

I didn't spend all of my time at the library. I also began what would be more than 900 interviews with athletes, coaches, trainers, sports officials, team physicians, pharmacologists, and endocrinologists, to learn exactly

- when anabolic steroids were taken;
- who took them;
- why they were taken;
- how much was taken;
- the kind and frequency of side effects;
- how athletes felt about them; and
- what was being done to control them.

As I began talking to athletes about anabolic steroids, both to get information and to convey my concerns about the drugs, they began to ask me, "Bob, how do I know if I'm O.K?" Even the girl friends of athletes began to call me, questioning me, expressing concern, asking me to try and talk their boy friends out of taking anabolic steroids.

The more I learned, the more concerned I became. Not only were more athletes taking anabolic steroids, but they were being taken by younger athletes. And, although most seemed to have at least some private reservations about taking drugs, especially over long periods of time, their lack of information was frightening. Young athletes were using the fact that older, respected athletes were taking the drugs as a rationalization for their own use.

I knew that I had to tell what I had learned. I further postponed my medical studies to write this book. I drew upon the voluminous scientific library I had amassed, my hundreds of interviews, and reports in the lay press. My goals were to provide information, alert athletes, and warn the families of athletes about these dangerous drugs that are endangering the health and lives of young athletes all over the world and that pose a real threat to athletic competition itself.

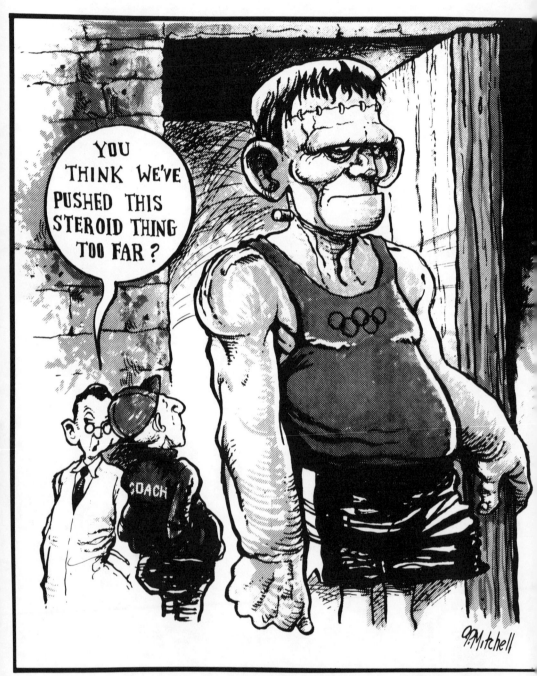

Reprinted with Permission from USA Today.

2
DRUGS IN SPORTS MEANS THE DEATH OF SPORTS

Bodybuilders don't like using them [steroids] because it lays them and the sport open to the use-one-use-them-all criticism often insinuated by people who don't know any better. Mostly, they don't like using them because they sense that in an oblique way, doing so gives some weight to one of the most abhorred of all the many public discomforts about them; that there is something as synthetic, unhealthy, useless, and faintly sinful as plastic flowers about what they do and the way they look; as though all the discipline, sacrifice, and work of their training, and the organic balance of exercise, feeding, and rest that has to be found and struck exactly right inside the body before the outside becomes a proper medium, and the sure, satisfying connection between the body's health and its beauty, and how good they feel all the time, how good the lungs feel, and the skin... as though all those things counted for nothing, could be reduced to something the size of a pill.

Charles Gaines
Pumping Iron

A FABLE

THE USE OF ANABOLIC STEROIDS IN SPORTS HAS ALWAYS REMINDED ME of a story I once heard about three men who kept sheep. Each man had one sheep, and they shared a small pasture. The sheep were fat and healthy, and the men competed with each other each year to see whose sheep would take the blue ribbon at the county fair. One day, however, one of the men had an idea. He figured if he got two sheep, then he could be more successful than the other two men and in-

15

crease his chance of winning the coveted blue ribbon. And so he brought another sheep to the pasture. As you can imagine, the other men were quick to see the advantage of having more sheep, and so the competition began, with one and then another trying to gain an advantage by adding to his herd in the pasture. At first it did seem an advantage to have the most sheep, but then something disturbing began to happen. They began to run out of room in the pasture. There wasn't enough grass to go around. The sheep became thin and sick. No longer was there a single sheep that was worth shearing, let alone showing at a fair. When one former winner tried it, the people just pointed and laughed behind their hands. But no man would decrease his herd. Each continued to try and gain an advantage over the others, until eventually, sadly, all of the starving, weakened sheep became ill and died, and with them the dreams of applause and blue ribbons.

This story of the three foolish shepherds with their singular pursuits of advantage that leads them to their mutual destruction parallels the dilemma of drug-taking athletes. Each takes drugs because he believes that his competitor is doing so. Each takes more than he believes his competitor takes so that he can have the advantage over his competitor. Each endangers his own health, but beyond this, he endangers the very arena, the very sport, for which he risks so much. For none are likely to admire, few will come to see, none will want to emulate, those whose strength or skill is believed to come from a bottle of pills or a hypodermic needle. If athletes continue down this perilous path of mutual destruction by synthetic chemicals, they will be denigrated, sneered at, diminished, and viewed as curiosities like freaks in a side show. Athletics, with its long and glorious traditions of hard work and fair play, of strong bodies and spirits, of professionals helping novices, of clasped hands across age, class, and cultural boundaries, will become little more than another commercial attraction.

THE FICKLE AUDIENCE

Much of athletics depends on the support of an audience of fans. But what kind of fan would support an athlete whose competitive edge came from taking 500 mg. of chemical bodybuilders two to three times a week over several years? I have already overheard in an audience watching an amateur wrestling match, "Hey, look at that guy; he's nothing but muscles and pills." Make no mistake about it, audiences are not able to distinguish between those whose current physical states derive from a combination of natural ability and years of drugless painstaking training, and those who have augmented their training with drugs. The remaining audiences will come to watch the circus, not to show their children what clean living, self-regimentation, and devotion to a goal can produce.

In the long run, public opinion and support are critical to athletics, whether sports are largely supported by donations, ticket purchases, and commercial television and radio sponsors, or by academic institutions and governments. Even in those countries where athletics is heavily subsidized, tax dollars will soon dry up if sport falls into disrepute, and audiences begin to laugh instead of clap. Audiences are fickle, and taste and fashion change like the colors on a chameleon. The public is against drug taking. Stadium seats may well remain empty if people begin to believe that athletes have bypassed or cheated on training. Athletes must remain admirable, suitable role-model figures to sustain the loyalty and support of the public. The public does not think that drug-taking is admirable.

Ironically, much of the reason athletes take drugs is to earn the super-adulation of audiences. Top athletes are known around the world; their names are household words; their faces stare at us from magazines; we watch them for hours on television; they earn enormous salaries; they lend their names to a variety of commercial products from beer to tennis balls; when they retire they become movie stars and sports commentators. Beyond this, they have increasingly come to represent our national honor.

In international sport, original concepts of competition have vanished. At one point in history, international competitors were believed to increase international understanding and friendship. In sport, with individual athletes competing against each other, national chauvinism was believed to disappear. The example set of sportsmanship and fellowship was supposed to moderate international relationships. Individual, not national, skill and honor were supposed to be at stake.

There has been a change. Now it is the United States versus the Soviet Union, or England versus East Germany, and so on. The number of gold medals accumulated by each country are carefully counted and bragged over. If you can't push them around in the world, you can at least beat them on the playing fields and gym mats.

International games have become a substitute for war, a pawn to

use, a bargaining chip in world politics. Those athletes, those winners, who must carry our national honor, are our new war heroes.
They are afforded all the adulation once reserved for great military
victors and political leaders in addition to that historically afforded
to athletes. And they are brought to us in our living rooms in full living color. We can see their successes, and we are proud of them. We
treat them like heroes. When they succeed, we reward them hand-
somely. When they fail, we weep with them.

Because the rewards are so great, athletes will do almost anything
to gain the edge that will make them into winners, stars, heroes, instead of also-rans. Unfortunately, that "almost anything" now includes injecting and swallowing dangerous drugs, a behavior not
approved by the public.

If drug taking in sports continues, I predict that athletes will stand
bewildered before public opinion crying, "I did everything possible
to win including risking my health and even my life. Why have you
abandoned me?" And the audience, if it could speak with one voice,
would answer, "Because you destroyed our idealism with a hypodermic needle."

Who will suffer the most in the long run? Certainly the athletes
will suffer because it is their health and their lives that are damaged.
But all of us will suffer since sports have been one of our few escapes,
a common denominator among men, and the common cement of
friendship and brotherhood among social classes, as well as the nations of the world.

THE STEROID EPIDEMIC

There should be no doubt in anyone's mind that drugs are widely
used by competitors in various sports, as the following statements at-
test:

> In a survey of twenty track and field [athletes] and weight lift-
> ers, it was reported that nineteen had taken steroids in prepara-
> tion for the 1968 Olympic Games.
>
> L. C. Johnson
> *Journal of Sports Medicine*

I guarantee that at least sixty percent of the contestants are on tissue drugs [anabolic steroids] of one sort or another.

> Dave Prowse
> *Power Magazine*

Look around at certain Americans and Central European weight lifters who, having had static poundages for years, have suddenly increased body weight and moved up a class [sometimes as many as two or three] and produced a fantastic improvement in poundage. I wager this was not done on Epsom salts.

> David P. Webster

I told the Russians, particularly in dealing with females, that they were going against strong medical evidence if they encouraged their athletes to take steroids.

> Dr. Clayton Thomas
> Harvard School of Public Health
> Soviet-American Symposium on Drugs
> Leningrad

They [the Soviets] are under more pressure. The real difference in the Soviet and Eastern European society of athletes is that there is no room for failure because failure means not making the team and not having the creature comforts that go with success.

> Dr. James Wilkerson
> Indiana University

If they could be sure East Germany and the Russians aren't taking anything, our athletes would stop.

> Dr. Anthony Daly
> Chief Physician, U.S. Olympic Team

The most popular story of the 1976 Montreal Olympics involved the success of East German women swimmers. When asked why so many of their women had deep voices, an East German coach replied, 'We have come here to swim, not sing."

> *New York Times*

The trouble was that the men went crazy about steroids. They figured if one pill was good, three or four of them would be better, and they were eating them like candy. I began seeing prostate trouble, and a couple of cases of atrophied testes.

> Dr. John Ziegler
> U.S. National Weight Lifting Team
> Physician

When the shocked doctor in charge of the tests at the world weight-lifting championships in Columbus, Ohio, reported finding positive results, an even more shocked committee of the International Weight-Lifting Federation called an emergency meeting, and voted unanimously to invoke their own rules: "Competitors whose doping test proves positive shall be disqualified." Five athletes were disqualified and two days later four more, thus removing four Poles, three Hungarians, one Russian and one Japanese—the most wholesale disqualification ever made in any sport, and the first time that competitors from Communist countries were involved.

World Sports

Let me put it this way. If they had come into the village the day before competition and said we have just found a new test that will catch anyone who has used steroids, you would have had an awful lot of people dropping out of events because of instant muscle pulls.

Dave Maggard
Olympic shot-putter and
University of California track coach

I guess this anabolic steroid thing must have started on the Chargers around 1963 or right in there somewhere. One guy I can remember who got involved was Howard Kindig. He came to us as a highly touted center and linebacker from Los Angeles State. He was long and lean and very quick, and they wanted to put some weight on him, so in addition to using the weight program run by our weight coach, Alvin Ray, they started pumping him full of Dianabol [a popular anabolic steroid], and sure enough, he gained about thirty pounds.

They were passing out the stuff to the rest of us. They called it just "pink pills." We started taking it as a matter of course.

Dave Kocourek
Offensive End, Oakland Raiders

It is an assumption based on reasonably good but unverified reports that some players in almost every NFL and AFL team have used anabolic steroids. It is a fact according to physicians or players, that, in addition to the Chargers, members of the Kansas City Chiefs, Atlanta Falcons and Cleveland Browns have taken the drug.

Sports Illustrated

I'd say anybody who has graduated from college to professional football in the last four years has used them [anabolic steroids].

Ken Ferguson
Canadian professional football player
(formerly of Utah State College)

It's an epidemic.

> Dr. Clayton Thomas
> Sports Medicine Task Force, U.S.
> Olympic Sports Medicine Council

The problem is worse than it's ever been.

> Dr. Daniel Hanley
> Sports Medicine Task Force
> U.S. Olympic Committee

I do not like the way we are going. We see small girls who I suspect are being controlled by drugs...They are being stopped from being women.

> Niels Peter Nielson
> President, Danish Gymnastics Federation

Evidence compiled by the Washington Post in recent months suggests that the use of steroids and other additive drugs [those intended to improve performance beyond the level the individual normally is capable of] and restorative drugs [those intended to treat injury and pain in order to permit the athlete to compete at or near his normal level] is more widespread now than ever before.

> *Washington Post*
> May 27, 1979

I suppose there are some sports that don't have any drug problems but most do—professional and amateurs, from high school age on up.

> Dr. Irving Dardik
> Sports Medicine Task Force
> Chairman, U.S. Olympic Committee
> on Sports Medicine

I honestly cannot name one guy, and I know just about all of them personally, who is not using some steroid.

> George Frenn
> Olympic hammer thrower

By 1968, athletes in every event were using anabolic steroids and stimulants. It was not unusual in 1968 to see athletes with their own medical kits, practically a doctor's, in which they would have syringes and all their various drugs...I know any number of athletes on the 1968 Olympic team who had so much scar tissue and so many puncture holes in their back sides that it was difficult to find a fresh spot to give them a new shot.

I said to myself nothing has really changed since '73 [the year of U.S. Congressional subcommittee investigation], except that athletes now are taking doses that would have blown our minds, and kids are taking them younger.

> Harold Connolly
> Four-time Olympian,
> 1956 gold medalist in hammer throw

...the athletes don't know what they take. They are given pills as part of the training program. The pills are in a little bottle marked "vitamins," without any ingredients named. I was given two pills a week, but after I had a physical reaction [hardened leg muscles, occasional loss of voice, growth of hair on upper lip, disruption of menstrual cycle], I stopped them.

> Renate Neufeld
> East German sprinter who defected to the West

In a year, part of 1978 and part of 1979, five European athletes lost their titles in major competitions because they were caught doping. Four Russian and one Bulgarian track-and-field athletes showed positive urine tests for anabolic steroids at the European Championships and were barred from competition for eighteen months. Nadechko Tkachenko of the USSR was ordered to give up her gold medal won in the pentathlon, and her teammate, Yevgeny Mironov, was not allowed to keep a silver medal in the shot put. Steroids were found in Viktor Kuznetsov's drug tests after he won a bronze medal in the 100-meter backstroke at the West Berlin world aquatic championships. A woman shot-putter, Ilone Slupianek, from East Germany, lost a gold medal in the European Cup, as did Markku Tuokko, a Finnish men's discus thrower. They, and three other athletes, were suspended from international competition for eighteen months for using steroids.

One of the largest scandals of its kind took place in late August 1983 in Caracas, Venezuela, when fifteen athletes from ten countries (the United States, Cuba, Canada, Colombia, Nicaragua, Argentina, Puerto Rico, Venezuela, Chile, and the Dominican Republic) were disqualified and stripped of twenty-three medals. Close to 100 drugs were being tested and resulted in the biggest doping bust in the history of international sport. Among the athletes stripped of medals was Jeff Michels, America's finest weight lifter and winner of three gold medals in Caracas, who tested positive for exogenous testosterone. Moreover, when told of the sensitivity of the tests—able to detect traces of scores of drugs used months, even years, before the test—twelve American athletes withdrew from the competition and went home. Hoping to leave Caracas quietly, these men were subjected to interviews virtually from the time they left the athletes' compound. None admitted to the use of steroids, although several claimed to have used various antihistamines and other medicines and said they were unwilling to lose their Olympic standing by testing positive in Caracas. Many were bitter that they were not backed up more by the United States Olympic Committee. USOC President William E. Simon retorted, "It's about time the athletes understand we mean business. This is a problem that is going to destroy the international Olympic movement if we allow it to continue. It's an evil and we are going to stamp it out. The athletes are going to find out that the game is over."

Evie G. Dennis, the U.S. team's chief of mission, said, "They [the athletes] asked me what the USOC was going to do so they could keep up with the Russians and others. I said we were going to do nothing, because we don't condone these drugs." Noting that there is no drug testing in U.S. track meets, Mrs. Dennis, chairman of the women's committee of The Athletics Congress, which governs track and field in the United States, said her committee had voted unanimously at their congress's past two conventions to test for drugs at national championships—and each time, the proposal was voted down. She assumed that the chief reason was the cost of testing, which was and is quite high.

In Caracas (and in the 1984 Olympics in Los Angeles), testing begins immediately after an event. The top four finishers and several others randomly selected are taken to a room and handed a bottle for a urine sample. They are watched while providing the samples, so there will be no substitutions. The samples are then covered, sealed, and taken to the lab, where they are put into two containers, one for immediate test analysis and the other for storage in case the first comes out positive; this second vial will then be tested in the presence of the athlete and his or her country's Olympic representative. The first sample is separated again, and the first part is tested for steroids, the other for a number of other illegal drugs (there will be at least 100 drugs tested in the '84 Olympics). The sample to be tested for steroids is broken into organic and inorganic layers, with the fatty organic layer eventually tested for the drug. The machines used in these tests are sophisticated, state-of-the-art gas chromatographs and mass sep-

trograph. Fewer than ten such machines exist in the world and are accredited by the IOC to do this work; the United States has only one
international Olympic accredited lab—at UCLA, to be used during
the 1984 Olympic Games.

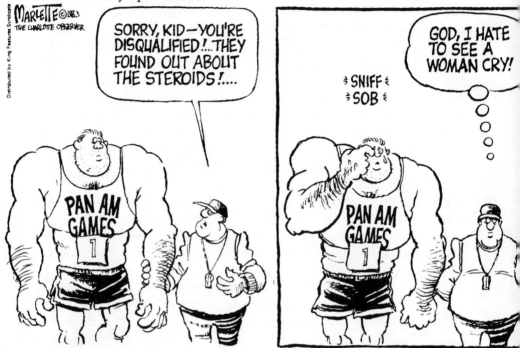

Pictorial Parade photo reprinted with permission from Marlette and the
Charlotte Observer.

   The Soviets have been heavy into hormonal experimentation since
the 1950s, when anabolic steroids were first noted to be used by athletes. Many of today's fans can remember some of the grossest examples from this period—European 200-meter dash Maria Itkina,
Romanian world-record high jumper Iolanda Balas, and, especially,
the Press sisters, Olympic champion pentathlete Irina and gold medalist in the shot put and discus, Tamara, "the flower of Leningrad."
All four of these women disappeared at high points in their careers
after Polish sprinter Ewa Klobukowska ran afoul of the tests following the 1967 European track-and-field championships, when her
chromosome count cast doubt on her femininity. Anyone taking a
look at these "women" would be hard pressed to remember in them
the girl next door (unless you lived next door to the New York Jets, of
course).
   Such cheating is assumed for the Soviets, whose reputation for

routinely providing such drugs to their athletes was not enhanced when recently four Canadian weight lifters were caught at the Montreal airport with 22,515 capsules of anabolic steroids and 414 vials of testosterone, purchased for virtual peanuts behind the Iron Curtain.

As for Caracas, perhaps we should reserve the last word for Dave Maggard, a former world-class shot putter, who had tried using steroids in the past, who said that once the shock wears off, "this may be the greatest thing that could happen to all sport." Maggard, now the athletic director of the University of California, said while he didn't like to see athletes disqualified, "this is going to take the huge burden off many athletes who felt they had to take steroids to compete."

When the officials are informed that an athlete's test is positive, they must vote on his suspension and whether to revoke his title if any. These votes frequently and unfortunately follow East-West lines. For example, all eight of the Western country representatives voted to ban the five athletes caught doping at the European Championships, while the six representatives from the Eastern countries voted against the banning.

> That's a dangerous thing. All of a sudden there's not going to be anymore fairness to the athlete. I don't know what to think. The East-West thing is the big thing now. There's no more true sport involved.
>
> Al Fuerbach
> U.S. Olympic shot putter

DOPING DOWN THE AGES

Although drug-taking to increase one's chances of winning is more prevalent now than ever before, and more dangerous because of the severe long-term effects of the current craze for anabolic steroids, athletes in the past also tried the drug short-cut to fame and fortune.

Among drugs that have spread through the athletic community in the past are uppers such as cocaine, amphetamines, strychnine, caffeine; downers such as muscle relaxants, tranquilizers, barbiturates, narcotics (morphine, heroin, Demerol); enzymes; vitamin B_{12} injections; antiinflammatories such as cortisone, butazolidin, DMSO; ether; diuretics; bronchodilators; and adrenalin.

Once an athlete takes a drug and is perceived by other athletes to perform well on it, the practice becomes almost impossible to stop, even though sports' officials roundly condemn it and pass rules against it.

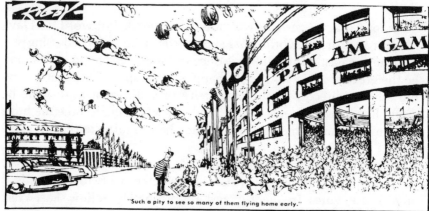

"Such a pity to see so many of them flying home early."

Drug use has been documented in all of the sports in which weight, speed, nerves, and endurance are factors. This takes in most sports, so drug use has been documented in sports ranging from swimming to wrestling to cycling to golf to track-and-field events.

Verified cases of doping, the athletes' word for drug-taking from the Dutch word *dop*, go back over a hundred years. The word *doping* appeared in an English dictionary in 1889, defined as a narcotic mixture of opium used for race horses. In the native Kaffir dialect of South Africa, *dop* refers to the stimulating hard liquor used in religious ceremonies. Through adoption into the Boer language, the final "e" was added to give the word *dope*.

The earliest reports of drug-taking by athletes in competition were in Amsterdam in 1865, when swimmers in canal races were charged with taking dope. It was also about this time that the first evidence of doping among cyclists appeared. In 1869, the coaches of teams of six-day bicycle riders were widely known to be giving the heroin-and-cocaine mixture called *speedball* to increase the endurance of team members. The practice caught the attention of the sports world when the first recorded drug-related death in sports occurred to a cyclist in a bicycle race in 1886.

Drug-taking in sports cropped up repeatedly to the end of the nineteenth century and on into the twentieth. The Belgians were said to be taking sugar tablets soaked in ether, the French to be taking caffeine tablets, and the British to be breathing oxygen and taking cocaine, heroin, strychnine, and brandy, all in frantic attempts to gain competitive edges that would return the coveted laurel wreaths of victory.

The quadrennial Olympic Games, which bring athletes from all over the world, began to serve as an exchange for drug recipes and helpful hints on how to win through chemistry.

In 1904, the games were in St. Louis, and it took four frantic physicians to revive Tom Hicks, who collapsed after he won the marathon. The physicians discovered that Hicks had taken a large dose of strychnine and brandy before he went out on the track.

The first dope testing was performed on animals. The testing of the saliva of race horses for the presence of alkaloids in 1910 was soon followed by similar tests in racing dogs after and to prevent further scandals at the dog tracks.

Despite Hicks, the early part of the twentieth century was relatively quiet in terms of drugs in people sports. And then came the forties, World War II, and the widespread craze for amphetamines. By the fifties, amphetamines were one of the most widely used and misused group of drugs, both in and out of sports. The word was out. "Want to study all night, drive all night, work all night, lose weight, jump higher, run faster, be more aggressive? Take amphetamines and succeed."

Cyclists in the fifties were known to carry amphetamines as they cycled over the hills and dales. The finding of numerous syringes and broken ampules in the locker room of a speed skater at the Oslo games in 1952 brought a new meaning to the words *speed skater* and engendered a great deal of controversy. Although revelations such as this precipitated considerable shock and dismay, there was no concerted action until 1965, after three fatalities.

The Danish cyclist, Kurt Jensen, died at the 1960 Olympic Games in Rome as a result of taking the combination of nicotinic acid and amphetamines that was given to him by his training manager. Heroin claimed the life of 400-meter hurdler, Dick Howard, at the same games. In 1963, drugs killed welterweight boxer, Billy Bello, who died of heroin poisoning.

Although these deaths, and the common knowledge that drug taking among athletes was increasing, and increasingly dangerous, stimulated the passage of tough antidoping laws by France and Belgium in 1965, these laws weren't enough to prevent the death in 1967 of Britain's Tommy Simpson, the best professional cyclist of his day, during the Tour de France. Nearing the end of the thirteenth lap, a lap involving a brutal 6,000-foot climb up a mountain in 90° heat, Simpson began to wander back and forth across the road, and eventually collapsed in a coma, from which he never recovered. A vial of methamphetamine [speed] was found in his pocket, and the drug was found in his body by the pathologist who performed the autopsy. The year before he died, Simpson was reported to have defended his use of amphetamines: "When you get up in the morning, do you need a cup of coffee to get started? Well, after cycling 150 miles the day before, we might need three or four 'coffees.'"

In May 1966, Jacques Anquetil, who has won the Tour de France five times, forfeited his victory and prize money rather than submit to a test of his urine for amphetamines. Said Anquetil, "I dope myself. Everyone, that is everyone who is a competitive cyclist, dopes himself. Those who claim they don't are liars. For fifty years bike racers have been taking stimulants. Obviously we can do without them in a race, but then we will pedal fifteen miles an hour. Since we are constantly asked to go faster and to make even greater efforts, we are obliged to take stimulants." In the following year, two cycling deaths were attributed to amphetamines, and in September 1967, Anquetil again forfeited a world speed record in Milan rather than submit his urine for a doping test.

In November 1968, Yves Mottin won a cross-country bicycle race in Grenoble, France. Two days later, he collapsed and died. In the following year, two of his friends, both French cyclists, were indicted on a charge of having given Mottin the amphetamines that caused his death.

Amphetamines were also the drugs involved in the death of Jean-Louis Quadri, a soccer player who collapsed on the field in Grenoble in 1968.

In the past, the drugs that athletes took—the amphetamines, the heroin, and the strychnine—brought on rather sudden collapse or death, usually from cardiac or respiratory arrest. If an athlete who took these drugs survived, the long-term effects on his body were believed to be small. The new drug darlings, the anabolic steroids, are another matter. Although there is some risk of sudden death accompanying injection due to anaphylactic shock, an athlete who takes an anabolic steroid is unlikely to suffer a sudden collapse on the playing field. The risks of these drugs are insidious and long term. Death by kidney failure or liver tumor is a slow process that may occur long after the athlete has hung up his track shoes.

NEW KINDS OF COMPETITION

There are two new kinds of international competition besides those in which athletes win over each other individually or on teams. One kind is where one bloc of countries has more votes than the other bloc, and so it can decide to suspend or to reduce the time of suspension of an athlete caught violating the antidoping rules. A reduction in the suspension time can allow an athlete to compete in an important competition occurring before the customary eighteen-month suspension time is up. In this international sports competition, the bloc with the most votes wins.

The second new kind of international competition consists of a race to find new drugs that can give an athlete a competitive edge but that can't be detected by existing testing methods and to find drugs that can render drugs now in use undetectable.

It is universally believed among athletes that the other side uses drugs, and that its drugs are better than our side's drugs. The Westerners believe that the Easterners, particularly the Soviets and the East Germans, have made a science out of it. The Easterners believe that the Americans are a pill-taking society and so, of course, all American athletes take drugs.

The only problem with these new kinds of international competitions is that the winners turn out to be the losers.

But, let's face it, drugs are only a symptom of the real disease. The true illness is the way we view sports—win at any cost, you're a bum if you lose. We must seriously look at ourselves to cure the illness and not just mask the symptom. Like a cancer, this sickness eats away at the very virtues and benefits of sport competition and further perverts and destroys it for our young people and children.

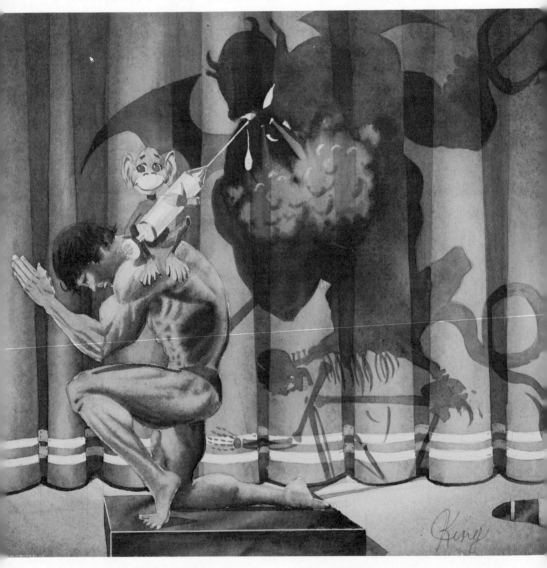

Drawing by Myron King.

3
THE HOOKED ATHLETE

The merciless rigor of modern competitive sports, especially at the international level, the glory of victory, and the growing social and economical reward of sporting success (in no way any longer related to reality) increasingly forces athletes to improve their performance by any means possible.

Manual on Doping
Medical Commission
International Olympic Committee

MANY ATHLETES ARE SINGLE-MINDED DRIVEN INDIVIDUALS. THEY DO not seem to perceive they have lives beyond some future sports event, perhaps the Olympic Games. Olympic gold looms so large and bright, is so tangible a goal, so dominates their lives, that it effectively shuts out any vision of a world beyond it. The future beyond the Big Win is misty and clouded, so nebulous that it is hardly worth mentioning let alone planning for. The present is a set of stair steps of relatively minor competitions leading up to the golden moment when the trumpets sound, the national anthem plays, time stops, and world stands in awe before THE WINNER.

The imagined magnificence of this moment and uncertainty about life-beyond-victory have produced athletes with mind-sets that in any other area of human endeavor would be called fanatical.

Dr. Gabe Mirkin, author of *The Sportsmedicine Book* and a de-

31

voted runner, said that a few years ago he polled more than a hundred top runners and asked them this question: "If I could give you a pill that would make you an Olympic champion—and also kill you in a year—would you take it?" Mirkin reported that more than half of the athletes he asked responded that yes, they would take the pill.

I was stunned by Mirkin's survey and wondered whether the indicated willingness to die was universal among athletes; perhaps it was idiosyncratic to runners. So I decided to repeat the poll with athletes I knew best, mostly weight lifters and field competitors—discus throwers, shot-putters, jumpers, etc. To my consternation, I was forced to conclude that weight lifters and field competitors were just as crazy as runners.

I asked 198 top world-class athletes a question similar to Mirkin's, "If I had a magic drug that was so fantastic that if you took it once you would win every competition you would enter, from the Olympic decathlon to Mr. Universe, for the next five years, but it had one minor drawback—it would kill you five years after you took it— would you still take the drug?" Of those asked, 103 (52 percent) said yes, that winning was so attractive they would not only be willing to achieve it by taking a pill (in other words, through an outlawed, unfair method— that is, in effect, cheating), but they would give their lives to do it.

Now it can be argued that it is only because the athletes knew there is no such magic medicine that they indicated their willingness to commit Olympic hari-kari. That faced with such a real-world magic medicine, they would have second thoughts. Perhaps this argument is correct, but the evidence suggests otherwise. The evidence suggests that athletes will take anything or do anything to their bodies to win, with no assurance of winning, and in apparent disregard for their lives beyond Olympia, or sometimes beyond the next major competition.

There is another group of athletes who are as willing to risk this contemporary version of selling one's soul to the devil. These are the big-money team-sport players. Not only is theirs the glory and status that comes with appearing via television in the homes of sports-loving Americans across the land, but they are accorded exceedingly good incomes. Some professional basketball players earn from half to a million dollars per year. Some football, hockey, and baseball players earn $1 million per year. Even an average professional team player in many sports receives over $100,000 per year. And these salaries don't include the extras that come from commercials or having your name on a racket or a shirt or a ball, or the special internal reward that comes from knowing you had the right stuff to make the team and then the right stuff to stay on it. It's little wonder that an individual will turn to whatever he thinks might possibly give him an edge so that he'll be the one to be noticed by the scout from the pro team or the one on the farm team who's tapped for the big time or the one who can keep going game after bone-pounding game. Too often that something he turns to is drugs.

Remember too, that these visible, successful athletes did not arrive where they are on their own. No indeed. Behind every successful athlete is, not the proverbial wife although she may be there too, but a small army of coaches and trainers and promoters and owners and families and neighbors and friends—all of them urging and cheering and cajoling and threatening and begging and supporting and criticizing and pushing the athlete onward. All in his best interest, of course. But when (and if) the goal is attained, many of the athlete's entourage share in the money, and all bask in the reflected glory.

It is not too surprising then that some of these "friends" are quite willing for the athlete to do whatever they can to gain that edge that will so enhance their own, as well as the athlete's future. Some of the friends are the purveyors of tablets and needles, and some of the others simply look the other way.

Down the road, after the trumpets have sounded and the tarnishing trophies are beginning to gather dust, is another group of athletes who are vulnerable to drug use. This is the group to which John belonged. The fading has-beens who aren't aging gracefully, who don't know quite how to live in a world where people they meet no longer recognize their names, where promoters and reporters and journalists no longer line up at their doors to ask them to play on their teams or lend their names to products or grant interviews. The group unprepared for life beyond victory.

Some of the ex-stars try to cling to that physical state where in a white moment of perfection everything came together and it seemed easy, natural to be better than all the others. Just beyond the peak, it seems possible to regain what they had before. If they only train a little harder, take care of themselves, and if that isn't enough, why not turn to the little bottle of magic helpers? After all, everyone knows everyone else is doing it. In fact, athletes can rationalize that the drug-taking of others is the reason they no longer are front runners.

TWO TYPES OF SPORTS DRUGS

A sports drug (or medicine) is any natural or synthetic substance that is taken solely because the taker is an athlete. The key is motive. Other people take drugs to prevent or cure illness. An athlete takes or is given a sports drug because he, she, or someone believes it will improve his or her performance, either immediately or in the future.

There are broadly two classes of sports drugs. One class is *restorative.* It consists of the drugs taken for some kind of injury or stress that enable the athlete to compete despite his condition. The intent of restorative drugs is to return the athlete to his normal or near normal state at the level of performance he had before he became incapacitated. Drugs in this class include painkillers (from aspirin to morphine), muscle relaxants, tranquilizers, sedatives, anti-inflammatories, enzymes, and topical anesthetic sprays and ointments.

The second class of sports drugs is *ergogenic* (additive). The intention of using drugs in this class is to increase performance beyond what would normally be achieved without them. In this class are the most controversial and dangerous drugs—amphetamines and anabolic steroids—as well as the most benign, such as vitamins and fruit juices, should all be in a class with drugs.

The broad range of substances taken by athletes, whether for restorative or additive purposes, complicates the issue of drugs in sports. Few people would argue that for an athlete to take an aspirin or a megavitamin or to eat a lot of carbohydrates before or during a competition (no matter what his intent) was wrong. And few people would argue that taking cocaine or anabolic steroids was right. But what about the area in between? What about taking codeine to stop a cough or lidocaine to stop the hurt of a pulled muscle? What about taking butazolidin, an anti-inflammatory drug? Or caffeine tablets? Or Valium? Or blood transfusions? The highly competitive athlete will try anything, whether restorative or ergogenic, if he thinks it might—just might—give him that little edge, that tiny little bit extra, that final surge that means he touches first or lifts five pounds more or jumps an inch farther or higher, and is flung from obscurity into being a CHAMPION instead of an also-swam or -ran or -jumped or -pushed or -threw.

When Alice went down the rabbit hole, she found a tiny cake that said, "Eat Me." When she obeyed, she grew and grew until she threatened to outgrow the room she was in. Just in time, she found another cake that shrunk her down to rabbit size. Many athletes seem to have acquired the Alice syndrome, behaving as if they can take some magical substance that will make them grow bigger and stronger. They haven't realized that there isn't any magic substance that can reverse the process. When your liver is shot and your kidneys are damaged, you can't easily get new ones or get them fixed. Impotence and sterility are difficult to treat and psychologically damaging. If your child is born with birth defects, you aren't allowed to give it back and get a better one.

Part of the attraction in taking ergogenic drugs is that, unlike Alice, who more than doubled in size, it is not necessary to be very much bigger or stronger to be a winner. In serious competitive sports, the top athletes are usually so nearly matched that a 2-to-3 percent advantage will ensure the gold.

Said Dr. Alois Marder, a former East German sports physician, about the East German use of drugs, "Seventy to 80 percent is talent. Twenty or 25 percent is training and maybe 5 percent is attributable to other influences, including drugs. True, if you can improve by one or two percent, you can go from sixth to first place." Others have suggested that if a whole team takes drugs, it will have about 10 percent advantage over teams that don't take chemical aids.

THE PLACEBO EFFECT

Although there is some scientific evidence suggesting that drugs may improve performance, it is not necessary that drugs *actually* help for performance to improve after drugs have been taken. It is only enough that people *believe* drugs improve performance, for a strong enough belief often can increase performance far beyond the sought-after 2 to 3 percent needed by winners. That amount that results from belief rather than chemicals is known as the placebo effect.

Athletes, if not physically addicted to drugs, are at least psychologically addicted. Because they believe their competitors are taking drugs, they feel they must take them too. Once having made the decision to take them, they become convinced they cannot do without them. An individual might start out with a relatively small dose, say five milligrams, and soon he has increased his dosage to fifty milligrams. Then, if he wins a big event, he attributes it to taking drugs. So he is afraid to stop taking them and may even take more to ensure his chances of continued success. He may even look at the cost as a saving on food and the other nutritional aids that can be a very costly part of serious training.

But much of the improvement that athletes believe came from a drug or a special food or vitamin did not come from that at all, but from the extraordinary power of the placebo effect.

Said Bob Bauman, a trainer for the St. Louis Cardinals, "In 1964, I devised a yellow RBI pill, a red shutout pill, and a potent green hitting pill. Virtually every player on the team took them, and some wouldn't go out on the field until they took my pills. They worked so well that we won the pennant. We used them again in 1967 and 1968 and also won the pennant.

"They worked because I never told them that the pills were placebos." In other words, grown men improved their performance, indeed became psychologically addicted to pills made of sugar, because of their belief that the pills contained some active chemical ingredient that would make them play better.

The placebo effect works because inside every person is an insecure dependent child who is not fully convinced that by his own capabilities he can succeed.

The demands of sports on a competitor's reservoir of confidence are great. The athlete must not only be as good as others; he must beat them. The combination of insecurity, which to some extent, all individuals are subject to, and the lure of rewards earned by the successful competitor combine to create a situation in which the placebo effect has its greatest chances of success.

Consequently, scientific, controlled studies have not found a single athlete to make the phenomenal gains that some individuals claim, yet athletes the world over have fallen for the wild stories told by some drug proponents of putting on pounds of muscle in almost no time and unreal performance gains. The stories do not fade out because an *individual* cannot distinguish between a pharmacologic effect and a placebo effect. The placebo effect can only be determined by comparing a *group* of individuals who have taken a drug with a *group* of individuals who have not taken the drug in question, and both groups must be evaluated under the same *controlled* conditions.

Moreover, merely comparing the groups is insufficient for making conclusions. It is essential that neither the individuals in the group who have taken the drug nor the group who has not taken it know which group they are in. Nor can the persons who give the drugs to the athletes know which ones are getting the active drug. A placebo must be made up that appears to be identical to the one containing the real thing, so that neither the athlete nor the persons who are conducting the evaluation can tell who is really taking the drugs. This can be accomplished by creating a code kept by a person making up the dosages that can be broken when the evaluation is over, and by handing out the real drug and the fake drug to experimental subjects selected at random.

This situation where neither the experimental subject nor the experiment's evaluator knows who is taking the real drug or who is taking the placebo, is known as a "double-blind" experiment, and it is the only kind of drug evaluation that produces evidence that is acceptable to scientists.

The word *placebo* comes from the Latin verb meaning "to please." A placebo is a fake medicine—usually a tablet or a capsule containing nothing but sugar or an injection containing nothing but a salt solution.

Strange as it seems, these fake medicines do work. When they are given by doctors to treat illnesses, placebos can be very powerful. However, doctors don't give them very often. Doctors don't give plain sugar pills because patients get angry if they find out and because doctors can't predict when and how much they'll work or which patients they'll work on. Moreover, in this scientific era, a doctor is supposed to find out what's really wrong and to prescribe a drug that's specifically formulated to treat the problem. A doctor charging patients for sugar pills would be considered a bit of a quack.

Just because doctors don't prescribe sugar pills doesn't mean they're not aware of the placebo effect. Today, the placebo effect is receiving very serious attention by medical scholars, and the meaning has extended far beyond the sugar pill. A placebo effect is any effect attributed to a pill, potion, or procedure, but not to its pharmacodynamic or specific properties. This definition has been expanded to mean any effect associated with the color or size of a drug, or associated with the environment (including the personality of the doctor) in which the drug is taken. What this really amounts to is that a drug can have an effect because the patient wants and expects it to, and this desire and expectation can be increased or decreased by all sorts of factors that don't have anything to do with the chemical properties of the drug.

The expectation of a drug's effect can be amazingly strong. Persons have actually had to be withdrawn from experiments because they have had dangerously violent reactions to totally inert pills. In some other cases, the usual effect of a drug has been completely reversed. Subjects have said they were stimulated by sedatives when they were told they were taking stimulants, and the reverse situation has occurred also, where stimulants sedated people who believed the drug they had taken was a sedative. If belief is so strong that it can completely reverse the usual activity of one of our strongest classes of drugs, it is not very surprising that athletes, who want so hard to believe, find that magic medicines are making them bigger and stronger. And never mind some potential harm to the body which might not happen, and in any event, is surely a long way off.

Berton Roueche, author of many popular books and articles about medicines, wrote in *The New Yorker* in 1960, that the placebo effect works because of the "infinite capacity of the human mind for self-deception." The mind exerts very strong control over the body. An expectation of harm or threat mobilizes the body into a fight or flight stance, the adrenalin fairly pours through the body, the heart rate increases, the breathing rate increases, the fear that one is about to make a fool of oneself produces the well-known and sometimes paralyzing phenomenon of stage fright with its attendant sweaty palms, faintness, and heart palpitations. We know now that people can will themselves into control over body processes once believed to be totally a matter for the unconscious mind. For example, people are learning how to raise and lower their own blood pressures, body temperatures, and to control their heart rates—all through a process called *biofeedback*. In biofeedback, people are hooked up to machines that record their body processes. When the individual is successful, for example, in lowering his blood pressure, the machine lets him know it. Apparently, the pleasure he feels—even at pleasing a machine—is a reward that reinforces whatever steps the body took to lower the blood pressure, and with practice, he can will his body into taking action that results in a more healthful state.

The placebo effect in healing works because it triggers specific biochemical processes in the body. It translates the will to live and to be well into specific actions. Totally inert substances have "cured" fever, headache, coughs, colds, insomnia, angina (heart muscle pain), postoperative pain, and even warts. They have affected processes such as blood cell counts, gastric juice secretions, pupil dilation, blood pressure, and respiratory rates. It is now believed that thinking and beliefs in therapy can help the body fight even diseases like cancer, by mobilizing the body's natural immunological system.

There is a great deal of exciting research going on right now with respect to alleviation of pain and endorphins, which are naturally occurring substances in the body. It has long been know that placebos work especially well in controlling pain. It appears that the body's expectation of help promised by taking what is believed to be a legitimate medicine triggers the release of endorphins, which are chemically similar to the strong opiates, morphine and heroin.

If placebos can trigger the release of narcotic-like substances, they may also stimulate the release of chemicals that take part in other body processes—even growth.

Doctors have believed for years that the proper attitude can work miracles in some people, and attitudes of hopelessness and giving up can literally kill. In African and Caribbean societies, people have died when they have become convinced that another, more powerful person has put a curse on them from which there is no escape. An athlete who believes that another person is taking powerful medicine and gaining an advantage over him may experience a negative placebo effect, his attitude of hopelessness literally weakening his body. Thus, we see that the placebo effect can be not only extremely powerful but a force for harm.

For the placebo effect to help, the athlete must have faith in the drug and, if someone else has given it to him (e.g., a doctor or trainer), faith in that person. If that trusted person believes in the drug as well, he will send a message to his "patient," a signal that says, "I can help you. This medicine will make you into a winner. I know what I'm doing. Your faith and hope are not misplaced." The athlete's belief and faith mobilize his body into exerting its utmost. The athlete succeeds and believes that the drug was responsible. He tells others about the "wonder drug," and they begin to take it too. And none on his own can tell if the drug had any real effect at all.

WOMEN ATHLETES & DRUGS

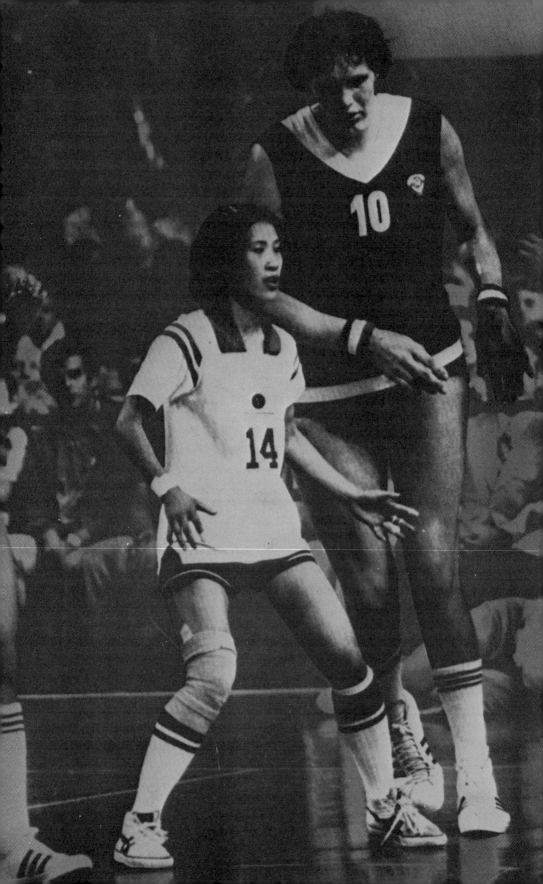

The USSR's 7'4" woman basketball player Semenova dwarfs Japan's Sachiyo Yamamoto during the 1976 Olympics. The Soviets won 98-75. While it becomes increasingly difficult to get actual steroid consumption data out of the Soviet Union, it is a fact that steriods critically affect the endocrine glands, which dictate abnormal growth patterns.

4

THE NEW UNISEX—FEMALE ATHLETES TURNING MALE

Steroids scare me for what they can do over the long term. And for what they can do to women.

Professor Arnold Beckett
University of London

YOU'VE SEEN HER STANDING ON THE BLOCKS AT THE END OF A POOL waiting for the starting gun, or running down the field, or into the spin that hurls her discus farther than the others, or standing at rest at the side of a track with a javelin in her hand, or walking away from you in her running shoes and warm-up suit. And you've said to yourself, "My god, is that a woman? Look at those great hulking shoulders and those arms. Why, she looks more like a man than half the men I know."

If you had seen her earlier—a month, six months, a year, three or four years, or more—in the privacy of her locker room at her home gym, you would have seen her drinking a white powder mixed in juice or swallowing tablets or taking an injection in her behind.

If you had asked her what she was taking, she might have been able to tell you, but she was more likely to answer, "Oh, just some powder to make me stronger. All the girls take it."

"Just some vitamins that the coach gave me."

"Some growth stuff that all the East German girls are taking."

If you had suggested that she was taking a drug that might be harmful, she would probably have dismissed your concern.

"I know that, but I need it so I can break the record," or "win in

43

Mexico," or in wherever the next major competition was scheduled, or

"Well, maybe. But I'm going to stop taking it when I retire and then I'll be O.K.," or

"I don't think my coach would give me anything that would really hurt me, and besides, it's worth it. Do you know I've taken nearly three seconds off my time since I started taking those drugs?" or

"I get a lot of exercise and I don't drink or smoke or take birth-control pills, so I don't think I'll get any bad effects from this stuff. It's only helping me get stronger like steak or supervitamins or something," or

"Listen, when everybody gives up booze and Valium, come back and tell me about it."

The participation of women is the newest and most exciting aspect of bodybuilding competition. My first exposure to real, honest-to-goodness female competition was at George Snyder's Best in the World contest, where the women competitors were all taken very seriously by the audience and the judges. The evidence of the hours of hard work, dedication, and physical excellence shone forth from these exceptional female specimens of health and fitness.

As I sat in the audience, troublesome thoughts entered my mind. Shades of past Olympics—incidents where sex tests and chromosome tests had to be performed to fully identify the sexual gender of the competitors. Visions of the seven-foot-four-inch woman basketball player from the Soviet Union—the East German swimmers with the deep voices, and the facial hair and massive arms of the Bulgarian female shotputter. I began to worry that the drug bastardization of the female form could also enter and destroy the beauty of this new area of competition.

Women are like men athletes in two respects. Both have their heads full of information about their sports. They can tell you who won what and where and their times for ten years back or more. They can tell you all about the places they competed—how they did, how they felt, why they won or lost, what they'd done to train. They can tell you how much they weigh, and what their measurements are, and what they think they should be. They can discuss strategies of winning, wind friction, temperature control, special foods, tough judges, good luck talismen, athletic shoes, whirlpool baths, ace bandages, variations in coaching styles. They know all about psychological readiness, looseness, tightness, psyching up.

The other respect they share with men is that neither knows totally about what they experience. They hurt. They mature. But they don't fully understand the metabolic processes that make these things happen. Lacking knowledge of the incredible interrelated homeostatic systems that are their bodies, that are far more sophisticated than the most advanced computers now envisioned, that become more awesome to biologists the more they are understood, it is perhaps not surprising that athletes are willing to take strange chemicals into their bodies. They need not concern themselves with the digestion, metabolism, and excretory products of a meal of spaghetti, salad, and apple pie. Bodies hum along efficiently taking care of things with little conscious effort by their owners and, considering their tasks, making few demands. In this respect, they are like the mysterious black boxes that physicists are so fond of. Physicists know what black boxes can do, but they don't care at all about what's going on inside them that makes them do it.

What information athletes do pick up is often confusing and contradictory. "Take massive doses of vitamin C." "You get all the vitamin C you need in a normal diet." "Don't eat foods with cholesterol." "Forget about cholesterol in foods; your body makes its own." "Don't eat salty foods." "Take salt tablets when it's hot." "Drink six glasses of water a day." "Drink only when you're thirsty." "Chocolate causes acne." "Chocolate has nothing to do with acne." "Carrots make you jaundiced." "Carrots make you see better at night." "Oysters are brain food." "Oysters give you hepatitis." "Smoking preserves meats." "Smoked meats give you cancer." "Vitamin E has no function in adults." "Vitamin E is an aphrodisiac." "Green peppers contain vitamin C." "Green peppers are indigestible." "Plain aspirin is best for minor aches and fever." "Aspirin makes your insides bleed." "A normal person moves his bowels about the same time every day." "People should let their bowels take care of themselves." "Red meat builds up your blood." "Red meat is bad for you." "Women need extra iron." "Women get all the iron they need in green salads." "Eat eggs and drink plenty of milk." "Cut down on eggs." "Adults don't need milk." And so it goes.

The amount of controversy over the effect of even simple foods on the human body tends to make athletes suspicious of messages telling them that drugs are bad. They've heard it all before, and they know that for certain drugs, for example, marijuana and cocaine, the dangers have been blown all out of proportion to the actual risk to health of minor and transient use. They feel that the consequences of getting caught breaking the drug laws are greater than the potential threat to their health.

These feelings—confusion and suspicion—coupled with the incomplete understanding of the workings of their bodies, are especially threatening to women, especially considering the nature of the drugs they are now taking to build strength and endurance.

WOMEN AT GREATEST RISK

"Giving male hormones to a male may not be a very nice thing to do, but at least you are giving him more of something his body produces naturally. But if you start giving a female that same male hormone, it's going contrary to her whole endocrine make-up," said Dr. Clayton Thomas of the Harvard School of Public Health, and a member of the U.S. Olympic Committee's Sports Medicine Committee, in an interview given to *The Washington Post* in 1979. Thomas went on to say, "I don't think you could do this for an extended length of time without running a great risk of doing permanent damage to her endocrine normality as well as her long-range potential for childbearing."

"I think you even run the risk of causing neoplasms [abnormal growths] or cancers in some part of her body that would not have developed if she hadn't taken these steroids. That may be a rather freewheeling statement, but I feel strongly about it—particularly in light of the problems we have seen with a female hormone that was widely used and thought to be completely safe; the oral contraceptive pill."

Women's bodies produce many steroids normally. Steroids are responsible for growth and metabolism, and some of a women's sex hormones, the estrogens, are steroids too. The problem with women taking anabolic steroids is that they are synthetic derivatives of the strongest androgen, the strongest male sex hormone, testosterone.

It is true that women's own bodies produce small quantities of testosterone naturally, and it is generally conceded that testosterone is responsible for a woman's sex drive. A woman's natural testosterone is in a delicate balance with her own estrogens that govern her reproductive cycle and feminine characteristics—breasts, distribution of body hair, and adipose tissue.

Women are not as big or as strong or usually as sexually aggressive as men because of the dominant relationship of their estrogens relative to their androgen, their testosterone.

Said Pat Connolly, former women's track coach at UCLA, "It's sad, because the use of [anabolic] steroids does—I hate to say this, but it's true—it makes freaks out of women. Women are beautiful creatures the way God made them, and they can do a lot of things tremendously well. We don't even have any idea of how well we can do some things because we haven't been trying very long. But by taking a male hormone, a woman is really changing what she is all about.

"I've seen some women who have been taking them, and their personalities change. It's just really sad and depressing that steroids are part of the scene, and that a woman instead of perfecting her body the way God gave it to her, has to make herself into some creature that's not really a woman and not really a man."

Anabolic refers to a substance that promotes growth or repair. *Androgen* refers to steroids that produce or stimulate male characteristics. An androgen produces male sex characteristics and has a second major effect, body building. Androgens are in a biological antagonism with estrogens. In men, androgens develop men's sex organs, beard growth, skin thickness, body hair, and depth of voice. Androgens also develop weight and muscle mass by increasing protein assimilation. There is no such thing as a strictly anabolic steroid, meaning a strictly bodybuilding drug. Anabolic steroids are androgenic and are masculinizing. All affect sexual processes and characteristics. When a woman takes an anabolic steroid, she is taking a masculine growth substance that is antagonistic to her own estrogens.

She is a female turning male.

And she is taking a very great risk.

When the American College of Sports Medicine issued its position paper on anabolic steroids in 1978, it said:

> The use of anabolic steroids by females, particularly those who are either prepubertal or have not attained full growth, is especially dangerous. The undesired side effects include masculinization, disruption of normal growth patterns, voice changes, acne, hirsutism and enlargement of the clitoris.
>
> The long term effects on reproductive function are unknown, but anabolic steroids may be harmful in this area. Their ability to interfere with the menstrual cycle has been well documented.

> For these reasons, all concerned with advising, training, coaching, and providing medical care for female athletes should exercise *all precautions available to prevent the use of anabolic steroids* by female athletes [emphasis added].

The risks that women take are especially great because there has been little research into the effects of anabolic steroids on women's bodies. As documented in the appendix, there have been dozens of investigations into the effects of anabolic steroids on males, and although much remains to be studied, something is known about what happens to men when they take moderate doses of these drugs. But scientists believe that the potential of anabolic steroids to harm women, both short- and long-term, is so great, scientists will not even take the risk of performing experiments to see if anabolic steroids improve women's athletic performances.

Any biologist, any physiologist, any endocrinologist, any pharmacologist knows that he is giving directly against nature if he gives a woman an anabolic steroid, i.e., a male growth hormone. Any team physician, coach, or trainer worthy of the title knows it too, and every female athlete and parent of a budding female athlete ought to know it.

The dangers of anabolic steroids to women are especially great in adolescent women and in those women who are also taking oral contraceptives. It is difficult to imagine a greater assault on a woman's natural hormonal system than the double whammy of synthetic estrogens (oral contraceptives) and synthetic androgens (anabolic steroids).

The risk of getting breast cancer in the normal population of women is 10 percent. Anabolic steroids will increase this risk many times. It is true that certain steroids are used in cancer therapy, but in most cases they are more likely to induce a cancer than cure or prevent one, especially in a healthy individual.

If you want to get an idea of the risks of women taking anabolic steroids, all you have to do is read one of the manufacturer's inserts that is sold with each package, Dianabol for example, and reprinted in the *Physician's Desk Reference*. It states in the section called "Contraindications":

"1 Carcinoma of the breast in females;

2 Masculinization of the fetus;

3 In females: hirsutism, male pattern baldness, deepening of the voice, clitoral enlargement.

THESE CHANGES ARE USUALLY IRREVERSIBLE EVEN AFTER

PROMPT DISCONTINUANCE OF THERAPY AND ARE NOT PRE-VENTED BY CONCOMITANT USAGE OF ESTROGENS."

Female athletes on oral contraceptives have been excused from the doping tests because the persons responsible for the testing have sometimes been unable to distinguish between the metabolic products of these two kinds of drugs in the urine. Thus there is a strong incentive for women taking anabolic steroids also to take oral contraceptives. It all comes down to an incredible risk.

EFFECTS OF ANABOLIC STEROIDS ON FEMALE METABOLISM

Metabolism is the sum of all chemical and energy processes, those that build up and those that tear down, in reference to living cells and their exchange of energy. It is the working of life from the smallest to the largest of living things. It represents an interlocking network of cellular functions.

Anabolic steroids have a variety of effects on female metabolism. They regulate the protein in connective tissue and bone. They inhibit the pituitary gland's ability to produce the hormones that stimulate the ovaries into producing estrogens. They affect the development of internal and external female organs. If a woman, pregnant with a female child, takes anabolic steroids, these drugs will have a masculinizing effect on her unborn baby. A female baby still in the uterus whose mother takes anabolic steroids will develop some male traits, extra hair, and clitoral enlargement.

Even in an adult woman, these undesirable effects can be irreversible. Many of the Soviet and East German women who took anabolic steroids and developed low voices and beards are stuck with them.

The effects of anabolic steroids on a woman's reproductive system and secondary sexual characteristics are in addition to those which also occur in men. In both men and women, anabolic steroids increase the body's normal insulin activity, upset the body's enzyme systems, break down genetic patterns in the nuclei of the body's cells, affect the absorption of calcium in the bones, stop bone growth in young persons who have not reached their full height, cause the body to retain water, produce the typical "moon-faced" appearance, produce acne, and destroy the kidney and the liver whose job it is, among others, to detoxify alien synthetic chemicals such as anabolic steroids.

Because of the potential damaging effects of anabolic steroids on the genetic material in the nuclei of the cell, many women athletes who took anabolic steroids are now afraid to have children. Says twenty-five-year-old Renate Vogel Heinrich, who nine years ago was a champion East German swimmer and who was brought up on anabolic steroids: "I would love to have children, but I am afraid that I would bring them into the world handicapped."

Warned Dr. Thomas, a consultant on human reproduction at the Harvard School of Public Health, "Supplying such drugs [anabolic steroids] to women may in the future be reclassified from unethical to criminal" (See Appendix on birth defects).

Despite warnings from concerned doctors like Dr. Thomas, anabolic-steroid use is reported to be on the increase among women competing at top international and collegiate levels. Many women have been caught doping and disqualified in the last few years, and many women have "taken and told."

EVEN WOMEN GET CAUGHT

At the Winter Olympic Games in Lake Placid in 1980, doping tests were administered to two athletes picked at random from every team event, the first four finishers in every individual event, and every athlete whose performance was much better than expected. The women were not excepted. They too gave about two ounces of urine to the Olympic drug watchdogs who were looking for athletes who had taken stimulants, narcotics, anabolic steroids, and other banned substances.

Said Olgo Fikotova Connolly, a 1956 gold medal winner who has participated in five Olympic Games as a discus thrower, "There is no way in the world a woman nowadays, in the throwing events—at least the shot put and the discus—I'm not sure about the javelin—can break the record unless she is on steroids. These awful drugs have changed the complexion of track and field.

"It's a terrible thing, but it's true. Once a girl has developed her natural powers to the utmost, she has to start taking something that will alter her natural endowments of strength in order to continue the quest for a world record. She sees these big balloons competing, and she thinks she must become a balloon too."

But with all the testing, how do they get by with it? Well, doping tests are not done at all sports events. And sometimes, as mentioned before, women have not been tested because they said they were on the pill, and the tests were not sensitive enough to distinguish between anabolic steroids and oral contraceptive steroids. Then it's possible to take anabolic steroids and go off them in sufficient time before a sports competition so that they won't show up in the urine.

But not all women have got by with it. In 1979, seven top women were banned from Olympic competition *for life* by the Amateur Athletic Federation because they were caught taking anabolic steroids. This means that the top three 1,500-meter runners of 1979 could not take part in the 1980 Moscow Games, even if their sentences were commuted to the eighteen-month disqualification period that commonly results from an appeal.

Banned for life were two Romanians—Natalia Maracescu, who holds the world mile record for women, and Ileana Silai, the 1968 Olympic 800-meter silver medalist—and a Bulgarian—Totka Petrova, who won the World Cup for 1,500 meters in Montreal in 1979. Also penalized were two junior discus throwers from the Soviet Union.

Dr. Tony Daly, a member of the International Amateur Athletic Federation, said he had been unaware before the banning that middle distance women runners were using anabolic steroids.

Other women caught doping at the European Championships were Nadechko Tkachenko, who forfeited her pentathlon gold medal in 1978 at Prague, and Ilone Slupianek, an East German who lost her gold medal in the shot put at the 1977 European Cup.

Although Slupianek was banned for eighteen months, her sentence was appealed and reduced to a year so that she could participate in the European Championships in Prague—the same games where Tkachenko lost her medal.

It is generally believed that the most recent group of banned women athletes got caught because their trainers had not realized that the tests for anabolic steroids had become more sensitive and specific. Athletes used to believe they could stop taking the drugs two to three weeks before a test, but now sophisticated equipment can detect anabolic steroids taken as far back as two months.

Some cynics believe that catching Ileana Silai doping will increase anabolic steroid use by track and field women athletes. At thirty years of age, Silai broke four minutes in the 1,500 meter race, a feat that is seen by many as proving that steroids work and that if women want to break records they had better climb aboard the drug bandwagon.

RENATE'S STORY

Now when Renate Vogel Heinrich looks at pictures of herself, during her competitive years, she says, "I get sick. We never really noticed what we looked like, because swimmers were always kept together. It didn't hit me until an old friend said, 'Wow Renate, you speak like a man, and you've got those unbelievably broad shoulders.' "

Renate was relatively lucky. Her weight has dropped from 155 to 130 pounds well distributed over a five-foot-eight-inch frame, and her voice has risen to its normal pitch. Renate managed to flee from a training environment where anabolic steroids were handed to her like morning orange juice. "It was just given to us along with the vitamin pills," she relates.

Ms. Vogel Heinrich is not so confident about the long-term effects that taking anabolic steroids for so many years may have had on her body and freely admits her fear of having children. Concerned about her husband who is still behind the iron curtain, she does not freely admit how she escaped to Stuttgart in West Germany in the late summer of 1979. When she left, her husband, Volker Heinrich, was immediately arrested by the East Germans.

Now Renate spreads her story about East German training camps and drugs, a story that has done more than catching a few athletes taking drugs, to convince sports authorities that doping is a methodical, covert practice in the state-supported training camps of East Germany.

In 1974, Renate Vogel held the world record for women in the 100-meter breaststroke. She was a national heroine, which meant that she enjoyed privileges denied to most East Germans: a luxury apartment, choice goods, and foreign travel. It was the foreign travel that opened her eyes to the intellectual restrictions of the East German Communist Party. Renate, like many tourists, enjoyed taking photographs on her trips, but when she returned to her home land, she found her slide shows were censured. Said Renate, "They let me show my slides of Hiroshima but not of Disneyland or Hollywood."

Renate quit the drugs—and perforce her training—but when she defied the authorities, she lost a special privilege. She was not able to participate in the program run by medical specialists that slowly decelerates an athlete who is coming off training and training drugs. Renate went "cold turkey," which worsened her already bad health.

"When I stood up," she says, "I often lost consciousness. If I moved my head too quickly, I blacked out." Her health and the social censure and ostracism in her native country were finally too much, and Renate went AWOL to provide us with a firsthand account of programmed athletic training in Eastern Europe where "success is as exactly planned as is production out of a nationalized factory."

DOSAGE

Most women in the West who try to increase their strength and endurance with anabolic steroids know that they are corrupting their natural hormone systems, and they are concerned about "the right amount," which they believe is an amount that helps them win without permanently damaging their health.

In general, women athletes who dope do so in lower doses and for shorter periods of time than their male counterparts. Said Pat Connolly:

> Women who start with a very small dose for four or six weeks, train on it, and then go off the drug and let their bodies get normal again still have the benefit of that training. They have taught the muscles to do new things, and the know-how remains. They can continue to compete at a higher level even though they're off the drug.

I think women coaches feel a lot differently about it than males who coach females. There are some highly principled male coaches who don't want their girls fiddling with that stuff, but there are others who let their egos get in the way. All they care about is performance, and when that happens, there doesn't seem to be any ethics anymore.

> Very few of the girls taking steroids have good medical supervision. No doctor would prescribe them for a woman. A few "understanding" doctors say that, while they are "unaware" a patient is on steroids, they will do regular blood, liver, and urine checks to watch for abnormalities.

What these "understanding" physicians should also be doing is explaining that by the time these so-called abnormalities show up, the female athlete who has taken anabolic steroids may have irreparably, irreversibly, damaged her body. These "abnormalities" are often signs of permanent underlying damage to the body's metabolic and excretory systems. In addition to menstrual irregularities and masculinization, there is no doubt that a woman who takes anabolic steroid drugs risks severe long-term effects—tumors, cancer, and babies born with birth defects.

There are no "right doses" of anabolic steroids for women, and no amount of medical monitoring by "understanding" physicians can make it so. There is no amount of informed consent that can make it all right for women to risk so much for athletics. There is no time in a woman's athletic career when taking anabolic steroids is worth it.

Some coaches believe that if women take anabolic steroids they should do it after ten to fifteen years of training, at the peak of their careers, and during their middle twenties. Although the side effects of anabolic steroids are somewhat less devastating at this age than during the growth period when bones are not fully developed, suggesting that it is better to take anabolic steroids at this time of a woman's life is rather like saying that lung cancer alone is better than cancer and tuberculosis.

No coach, no physician, should in any way, tacitly or otherwise, appear to condone anabolic steroids. Every parent of a young woman who is on a team should make certain that drugs are not a part of her training, and that she knows the special danger of anabolic steroids. Any woman who has taken anabolic steroids in the past should have her hormone levels checked and should have liver- and kidney-function tests.

Everyone (fans, athletes, and health professionals) should support an educational campaign to make certain that female athletes and female potential athletes know the special long- and short-term dangers than anabolic steroids pose to women.

DORIS' TESTIMONY

Truly one of the most exciting and dynamic sports to come into being in the past five years is women's bodybuilding. But here too anabolic-steroid abuse is very frightening. Women abusing such substances are at a much greater risk even than their male counterparts. Doris Barrilleaux, a 52-year-old grandmother with a stunning 20-year-old body, is the principal guiding force behind women's bodybuilding. As president of Superior Physique Association and chairperson of the women's division of the International Federation of Body Builders, she has seen first-hand the tragedies to befall certain women competitors.

The widespread misuse of steroids in the sporting realm becomes more prevalent with every passing year. Although male and female athletes in many sports admit and, yes, even boast about using these chemicals to enhance their performance, my personal knowledge stems only from my involvement in the sport of physique competition. And of all the athletes involved, it is most ludicrous for bodybuilders to resort to these tactics. They have no distance to cover, no clock to beat, no really strenuous performance of any kind to compete in their chosen field. Yet they risk their life and limb to achieve a certain "look" for a short period, sometimes a matter of hours. And why? To appeal to a panel of judges who may or may not *like* the way they look. Even though there are guidelines for judging physique competition, it is still highly subjective.

The reports I have heard concerning the use of steroids make one wonder about the people who have so little value for their health that they will risk their lives for the acquisition of a *trophy*. Some professionals compare these health risks to those of a race driver hoping to win a big purse. But the use is not limited to the professionals. I have attended many seminars given by top male professionals where the first questions asked by young boys were what drugs to take and what dosages. Everyone is looking for a short cut, an edge over the next guy. No one wants to wait the five or ten years it takes to build a championship body naturally. Sometimes their questions are answered in detail. Sometimes they are told, "I take them because I'm a professional, but you shouldn't take them." And other times I truly admire the men who state, "Ask me anything you want about training and diet, but drugs are bad news, stay away from them."

As a physique photographer, I was involved in men's bodybuilding long before organizing women's bodybuilding in 1978. My first introduction to the presence of drugs came one day as I walked into a local gym and witnessed a young boy walking out from behind the counter pulling up his pants. I innocently asked what was going on and was informed that the gym owner had just given him a steroid injection. Over the next few years I was to hear unbelievable tales related to drug use. Some have been related in various publications, but the saddest part is the fact that those who were most harmed by the drugs do not speak out to help educate others who follow in their path of destruction. I have seen an aspiring young hopeful with stars in his eyes take a year off work to train for the "big one." He dropped from sight, but I ran into him a few years later. He was reduced to a part-time gym instructor, now physically unable to hold a full-time job. I have witnessed one already on medication because of a serious medical problem using mega-doses of various drugs trying to balance and counterbalance their effects. I was even told of one who was warned before stepping on stage at a prestigious contest that "this injection can kill you" to which he replied, "I don't care. I've worked too hard to get here!" He was lucky that he only became violently ill. Had it been otherwise, would his wife and children reading his tombstone in the future care or understand the meaning, "I've worked too hard to get here?"

The hypocrisy of the whole situation is that these individuals, male or female, are not the perfect physical specimens they lead the world to believe. They are drug-wracked shells, products of the chemicals they pump into their bodies. If they were the ultimate physical specimens, then they could physically maintain a superior level of fitness at all times. They would not have to pick and choose a limited number of competitions to enter per year in an attempt to safeguard their lives. And between these times, they would not be considered fat or out of shape and ashamed to appear in public. Real peak perfection is permanent—not periodical. Bill Pearl, a legend in the sport, told me once at a contest that "none of those men on the stage are healthy."

I can only speculate about the lack of concern by these athletes. Perhaps we live in such a drug-oriented society with the epidemic numbers of people using cocaine, heroin, marijuana, etc., that by their standards, steroids are almost harmless. Concerning the men's sport, I can sum it up with an incident that was related to me. A top bodybuilder was dining in a restaurant with a group of other competitors, all known to be heavy steroid users. This particular man picked up the nondairy creamer and studied the contents, reading aloud "sodium caseinate, mono and diglyceride, dipotassium phosphate, sodium silicoaluminate, etc. etc." He blurted out, "*No way* will I put this stuff in my body!" The others chided him and said, "But you take loads of anabolic steroids and thyroid drugs. Why would you be worried about that?" To which he replied, "Well, you've got to draw the line *somewhere.*"

But drug use is not a laughing matter. It has been in the men's sport for years, and very little attempt has been made to discourage it. My primary concern is that it has already infiltrated the women's sport. It is sad enough that women will resort to its use to try to improve their physical performance. But why on God's earth will they resort to it to change their physical appearance? Where is it written that women bodybuilders must emulate male bodybuilders?

While it is true that for generations women were not encouraged to pursue physical excellence, those who did—gymnasts, dancers, and swimmers—improved their musculature, which is evident in the dancer's well-developed legs, the swimmer's superbly developed upper body, and the gymnasts equally balanced development from head to toe. These women athletes are seldom mistaken for males. With the drug use spreading into women's bodybuilding competition, some women are doing everything conceivably possible to mold themselves into minimen with wide tapering shoulders, flat chests, thick-waisted abdominals, bulging biceps, and hips devoid of curves. In fact, they diet so radically that at competition time, some can actually be mistaken for young males.

One psychiatrist stated that women who feel the need to excel at bodybuilding are dissatisfied with their feminine identity. I disagree wholeheartedly. But from my observations there are several distinct reasons why some women will resort to drugs. The first and foremost is the fact that many women, lacking the knowledge, will succumb to pressure and encouragement from men in the field. These husbands, boyfriends, trainers, and gym owners who think nothing of prescribing steroids to men, do not hesitate to push them on the women. Secondly, many young and impressionable women do not have the guts, integrity, independence, and backbone to *refuse* their use. And thirdly, women who were never able to excel or be recognized in other ways seek attention even if it comes from an unusual or unnatural appearance.

Ironically, many women confide to me that they do not like the way they must look to win or even to enter competition. Therefore, it is even more confusing to learn that more and more women are resorting to the use of drugs to bring about these physical changes.

One top female competitor, who had vowed vehemently and repeatedly that she would *never* touch drugs and opposed the look of other women known to use them, confessed that six weeks before a major competition she finally succumbed to the temptation to try them. She took Maxibolin, which was supposed to give her size. When she ran out of that drug (supplied to her in Europe), she switched to Anavar. The dosages prescribed were in such excess from what a doctor had prescribed that she took 1/2 the dosage. Then, in addition to the Maxibolin, she started on injectable Primabolin. At the same time she was taking oral Thiomucase. By the time she went into the contest she was taking two injectables and two orals every day plus vitamins and supplements. Her strength went up, and she looked like a different person (a look she did *not* like). She put on 10 pounds in six weeks. When she went off the drugs, she stopped completely instead of following instructions, and she suffered many ill effects. One was that she kept on getting bigger and bigger. She broke out with a rash all over her whole body, which turned to scabs. Every joint in her body ached so badly that she could not sleep at night. She had no sex drive at all, and she became very aggressive. She felt different and thought differently. She grew a moustache, which was very traumatic, and also her genitals began to enlarge. Within the six weeks, the muscles of her arms grew an inch and her deltoids showed marked development. It was frightening. There was a definitely different look and thickness, and she had to be doubly careful not to include any exercises to thicken her waist.

The doctor that she was forced to consult explained that when taking the artificial steroids the body sensed that these substances were not needed, so production shut down and the artificial drugs took over. She was lucky that eventually her body was able to reproduce the needed hormones. (I have heard of some women who must take medication for the rest of their lives.) The whole experience was entirely negative. This woman feels the way many others in the sport have come to feel—that until the judges begin looking for an athletic-looking woman and not a miniman, they will just stop competing.

A recent letter to me from a SPA member is instructive in this regard:

> I've been competing since 1980 and girls I used to beat have grown to un-GODLY proportions in three years time, much larger than their normal testosterone level would allow—a biological impossibility unless drug induced. Can't you help this time? Isn't there anything at all you can do to prevent us "women" from having to compete against these "men?"
>
> In 1981, I was accepted to compete in the America in Las Vegas. I wish you could have been in the dressing room to see these women(?) shaving their arms and shoulders, trying to hide their horrendous clitoral hypertrophy, and balding pates by 'fro-ing ' their hair forward. I came home with a disgusted attitude toward the abuse of steroids and wondered when it would all stop. Well, it *hasn't*—and I'm competing in the America again this year, still free from drugs, hoping for a chance at the top.
>
> I just became aware that the "surprise" urine test taken at last year's America was a farce in that the samples are *still* in the freezer. I've been fighting a losing battle.
>
> A girl I know who had pictures and article written about her in M&F this year, traveled to California and soon met many top amateur bodybuilders. She said they all go to one of three well known steroid doctors in California, and 90% were "going on" for the America *this* year. Fair? No way! Please do something now! You are my last hope, Doris.

Sincerely,
An Oldie, But Goodie

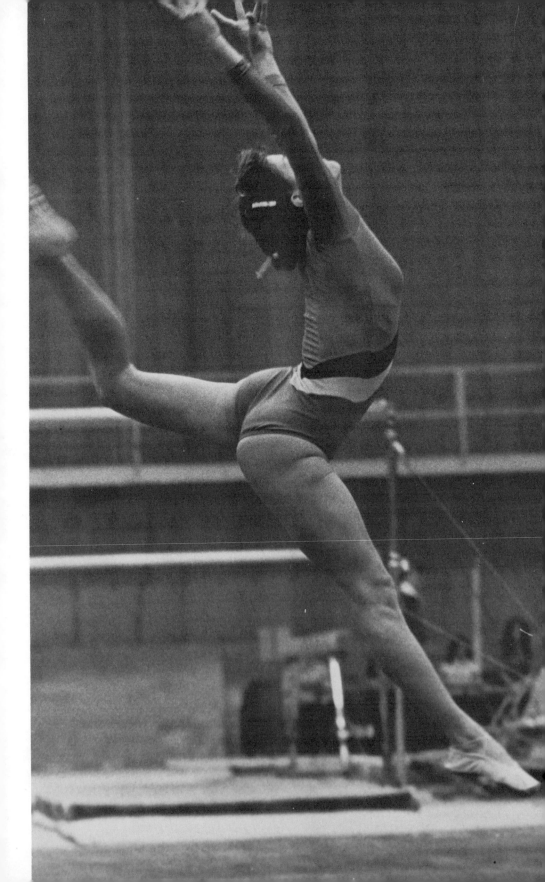

Photo courtesy of John Hansen, University of Illinois at Chicago.

5
BRAKE DRUGS FOR CHILD-WOMEN GYMNASTS

THE PHARMACOLOGISTS AND CHEMISTS WITH THEIR TEST TUBES AND spectrophotometry don't bother to check the urine of women gymnasts for anabolic steroids. The last thing gymnasts want is an extra pound. Nevertheless, if you listen closely at any gymnastic competition, you'll find drug rumors flying through the air as fast as the athletes.

In 1977, some Western coaches began to complain to the sports medicine task force of the U.S. Olympic Committee that Eastern gymnastics coaches were giving brake drugs to female gymnasts so they would not enter puberty but would remain small and childlike for more years of competition.

Everyone has begun to notice that the female gymnasts in international competition are smaller and lighter than they used to be. The little girls who look like they're about eleven or twelve years old are actually sixteen, seventeen, and eighteen. For example, three top Soviet gymnasts at the 1978 Gymnastic Championships in Strasbourg, France, were the following heights, weights, and ages:

Natalia Shaposhnikiv, 57 inches, 79 pounds, 17 years;
Maria Filatova, 53 inches, 65 pounds, 17 years;
Elena Mukhina, 60 inches, 92 pounds, 18 years.

Said Dr. Robert Klein, the official physician at the Strasbourg-based Gymnastic Championships and a member of the international Sports Medicine Federation, "We have no evidence that any teams are being given drugs or hormones to brake their growth. However, we can make certain observations."

Another physician, a pediatric endocrinologist at the University of Southern California in Los Angeles, has commented that there are drugs available that are sometimes given to young girls who are maturing at very early ages (four and five years), a condition known as sexual precocity, and that these drugs are capable of delaying maturity and the development of sexual characteristics, such as menstruation and breasts. This physician, Dr. W. Douglas Frasier, has suggested that these drugs or their analogs might be given to normal young girls to delay their growth. Dr. Frasier told *Sportsmedicine*, "There are a couple of drugs used to treat early puberty that slow down the rate of growth. They don't work very well, but it's conceivable that they might be effective in normal children at very high doses. Of course, you risk serious side effects when you interfere with adrenal, pituitary, and gonadal function, in terms of long term reproductive function."

Dr. Klein is convinced that the older female gymnasts are showing signs of having taken brake drugs. He has observed kyphosis (curvature of the spine), hirsutism, and signs of premature bone and muscle aging in eighteen- to twenty-one-year-old gymnasts, all of which may result from an imbalance of hormones.

Steroids in particular, when taken by a young person who has not attained her full height, causes premature epiphyseal closure. This means that the place at the ends of the long bones where new growth is made stops working, and the body becomes distorted. This phenomenon could account for the kyphosis that Dr. Klein has observed in older gymnasts; their long bones simply did not keep pace with the rest of their body growth, causing them to acquire some spinal curvature and to appear somewhat humpbacked.

Not all physicians agree that the physical immaturity of female gymnasts is necessarily caused by drugs. When the Romanian gymnastic team, whose Nada Comeneci electrified the crowd at the 1976 summer Olympic Games, toured the United States in the following year, it was observed that the team of young women subsisted on very little food. It was reported that they ate but five meals, mainly consisting of tomatoes and lettuce augmented with vitamin pills, during a two-week period. The training theory of the highly successful Romanian coach is to keep the proportion of body fat on the girls to less than 8 percent. If this semi-starvation is successful, the low fat content will delay the onset of puberty and the accompanying shift of gravity that is so unwelcome to tiny female gymnasts who have trained so painstakingly over so many years.

Said Gordon Maddux, a former gymnastics coach turned sports commentator for ABC, "There is no denying that the training regimen of Bela Karoli [Nadia Comeneci's coach] is completely productive, but is it ethical or humane?"

Even mature women have noted the relationship of eating to their hormonal cycles. Women who go on diets frequently find that their menstrual periods stop or are delayed, so it is not surprising that starvation of a young girl will delay onset of maturation altogether. It is nature's way of saying, "There isn't enough food for a baby coming into this body, so let's make it impossible for this woman to get pregnant."

Meanwhile the rumors continue, and many persons are convinced that there is no way the Eastern European gymnasts can remain immature at eighteen and nineteen years of age without some kind of chemical interference in the normal maturation process.

BRAKE DRUGS

The drugs that are most often mentioned as candidates for braking the growth of young women are medroxyprogesterone, an estrogen (female hormone), and cyproterone acetate, a drug available in Europe that has anti-androgenic (antimale hormone) properties.

Medroxyprogesterone acetate is a synthetic form of progesterone, a naturally occurring hormone, and is available under the brand names *Provera* and *Amen* in the United States. Its chemical structure is very similar to the naturally occurring steroids. Cyproterone acetate is an antisex drug used in Europe to treat hypersexuality in men.

When an adolescent girl begins her menstrual cycle, her pituitary gland sends a message hormone to her ovaries telling them to release an ova. When this occurs, the corpus luteum of the ovaries produces progesterone, which mainly functions to prepare and maintain the lining of the uterus for the implantation and nourishment of a possible embryo. If fertilization does not occur, the progesterone level drops, and the lining of the uterus is sluffed off in the process known as menstruation. If fertilization has occurred, the production of progesterone by the corpus luteum continues until about the third month, after which it is produced by the placenta. The continued high level of progesterone prevents ovulation and menstruation.

The synthetic medroxyprogesterone acetate differs from progesterone mainly in that it is active in the oral dosage form. Progesterone is poorly absorbed from the gastrointestinal tract when it is taken orally.

The theory of giving medroxyprogesterone to young gymnasts is that it will delay puberty by suppressing ovulation and menstruation in the same way it does during pregnancy. When ovulation is suppressed, there is also suppression of the hormones that are responsible for physical changes in the body. If there's no ovulation—hence no possibility of a baby—there's no incentive for the body to get ready for it, and there's no need for the hips to widen and the breasts to develop. A prepubescent girl given a progestin remains in childhood for a longer period of time than she would without the drug. That extra year or so can mean many more opportunities to compete. While the risk to her health is a certainty, many young girls are willing to trade a risk with the possibility that no permanent damage has been done (or is at least far in the future) for the certainty that her body will remain a little longer the familiar one she has been training with for so many years.

Cyproterone acetate is a true antihormonal drug. Its primary use to date has been to control hypersexed men, particularly those who have committed sex crimes such as rape, exhibitionism, and pederasty, but sometimes merely to suppress unwanted spontaneous erections. In some European countries, sex offenders are given the choice: Take cyproterone or go to jail.

After men take cyproterone, their testosterone levels fall to one-fiftieth of their former levels. They may become infertile and develop some secondary female characteristics—particularly gynecomastia (breast development).

Although in Europe, doctors recommend that cyproterone be given for cases of hypersexuality that result in compulsive masturbation, indecent exposure, exhibitionism, aggressive alcohol-related sex behavior, sado-masochism, hetero- or homosexual pedophilia, and possibly for instances where a husband is much more highly sexed than his wife, cyproterone is not specifically an anti-testosterone drug, but a general antihormonal drug. Therefore, if cyproterone were to be given to women, it would block their hormones the same way it blocks the hormones of men. It follows that if cyproterone were given to female preadolescents, it would dampen the production of the hormones that are responsible for their maturation and put off puberty, possibly long enough to permit a young gymnast to compete an extra season.

Many gymnastics watchers believe that the Eastern Europeans are experimenting with various drugs at the training camps they run for young athletes. There is a new class of cerebral wonder drugs that modify the action of neurotransmitters in the brain. For example, a drug called LRH (luteinizing release hormone) is produced naturally by the hypothalamus. It controls the production of LH (luteinizing hormone) and FSH (follicle stimulating hormone), which in turn controls the production of sex hormones, and thus the production of ova and sperm. LRH also has been linked to a mating center in the brain. When it has been given to men whose sexual appetites were depressed for psychological reasons, sexual desire and activity have usually returned.

In Europe, LRH has already been used to correct delayed puberty in young men, to induce potency in previously impotent men, and to increase male fertility. In women, it has been given to treat infertility. Because LRH is natural, it stimulates the ovaries into releasing but one ovum each cycle—unlike the fertility drugs on the market which stimulate the release of many ova and often result in multiple births.

Of course, LRH does exactly the opposite of what is wanted for female gymnasts. But with a breakthrough such as this by neurobiologists in the understanding of brain chemistry, it is a certainty that LRH blocking agents have also been found. A blocker might interfere with the body's natural production of LRH or a precursor of it, or it might take up the place of LRH at LRH receptor sites distant from the brain—perhaps the pituitary gland or the ovaries of women and the sperm-producing center of men. Indeed, the new male contraceptives work precisely this way. They are LRH antagonists and block the production of sperm. LRH antagonists may also be used to block the production of ova, and if long-acting ones can be found they may be marketed in contraceptive pills for women.

As can quickly be understood, drugs that block LRH could be given to young women to delay puberty. Because Europeans are at the forefront of sex-drug research, it is possible that young gymnasts are among the first on whom such brake drugs are tried.

If neurotransmitter-stimulating and -blocking agents have not yet been given to young women, there is little to suggest they won't be. In my experience, the power of the desire to win is so compelling that unless the dangers are evident and immediate, an athlete will risk the remainder of his or her life with hardly a thought. This leaves it up to mature individuals to make certain that a climate exists that rules out drug taking by athletes and makes it a *criminal* and *antisocial* act to give drugs to children. For children to be given drugs that interfere with their natural development and mortgage their futures by increasing the risk of cancer and other metabolic diseases—all for the pleasure of adults and the supposed glory of their countries—is an outrage against society.

Ask yourself. Would you want your daughter to be given a brake drug that blocked her normal development, a drug that suspended her in childhood but that would most certainly have a profound effect on her health, appearance, and childbearing abilities in later years? Even if such a drug gave her a moment on the victory platform (not at all a certainty because if she were taking drugs, so would the others), would it be worth it? When she came to you later and said, "What did you do to me?" could you answer?

DRUGS & SOCIETY

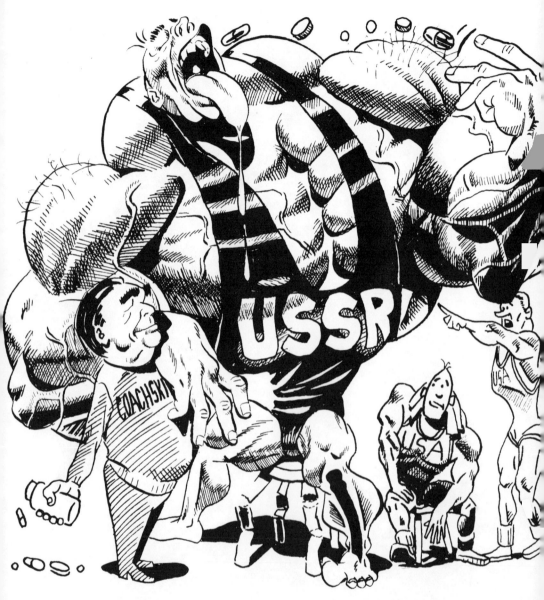

WOW! THEY MUST BE USING SOMETHING NEW!

Drawing by Myron King.

6

TEAM PHYSICIANS UNDER PRESSURE

Quackery. That is the bane of sports medicine. We've rid ourselves of some of the worst, but there are still many people handing out get-good-quick pills, touting machines that send blue sparks and make big muscles, or advising athletes to drink superduper seaweed extracts.

Dr. Daniel F. Hanley
Bowdoin College

MEMBERS OF THE SPORTS MEDICINE TASK FORCE OF THE UNITED States Olympic Committee have noted that a chemical technological race in sports has been under way for some time. The members say that athletes, coaches, and trainers are constantly experimenting with various drugs and their combinations, especially the banned anabolic steroids.

But nearly every team has a team physician. What about them? What part have they played, and what part should they play, in the dangerous and self-defeating drug epidemic?

The *Physicians' Desk Reference*, a compilation of drug manufacturers' package inserts, is the book most often turned to by physicians when they want information on prescription drugs. The PDR states unequivocally that "anabolic steroids do not enhance athletic ability." Moreover, every medical doctor is well enough trained that he knows about the workings of the endocrine system and the potential dangers of exogenous steroids causing liver damage and cancer.

The sad facts are that a few sports physicians are unethical and are full participants in the win-at-any-price syndrome. Others, dangerously ignorant, discount the dangers and believe that the benefits are worth the risks. Some doctors value the pleasure and excitement they derive from their association with sport and find it easier to look the other way when drugs are passed out than to do anything about it. Other doctors argue that they are powerless to stop drug taking and that it is better if drug-taking athletes are under their supervision. These doctors say that athletes are bound and determined to take drugs no matter who advises against it, and that a conscientious team physician can monitor the drug takers' health by testing blood, liver, and kidney functions. They say they are at least available to answer questions about drugs if they are asked and to pick up the pieces that represent the athlete who has taken drugs unwisely. If doctors quit their jobs over the drug-taking issue, they argue, the team will simply find another doctor who is more cooperative.

DOCTORS ARE HUMAN TOO

Sometimes people forget that doctors are human too and that they are just as big sports fans, and get just as excited about their teams' winning, as the most avid team boosters. The enthusiasm and pride that are part of being associated with a winning individual or team are much more powerful incentives than economic ones to doctors. They know that if they are not cooperative, but bite the hand that feeds them, that hand is likely to show them the exit door of the gym.

Said Dr. John Finley, a Detroit Red Wing team physician, "Exuberance, our own exuberance, is something we physicians in sports have to guard against. Most of us work with teams as a sort of labor of love, because we are fans. I know I am. I root hard for the Wings. I'm trying to think of what I can do to help them win. Maybe there is a drug that will help. I try to watch myself, not let my emotions influence my medical judgment, but it is something to keep in mind."

Certainly, the positivistic scientific era of the sixties and early seventies influenced many team physicians. Drugs, especially antibiotics, had been shown to make almost miraculous cures. Knowledge of the chemistry of the body was increasing by leaps and bounds. Although most doctors did not personally participate in the scientific search for knowledge, they came to have confidence that the new understanding of how the body worked meant that drugs could be found that could fix the body chemistry when it went wrong. This time of scientific positivism that put men on the moon also cranked up the drug companies and led to the pill-for-every-ill syndrome, a syndrome whose limitations have only recently begun to be fully appreciated.

To be sure, there were doctors even then who were suspicious of magic by chemistry. A few of these were therapeutic nihilists, more by philosophy than scientific reasoning; but some were suspicious because they were so well trained in biology and pharmacology. They understood that, despite magnificent gains in scientific understanding of the body, actually very little was known. They understood that the body is a complicated system of interrelated subsystems and that it is impossible to affect one part without affecting others. They understood that drugs lacked specificity. For example, if aspirin is taken for a headache, it does not speed to the site of the problem and fix it but spreads throughout the body, affecting the intestinal tract, the joints, the liver, the coagulation of blood, the enzymes, and so on. Moreover, these doctors understood that most drugs are palliative and do nothing to cure a disease but only make the symptoms more tolerable. They understood that pain can be useful and that if an injured athlete masks his pain so he can continue to perform, he may do himself permanent injury.

Only in recent years are most doctors and the public beginning to appreciate the limitations of medicines and to understand that such factors as heredity, nutrition, sanitation, work environment, air and water quality, and lifestyle have far more influence on health than any medicines.

Most doctors are interested in the application of medical knowledge and not the research process. Thus it is understandable how the can-do American spirit and enthusiasm for sports combined to make it a near certainty that sports physicians would give drugs to athletes to help them win.

Said a New York physician, "I obviously don't want to be quoted. However, as a generality, team physicians tend to be men of action, not scholarly, speculative types. They are interested in immediate problems making somebody strong, relaxed, mean, or quick, and in getting a player back in the game as soon as possible. If somebody tells them there is a drug that might do the trick, they are apt to try it. They are not likely to wait around for a double-blind control study to find out if the drug is effective or what it will do to the liver three years later. They are interested in today."

Even though sports doctors are not necessarily academic types, they realize that adverse effects rarely occur in 100 percent of the

people who take specified drugs. In fact, most drug-related side effects occur in a small percentage of people who take them. The
results of clinical drug trials are always reported in terms of the increased risks of taking a particular drug. And some of the reports refer to the results of giving drugs to rats or other laboratory animals,
and not people at all. This situation helps the doctor who wants to
administer drugs to athletes to rationalize in his own mind that even
though the drug increases the chance that the athlete will suffer an
adverse effect, there is still a greater chance that the athlete will not
suffer an adverse effect than that he will. The psychology of the situation leads the doctor to yield to the pressures to give drugs. "After
all," he says to himself, "these athletes are in peak physical condition. They want the drugs, and chances are the drugs won't hurt
them anyway."

Most of the drugs given by sports physicians are restorative—pain
killers to alleviate the hurt of turned ankles or muscle relaxants to
help with pulled muscles. For example, Dr. Daniel F. Hanley who has
been an Olympic team physician for three teams, gave an injection of
a local anesthetic (of the type used in dentistry) to Wayne
Baughman, a middleweight American wrestler on the 1967 Pan
American team. Baughman had severely pulled a chest muscle while
winning his semifinal bout and was virtually incapacitated from the
pain. Before his final match, Dr. Hanley gave him the injection, and
he went on to win a gold medal. Hanley said, "I am normally opposed to this type of treatment. I would never use it in high school or
college competition. But this was a special case. The injury did not
involve a weight-bearing area, such as a knee or ankle. There was little risk of aggravating the injury. And Baughman was a grown man
competing for an international gold medal, an opportunity he might
never have again. You balance risk against reward."
"Could he have wrestled without the shot?"
"No. He could hardly stand up," Dr. Hanley said.
Few physicians knowingly administer a drug that will harm a
player. As they say, when they take the Hippocratic oath, "I will use
treatment to help the sick according to my ability and judgment, but
never with a view to injury and wrongdoing. Neither will I administer a poison to anyone when asked to do so, nor will I suggest such a
course."
When harmful drugs are given by physicians, they are most likely

to be given from ignorance and the mistaken faith that drugs approved by the United States Food and Drug Administration and sold by reputable drug-manufacturing companies are safe to be used in a manner selected by the physician, most especially a physician with a frontiersman, can-try spirit and an overwhelming desire to be associated with success.

Some physicians, however, don't fall into the drug trap. Some won't even give pain killers to athletes if they intend to take them so they can compete. If the athlete is injured, many (probably most) simply say that the athlete doesn't play. Dr. W. Norman Scott, MD, who is the orthopedic assistant to Dr. James Nicholas, former New York Jets team physician and guardian of Joe Namath's knees, said to me in a phone interview, "I haven't been exposed to pressure from sports officials as of yet, but if I were, there is no way I would endanger the life of the athlete. . . . *No Way.*"

Broadly speaking, throughout the athletic drug-taking scene, there have been three kinds of sports physicians. One kind who believes that drugs, both restorative and ergogenic, have a place in sports. A second kind who supports only the use of restorative drugs, and a third kind who is reluctant to prescribe drugs of any kind to an athlete for use during competition.

When anabolic steroids first came on the scene, there were many physicians, including the father of anabolic steroids, Dr. John Ziegler, who cautiously embraced them and willingly prescribed them to athletes for whom they were responsible. These physicians were sincerely hopeful that a way had been found to bypass some of the long, arduous years of training and diet that are required to produce champions and near-champions.

Certainly, patriotism was a factor as well. Getting beaten on the playing fields, as well as in outer space and the Cold War, was a hard-to-swallow pill for American doctors who had been raised on American virtue-will-out based supremacy. The feeling of these doctors was that if they could in any way help an American athlete bring home the gold, they had somehow struck a blow for freedom. Moreover, these doctors were convinced that all of the Eastern European athletes were gulping Sputnik-era growth-and-strength steroids, thus gaining an unfair advantage over Western competitors. To the doctor who equated victory on the athletic field with a victory in the political arena, the choice seemed to be to give drugs or risk an American humiliation and open the door to Communism.

Said Dr. Ziegler, "I felt the Russians were going to use sports as the biggest international publicity trick going. . .and strength sports especially. . .They saw it as a political advantage 100 percent."

As time went by it became apparent that anabolic steroids were being taken in doses far, far beyond those suggested by any physician, and physicians began to gain an understanding of the potential dangers that so drastically modified the body's metabolic pathways. In some instances, the cry, "What kind of monster have we created," became more than a metaphor. A more cautious group of physicians began to emerge. These pragmatists took the view that their jobs were to accept reality, ensure that anabolic steroids were taken under medical supervision, monitor the athletes' blood, kidney, and liver functions, and stand ready to try and put the pieces back together.

This kind of sports physician is typified by Dr. H. Kay Dooley, director of the Wood Memorial Clinic in Pomona, California, and the doctor in charge of the medical services at the 1968 Lake Tahoe summer Olympic high-altitude training camp. Said Dr. Dooley: "I did not give steroids at Tahoe, but I also did not inquire what the boys were doing on their own. I did not want to be forced into a position of having to report them for use of a banned drug. A physician involved in sports must keep the respect and confidence of the athletes with whom he is working."

By and large, the doping sports doctor has given way to the doctor who provides restorative drugs when he believes they are indicated, and the doctor who abhors drugs as feeding the give-'em-an-inch-they'll-take-a-mile syndrome. Dr. Robert Kerlan exemplifies this kind of physician. "I'm not a therapeutic nihilist," he says. "Situations arise where there are valid medical reasons for prescribing drugs for athletes. There are special occupational health problems in some sports. However, the excessive and secretive use of drugs is likely to become a major athletic scandal, one that will shake public confidence in many sports just as the gambling scandal tarnished the reputation of basketball. The essence of sports is matching the natural ability of men. When you start using drugs, money, or anything else surreptitiously to gain an unnatural advantage, you have corrupted the purpose of sports as well as the individuals involved in the practice." Dr. Kerlan was formerly the sports physician for the Dodgers and a number of individual athletes in various sports.

In the late sixties, official bodies were reluctant to tell physicians what to prescribe. Wrote the director of the American Medical Association's Department of Medical Ethics, Edwin J. Holman, to a San

Francisco physician, "I have your letter of November 29 asking if it is legal and ethical for you 'to prescribe moderate doses of anabolic agents to weight lifters for two or three weeks prior to competition, followed by intervals of three months or more without these agents.' No categorical answer can be made to your inquiry inasmuch as this is basically a medical question. The physician must exercise sound medical judgment in prescribing any drug. Sound medical judgment is not determined by the courts, but rather by fellow physicians."

In the case of anabolic steroids, the hoping-to-dope physician had better be careful and keep his malpractice insurance up to date. It is highly unlikely that a fellow or any other group of physicians would testify in a court of law that it was medically sound to administer anabolic steroids to a healthy person.

DOCTORS AREN'T THE ONLY ONES

If team doctors won't dope, often team trainers will. Coaches and trainers who are on the firing line day after day hold the keys to the drug lockers, and there's a lot more incentive for them to dope than for doctors to do it.

A physician is rarely dependent for his entire livelihood on the money he earns from his association with a team. Physicians are in great demand and can always get other jobs. Most often, their athletic jobs are only part-time anyway. For many physicians, being against drug taking is easy. They're never under pressure if they've made their positions clear. The doping physician does so from his own exuberance, ignorance, and misplaced self-confidence.

Not so the team trainer. The trainer is entirely dependent on the team, and he is under almost constant pressure to make the athletes perform. If they don't, he, unlike the doctor, loses his job and what little status he derived from his association with success. The trainer is under real pressure from the coach, who is under severe pressure himself. Athletes don't win sitting on the bench with injuries. Some athletes don't win unless they are fired up enough to go out and tear into their opponents with total disregard for the possibility of injury to themselves. Some athletes have become psychologically dependent on drugs, and they can't play without them. When it becomes a matter of winning and losing, who plays and how they play, the trainer who has no formal training in medicine and surgery, nevertheless, will give almost any kind of drug to any kind of player.

Said Joe Kuczo of Georgetown University and once the head Washington Redskin trainer, "You do things in the big game you might not do otherwise. But the catch is that everything is getting to be a big game. The one you saw win or lose in September is just as important as the one in November. A pro football training camp used to be a fairly relaxed place. Now they are banging a week after they get there. What goes on in July or August is real important to a rookie trying to make the team or to an older fellow struggling to last one more year. The coaches get worked up to the point that it is a life-or-death matter whether Joe Zilch is ready for a Tuesday practice." There are two sources of pressures working here. One from the coach, owners, and fans, and one from the players who often beg for drugs that will fix them up enough to compete.

There is a foolish sense of false pride in playing injured. It's a macho thing. Peer pressure also comes in. If you don't play, your team looks at you as an outcast or traitor to the faith. I felt these same pressures during my amateur competitive wrestling and football years. Lord help those whose sport is their profession. When their team loses a game because of their illness or injury, the other guys on the squad really make life miserable—especially when the loss means money out of their pockets.

NO UPPER LIMITS

It's hard for football players to go out on a football field every Sunday and get into the mind-set that seems to be required to win. Some players think it's nearly impossible, so they take uppers (usually amphetamines, but sometimes cocaine) to get a jolt of get-up-and-kill.

Many spectators as well as team physicians have lost interest in watching drug-crazed men bloody each other every Sunday kickoff. The use of amphetamines by pro ball players is at epidemic levels. Dr. Arnold Mandell, speaking of these abusers said, "I imagine what it is like to gulp down thirty pills at one time. The result is a prepsychotic paranoid rage state. A five-hour temper tantrum that produces the late hits [in football or the fights], the unconscionable assaults on quarterbacks that are ruining pro football. They're at war out there, and the coaches, even if they're not aware [of the drug's effect] are the generals. Coaches know the game is ideally played in controlled anger. They hang up clippings and talk vendettas. Players get half-crazy anyway, and 60 percent of them have their heads filled with amphetamines. The injury rate is enormous."

Some players have been known to say to their team physician, "Doc, I'm not about to go out there one-on-one against a guy who's grunting and drooling and coming at me with big dilated pupils unless I'm in the same condition." At times the older players will confide in their team physician to the tune of, "Doc, I'm making $60,000 a year. It's easy for you to preach, but if I lose my spot, I will be walking the unemployment line, and I have a wife and two kids to support and a house to pay off."

Although officially there is no amphetamine use in the National Football League, the players tell a different story privately, and there are no doping tests in the NFL. Several Redskin team members told a *Washington Post* reporter in 1979 that up to a third of the players took stimulants every time they played. Players from other pro teams argued that amphetamine doping was about the same throughout the league.

Said one player, "What you've got to be concerned about is the amphetamine gap between you and the opposition. . .If their pupils are dilated, and they're jabbering away in paragraphs, fidgeting and ranting and licking their lips, those are pretty good clues there's an amphetamine gap. It's disconcerting to look across the line and see that."

Too bad. Amphetamines are among the most dangerous and damaging of all abusable substances. Tolerance to amphetamines develops rapidly so that higher and higher doses are required to attain the highs that are produced by the drug's ability to release and sustain adrenalin and adrenalin-related chemicals in the body. Even moderate chronic use can cause high blood pressure, abnormal heart rhythm, irritability, insomnia, and anxiety, in addition to the aggression that the football player is seeking in the drugs. As use continues and dosage increases, the user can develop marked personality change, severe weight loss, and paranoid psychoses with delusions and hallucinations. Many amphetamine junkies have a compulsion to engage in repetitive, bizarre, purposeless tasks like unfolding and refolding clothing for hours. Some amphetamine takers fall into a terrible cycle of taking uppers, which keep them hyperactive and awake, and then downers to get some rest, and then back to uppers and so on in a crazy drug-marked roundabout.

Some of the amphetamines are taken to counteract the bloated and sluggish feeling brought on from taking anabolic steroids to build weight. At first, an individual on anabolic steroids feels exhilarated and strong, but this feeling soon gives way to a constant, tired, dragged-out feeling. Instead of stopping the anabolic steroids, the athlete, on the advice of other anabolic steroid-taking empty-heads, begins to take more of them and to add amphetamines to overcome the steroid-induced lethargy. As his system develops a tolerance for anabolic steroids and his adrenals are damaged, he needs some amphetamines to feel like "himself." The next step is onto the upper-downer merry-go-round.

Said Jack Kvancz, Catholic University's basketball coach, "I know that the players of today have no fear of drugs, no damn fear at all. They've grown up in a generation that will smoke, swallow, or snort anything, I guess. I remember how scared I was of any kind of drugs, but nothing is foreign to the kids of today."

If athletes can't get drugs from doctors or trainers, they'll buy them on the drug black market, from friends, or salesmen who import them from abroad.

MEDICAL GAMES

Some believe winning at any cost is the way to go. This can be a confusing issue when we are talking about a child in a pee wee football game and not an Olympic gold medal finalist.

You can get these drugs from a physician, black market dealer, or even by mail order. Here's how *The Underground Steroid Handbook* advises young people:

HOW AND WHERE TO GET THEM
Well, it would be nice to get them from a doctor. A knowledgable [sic], kind, honest, humanitarian-type doctor who would give you a fair price on injectables, let you take them home with you so you could save time and gasoline by injecting them yourself, and would write you refillable prescriptions for your orals. He would be concerned with the progress you are making while on the drugs. We happen to go to such a doctor. Unfortunately, this is the exception. Most doctors have formed an opinion on steroids, which means that they don't like them. Lucky for us though there is a large number of what we call the 'businessman doctor'. These guys are out to hustle a buck.

We'd recommend that you first look for the young ones just out of medical school. Young doctors have a different morality than the older ones. Many do the standard recreational drugs and are open minded about steroids. Also, doctors just starting up a practice usually need instant money. Steroid users are regular, cash paying customers who take up little of a doctor's time. This is financially attractive to him as it frees him to make more money with other patients. Some of the most successful doctors on the West Coast who specialize in steroids have between 1000 to 1500 steroid patients. As you can imagine, this is a very lucrative sideline. You should ask the doctor if he has an interest in building up a steroid clientele as you should be able to pitch him a lot of business. Don't be indiscriminate though; don't send him a deluge of crazies, animals and loudmouths. We've seen that happen before, and what results is suddenly the doctor will not see anyone for steroids. So be careful; don't spoil it for yourself.

Most medical personnel refuse to prescribe anabolic steroids unless indicated for the sick or hormonally deficient patient. Then there are others who feel that since the athlete will use them anyway, it is safer to get them from a physician and be monitored instead of using black-market drugs (with unknown impurities) and self-administration (with its increased chance of infection, hepatitis, sepsis, etc.) I agree, it is, no doubt, safer when controlled by a physician, but this is where the personal medical ethics of the physician comes into play. The Hippocratic Oath states: "I will prescribe regimen for the good of my patients according to my ability and my judgment and never do harm to anyone. To please no one will I prescribe a deadly drug." Again we have to examine how different people interpret this oath. If you took a bottle of Winstrol it would not kill you immediately whereas a bottle of aspirin would. That is the insidious aspect of these drugs—the harmful manifestations are not evident until years later at times. These are wonder drugs for proper medical indications but could turn out to be the nightmare drugs for improper uses.

One such physician who feels he is performing a needed service for athletes is Robert Kerr M.D. of California. He has published a 92-page book in which he describes how he feels about drug use and how to use anabolic steroids. There he says: "I think that you'll agree that if the 'alteration from normal' is neither a true hazard for the patient, or others, and if the patient derives a certain amount of happiness or satisfaction from it, then perhaps it isn't so bad after all." Then he goes on to say that since athletes will take them anyway, he might as well give steroids to them. This is correct, but some patients "derive a certain amount of happiness or satisfaction" from heroin, morphine, amphetamines, and cocaine, yet dispensing these drugs, unless indicated medically is "bad after all!"

He goes on to say:

> In regard to.... "doping" what about those critics of anabolic steroids who still place these drugs in that category called "doping." To my way of thinking "doping" is a term for the use of medicinal agents that will cause an athlete to act or think in a highly abnormal manner. A drug that energizes the athlete by causing him to feel "high" or hyperactive, or to perform in an abnormal way before and during an athletic event, is not proper. A "natural high" should suffice, but something that causes the sensorium to function in an abnormal manner should not be used. Mind altering drugs of any kind have no place in athletics, and to be honest with you, I don't know any athlete who takes them.

Hormones clearly energize the individual and alter the mind (see chapter on withdrawal symptoms). Furthermore, the good doctor never must have met or heard of an athlete taking cocaine. Anyone who has their cortex intact is well aware of mind-altering drug abuse in sports.

His next line of logic infuriates me.

> New tartan tracks for racing have allowed runners to run faster; new running shoe developments have also increased the racer's speed. The flexible pole vaulting poles have allowed vaulters to reach new heights never imagined before. Well, I could go on reciting such examples of track and field innovations but I'd just as soon not—the point is, man is just not content with retaining old standards...If work-out or exercise aids are improper, then is not the Nautilus or similar type of exercise equipment cheating, after all this new technology was developed to give greater gains with less effort—isn't that why anabolics are taken?

You don't eat track shoes and you don't insert flexible pole vaults rectally as suppositories. How can one compare new athletic equipment with hormone drugs! You won't get cancer of the feet from new tartan tracks, nor prostatic hypertrophy from a Nautilus calf machine. Exercise and weight-resistance equipment and vitamins and nutritional aids, along with hard work and good coaching, are what sport is all about. Using healthful, clean and fair methods of training is the essence of athletic and personal growth.

Dr. Kerr has a family practice, yet he has been administering steroids to athletes for sixteen years. He claims that he has seen virtually no side effects in all those years. This is quite remarkable and should be documented in the literature. The disturbing fact is that his entire book is seemingly off the top of his head and devoid of any semblance of back up with medical published literature. Barely a reference is noted. He claims in some of his TV interviews he is not in it for the money. In fact he treats Olympic athletes for free. Well, for every Olympic athlete who walks through his door 100 plus would-be hopefuls will follow. He claims to monitor his athletes closely but does not go into the needed detail to prove that. His section on lab tests is sparse, and I had hoped he would have explored differential diagnoses so that others could benefit from his years of experience in this area. He tests his patients 3–4 times per year and just a simple CBC (complete blood count) and SMAC (blood chemistry profile) would run at least $50.00. Back in 1981 he had a mere 2,000 steroid patients while at the 1983 publication of Terry Todd's *Sports Illustrated* steroid expose, he claimed to have 10,000. I know he's not in it for the money, but you don't have to be a mathematician to see that just on laboratory tests alone, with no office visit fees or ancillaries, we are talking with the typical three testings per year times $50.00 times 10,000 patients equals $1.5 million a year! Not bad for a GP practice.

One last quote from Dr. Kerr's book:

> So, can our track men and power lifters abide by the code of conventionality and refuse to take the strength and speed gaining drugs and allow the other countries to defeat us—of course they can't. . . . Do we really want our international athletes to come in a far second, or third, or worse, behind athletes from other countries who do not have the willingness to refuse to take the drugs? I don't think in the long run that we do. We might say that we have certain standards that we feel we must follow, but in the end we really want to win at nearly any cost—and you know that's true. We've been witnessing today, and for the last number of years, how our female athletes are being defeated in certain strength and power sports by Russia and East German women who just seem to have an edge—*a masculine edge. Right now we don't want our women to be defeminized in order to win, but in the next olympics, or the next after that, will we still be willing to feel the same way?* I don't know, I hope in this case that we don't change.

Let us not confuse the Olympics with a junior-high-school girl's track team. I do not mean to castrate Dr. Kerr, but he is enjoying much visibility and financial success from his stand, and he must come to grips with what his actions might mean, even indirectly, to the youth of America ten to twenty years from now.

When the human body only produces 1700–3700 mg. of testosterone per year, and we have young people ingesting that much or more every month, something is bound to occur. Do we really want our children to win at any cost? I hope not.

WHAT'S A DOCTOR TO DO?

Here are some simple straightforward rules, don'ts and dos, that every sports physician should follow, and a list of suggestions that would help stamp out dangerous drugs in sports.

Don'ts
1. Don't *ever* give an athlete a drug that will change his or her growth, hormone cycle, or metabolism. If an athlete seems to have an abnormality in this regard, he or she should be referred to an endocrinologist. Female athletes who wish to take oral contraceptives should be referred to their gynecologists or family-practice physicians.
2. Don't give ergogenic drugs (other than foods and minerals or vitamins) to athletes.

Dos
1. Develop a sensible drug policy, print it, distribute it, and stick to it.
2. Educate the athletes and their coaches and trainers about drugs.
3. Acknowledge your biases against drug use, and fight against such use.
4. Seek out and offer tests to athletes whom you believe have taken anabolic steroids. These tests should include the following as a minimum:
   a. physical signs and symptoms: prostate enlargement, breast lumps, palpable liver, jaundice, elevated blood pressure, edema, Cushing's syndrome look
   b. complete blood work
   c. liver function
   d. urinalysis
      (See Appendix)

Suggestions
1. Join with other sports physicians to establish guidelines for drug use in sports.
2. Support drug testing programs.

3. Develop positive programs so that athletes feel they have alternatives to drugs.
4. Speak to community groups about the dangers of drugs in sports.
   (See Appendix)

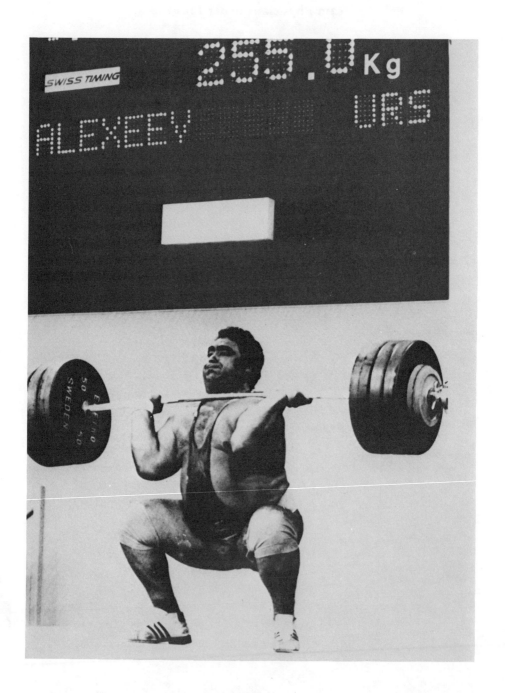

The Soviet's superheavyweight king Vassily Alexeev en route to his world record lift of 255 kg (490 lbs.) during the 1976 Montreal Olympics, July 28. Photo by Pictorial Parade.

7
DRUGS ACROSS THE BORDER: DANGEROUS ILLEGAL ALIENS

In the U.S. and some Latin American countries, the potential haz-ards—including growth stunting in children, jaundice, premature sex development in prepubertal males, testicular atrophy or impotence in older males and hirsutism, deepening of the voice, and menstrual ir-regularities in females—are disclosed in detail. In other Latin Ameri-can countries, they are minimized or ignored.

Dr. Milton Silverman
The Drugging of the Americas

STEROIDS, WHETHER THEY OCCUR NATURALLY IN THE BODY OR ARE made synthetically, are organic chemicals (meaning they are made of carbon and hydrogen with perhaps oxygen or nitrogen) and share the same basic structure. Take a deep breath and say, *perhydrocyclo-pentanophenanthrene*, which is a mouthful.

The drugs in the steroid group vary from each other by virtue of the chemical groups that are stuck on this basic structure. For example, the male hormone, testosterone, has the elements of water, a simple hydroxyl group (OH), and a hydrogen (H), stuck on the top of the five-sided portion at the upper right—where the chimney would be on a house. Progesterone, one of the naturally occurring female sex hormones, is exactly like testosterone except it has a more complicated group, a carbon (C) with a methyl group (CH_3) and an oxygen (O) stuck to it, instead of the water elements. Another naturally occurring anabolic steroid, the male hormone androsterone, has only a single oxygen (O) bonded to its top. Except for testosterone, having an oxygen group (or ketone as chemists like to call it) is a distinguishing characteristic of the anabolic steroids, so if you hear or see the word 17-*ketosteroid* (the 17 refers to the place on the structure, specifically the chimney-place top of the five-sided ring), you'll know that a sex hormone or hormone produced by the adrenal gland is meant.

The adrenal gland, lying just over the kidney, has two parts. The outer part, the cortex, secretes three kinds of 17-ketosteroids: (1) mineralocorticoids, which moderate potassium and sodium retention and excretion, (2) glucocorticoids, which affect carbohydrate (sugar), fat, and protein metabolism, and (3) androgenic steroids, which influence growth metabolism and masculinzation. Androsterone is an example. Unlike testosterone, the 17-ketosteroids, such as androsterone, which are produced by the adrenal cortex, are excreted in the urine.

By experimenting with the basic 17-ketosteroid structure, chemists succeeded in making many varieties (or me-too drugs) of androgenic steroids, which combine the sex effects of the male hormones and the growth effects of the adrenal steroids. *Voila!* The medical chemists produced a new growth industry—the synthetic anabolic steroids.

ANABOLIC STEROIDS AND PROTEIN SYNTHESIS

Androgens appear to promote protein anabolism (building up), along with nitrogen retention.

The importance of the Androgen Receptor—one of the first steps of androgen action is the binding of testosterone or dihydrotestosterone to an intracellular protein that is termed the androgen receptor. The presence of this protein in a tissue is a major determinant of whether it will respond to androgens. Following the interaction with testosterone or dihydrotestosterone the steroid-receptor complex binds to specific sites on chromatin called the nuclear acceptor. Interaction of the steroid-receptor complex with its acceptor results in a striking increase in nuclear metabolism. This includes an increase in chromatin template activity, an increase in the activities of RNA polymerases, increases in the number of initiation sites on chromatin, and an increase in the synthesis of all classes of RNA. These events lead to transfer of messenger RNA to cytoplasm, which results in protein synthesis. This process (along with DNA synthesis in some tissues) results in growth and development of differentiated function.

Williams' *Textbook of Endrocinology*

V. Rogozkin of the Scientific Research Institute of Physical Culture in Leningrad has performed important research exploring the effects of anabolic steroids on skeletal muscle. He found that the skeletal muscle of test animals was effected by anabolic steroids with changes in protein synthesis. His test results showed that anabolic steroids were engaged in transcription regulation in skeletal muscle. He states: "The essential feature in this process is the binding of the anabolic steroid-cytoplasmic receptor complex with the intranuclear structures of skeletal muscles." Rogozkin also found that the skeletal muscle of his test animals had receptor sites for synthetic anabolic steroids that compete with that site for testosterone.

Although anabolic steroids are imported illegally and sold on the black market like any illegal abusable substance, they are made by some of the world's most prestigious drug manufacturing companies—Ciba-Geigy, Winthrop, Searle, Organon.

The following table lists the generic (universal) names and their associated brand names (trademarked name owned by a drug manufacturing company) of synthetic anabolic steroids that are being manufactured today.

Generic Name	Brand Name	Manufacturer
ethylestrenol	Maxibolin	Organon
methandieone	Dianabol	Ciba
nandrolone	Deca-Durabolin	Organon
oxandrolone	Anavar	Searle
stanolone	Neodrol	Pfizer
stanozolol	Winstrol	Winthrop

Although only one of the companies (Ciba) is based in a foreign country, all are multinational companies and sell their products throughout the world. And here's where the problem lies. The manufacturers of drugs sold in the U.S. have to meet the FDA's requirement that any drug sold in the U.S. be safe and efficacious no matter where it is produced and, furthermore, that thorough "labeling" of the drug accompany each package that leaves the factory or laboratory. Some of these labels are the package inserts that make up the *Physicians' Desk Reference*, a book compiled by drug manufacturers as a service to physicians. However, other countries don't have nearly as restrictive drug regulations as the U.S. In fact, some foreign countries have virtually no drug regulations at all.

All of the anabolic steroids listed in the table above are sold legally in the U.S. and all have package inserts carrying information about their indicated and very limited uses, dosage, and side effects. There are copies of these inserts in the *PDR* for Dianabol, Winstrol, and Deca-Durabolin, but not for the others. It is a reprehensible truth that the drug companies that make these drugs, most of which are U.S. owned, have not supplied these package inserts as a matter of course in those foreign countries that do not require them. Thus, we have a situation where physicians and other health-care providers in foreign countries have a different (and inadequate) list of indications for use and precautions and warnings than have physicians in the U.S.

The accompanying table shows the variation in the information that was provided by Winthrop, the manufacturer of stanozolol in the U.S. and South American countries. Note that the table indicates there was not a single contraindication or warning or adverse reaction provided on stanozolol in Ecuador and Columbia, and few listed in Argentina and Mexico. Moreover, the listed indications for use in the U.S. version are almost completely different from those listed for other countries. For the U.S. market, the drug was labeled as indicated for protein synthesis (anabolic effect), aplastic anemia, osteoporosis ("probably" effective), and dwarfism—all problems occurring relatively infrequently in the population. In other countries, the drug was labeled to be useful for weight gain, strength gain, lack of appetite, preoperative and convalescent care, supportive care in acute and chronic illness, and tonic action—all indications that occur with great frequency in the population, thus providing a large and profitable market for sales of the drug.

	U.S.A.	Mexico	Central America	Ecuador, Colombia	Brazil	Argentina
INDICATIONS FOR USE:						
Protein synthesis increase, anabolic effect	✓	✓	✓	✓	✓	
Increase hemoglobin in aplastic anemia	✓					
Senile or postmenopausal osteoporosis, as adjunct	✓[a]					✓
Pituitary dwarfism	✓					
Weight increase		✓	✓	✓	✓	✓
Anorexia		✓	✓	✓	✓	✓
Strength increase		✓	✓	✓	✓	
Cirrhosis, chronic hepatitis		✓	✓	✓	✓	
Preoperative, postoperative, convalescent care		✓	✓	✓	✓	✓
Supportive treatment, acute and chronic illness		✓	✓	✓		
Tonic action in elderly					✓	✓
Gastrointestinal diseases						✓
Burns						✓
Renal disorders						✓
CONTRAINDICATIONS AND WARNINGS:						
Prostate carcinoma	✓	✓	✓		✓	✓
Breast carcinoma	✓					
Benign prostate hypertrophy	✓					
Pregnancy	✓	✓	✓		✓	✓
Cardiac disease	✓	✓	✓		✓	
Renal disease, nephrosis	✓	✓	✓		✓	
Hepatic disease	✓		✓		✓	
Edema	✓		✓			
Caution in coronary artery disease	✓		✓			
Caution in infants and children, check bone x-rays	✓	✓	✓		✓	
Laboratory test interference	✓		✓		✓	
Caution in patients on anticoagulant therapy	✓					
NONE LISTED				X		
ADVERSE REACTIONS:						
Nausea, vomiting, diarrhea	✓					
Excitation, insomnia, chills	✓					
Changes in libido	✓					
Acne	✓					
Premature closing of epiphyses in children	✓	✓				
Jaundice, rarely with hepatic necrosis and death	✓					

TABLE Continued.

	U.S.A.	Mexico	Central America	Ecuador, Colombia	Brazil	Argentina
Phallic enlargement in prepuberal males	✔				✔	
Inhibition of testicular function, impotence, gynecomastia, priapism, etc. in postpuberal males	✔					
Hirsutism, voice deepening in females	✔[b]	✔	✔[c]		✔[c]	✔[c]
Male pattern baldness, clitoral enlargement in females	✔[b]					
Menstrual irregularities	✔	✔	✔		✔	✔
NONE LISTED				X		

[a] "Probably effective."
[b] Usually irreversible even after prompt suspension of treatment.
[c] Reversible by reducing dosage or suspending treatment.

From Silverman, Milton: *The Drugging of the Americas.* (Berkeley, CA: University of California, 1976), 59–60.

As someone has pointed out, when economic theory addresses capitalism, it says nothing about morality. In competitive markets, morality is sometimes compatible with competition, but usually must be legislated. In the case of drug labeling, the U.S. Congress has not seen fit to regulate drugs that are exported, taking the view that protection of its citizens is a matter for each nation's own government. The companies have taken the view that the professional literature reporting results of research on anabolic steroids is available to physicians wherever they may be, and it is their duty to keep themselves informed and to act accordingly.

As the result of the publication of the book, *The Drugging of the Americas* by Dr. Milton Silverman of the University of California at San Francisco, the PMA, the association of U.S. pharmaceutical companies, has suggested that the same information be made available to other countries that is available in the U.S., regardless of the individual countries' legal drug regulations governing the amount and type of information that shall be supplied with drug products.

There is another, and more dangerous, aspect to foreign drug regulations (or lack of them) than inadequate labeling for physicians. In the U.S., anabolic steroids cannot be sold over-the-counter like aspirin but can only be legally sold on a prescription signed by a licensed allopathic (M.D.) or osteopathic (D.O.) physician, dentist, or veterinarian. But in many Latin American and some European countries, one may obtain anabolic steroids in pharmacies simply by asking and paying for them. Spain, for instance, and Yugoslavia, Hungary, and Mexico. In a televised incident, a reporter simply walked into an Eastern European pharmacy and asked for Dianabol. The pharmacist merely asked whether the reporter had a prescription. The reporter said, "No," and the pharmacist replied, "Never mind, I'll write you one." She did, and he walked out with a vial of injectable anabolic steroid along with the paraphernalia (needle and syringe) needed to use it.

Because steroids are sold over-the-counter to persons who ask for them, the drug advertising that is normally directed at physicians may also be directed at consumers in foreign countries. The *Medical Letter,* a prestigious, unbiased source of drug information for physicians, reported in 1973 that Winthrop, the manufacturer of stanozolol (Winstrol) had directed advertising at the parents of young boys. *The Medical Letter* said:

> Some drugs that are considered too toxic for all but the narrowest indications in the United States may be promoted for broad indications, without warnings, in Latin America. For example, a recent edition of *Medico Moderno*, Edicion Mexicana (July 1972) carried a two-page promotion for Winstrol Compound (Winthrop). The ad showed a picture of a healthy-looking boy about seven years old and recommended Winstrol Compound "if he complains of poor appetite, fatigue, or weight loss." There is no warning of any adverse effects. Winstrol Compound is offered in tablets that contain 1 mg. of stanozolol, an anabolic steroid, in addition to vitamins and iron.

The sad irony of Winthrop's blatant appeal to the macho image of Latin males is that anabolic steroids may actually stunt a child's growth by prematurely stopping his bone growth. There is no question that if a U.S. physician prescribed an anabolic steroid for a child because he was short for his age, and the child suffered an ill effect from the drug, that physician would be at high risk of having a malpractice suit filed against him. A physician in the United States is always at risk of being the target of a malpractice charge when he prescribes a drug for a nonapproved indication and the drug causes harm.

In the past, many sports journals were lulled by the lack of regula-

tion of anabolic steroids, into believing that they were not dangerous. For example, from a 1970 article: "Patients in hospitals who are
taking from 10 to 15. mg a day usually show few side effects...How-
ever, it is thought that dosages taken by many strength athletes may
be 20 times this amount."

The journals did not crusade against anabolic steroids or under-
take serious scientific investigations but merely reported what athletes were doing. The unfortunate result of this brand of journalism
was that many young persons began to use anabolic steroids because
successful athletes were reported to be doing it and anabolic steroids
are legal FDA-approved drugs.

Because of the differences in the information on anabolic steroids
provided by their manufacturers in Latin American countries and
their easy availability, the foreign connection is the major source of
anabolic steroids. Either an athlete goes himself or herself to an
"easy" country—from the United States, it's usually Mexico—buys
them, and smuggles them across the border, or a black-market sales-
man imports them illegally and makes his rounds of the gyms and
training camps. Occasionally, a physician prescribes them, arguing
that it is better if athletes get anabolic steroids, which they are going
to take in any case, from legal and controlled sources, than from illegal and uncontrolled sources.

Much has been made by the authorities and press of marijuana
smuggling. Planes and boats from Colombia and Mexico are stopped
and searched and their illegal cargo seized and burned on a regular
basis. However, little to nothing is being done about the illegal im-
portation and diversion of anabolic steroids. There are three principal reasons for this neglect. Anabolic steroids are legal drugs as
compared with marijuana for which there is only rare and experimental legal use; anabolic steroids are made by reputable drug companies as compared with marijuana; and anabolic steroids are not
psychoactive—they do not cause pleasure—as compared with marijuana, which is psychoactive and is used recreationally. The disinter-
est of the Justice Department in anabolic steroids is unfortunate in
view of their potential to do permanent damage and cause death, neither of which has been shown to be true for marijuana, the focus of
much of their efforts. Although, in general, education of the users is
the best way to assure responsible drug use, some potential young
anabolic-steroid users might be alerted to the dangers of anabolic steroids if some of these drug purveyors from foreign countries were

picked up, fined, and left to contemplate their unsold hypodermic needles in jail.

Meanwhile, the black market in anabolic steroids operates relatively openly abroad.

Tijuana, for example, has become for many athletes with Olympic dreams the shortest distance between themselves and Los Angeles. Although Tijuana is not the only black-market source for anabolic steroids for American athletes, it is certainly the most popular one. Nowadays, however, there are even mail-order catalogues that offer everything from human growth hormone (HGH) to serum made from hog thyroids. In Tijuana, steroids are sold over-the-counter at much lower prices than would be available in the U.S. (the Canadian weight lifters who had 414 vials of pure testosterone and 22,515 tablets of anabolic steroids seized upon their return from the world championships in Moscow were said to have purchased the tablets at $1 per 100 from Soviet athletes and intended to sell them for $35 per 100 in Canada; in Tijuana, they sell for between $17 and $22 per 100).

In Tijuana, the market for anabolics has skyrocketed—in some pharmacies, steroids account for 30 percent of the business. After all, controls in Mexico are not as strict as they are north of the border. One brand of steroids even advertises their product to mothers as a way to help lethargic children—like 1-a-Day vitamins.

THE ORIGINAL FOREIGN CONNECTION

One of the most unhappy and outspoken persons about anabolic steroids was the physician who (in the United States) is generally credited with being the father of anabolic steroids. The late John Ziegler introduced anabolic steroids with the best of intentions and had seen his "baby" grow into a monster that frightened him. When he heard about this book, he called from his retirement home in Olney, Maryland, and urged me to do whatever I could to stop this menace to the health of the athletes and the health of the sport, both of which he loved. Doc Ziegler said, "The body and its muscle system are sufficient. . . . If you want virility, work out hard, but don't kill yourself."

The introduction of anabolic steroids to U.S. athletes, by Dr. Zeigler's own account, as done out of patriotism following a dark period in U.S. history. In 1956, the decade of "McCarthyism," with its fears of Soviet expansion in Europe, was just ending. On the international sporting scene, the cold war was anything but cold. The Olympics had become the arena where winning was believed by many to be a reflection of the correctness of the winner's political system. Dr. Ziegler, like many others, was a victim of this misplaced athletic chauvinism. His intention was not to do harm, but to help his country out of loyalty. Doc Ziegler, a former World War II hero who was highly decorated, and who had special training in general surgery, neurology, geriatrics, and physical and nuclear medicine, was outraged by the success of the Soviets who he discovered were using male hormones to build weight and power, while our boys were slogging along with diets and workouts alone. While in Vienna, Dr. Ziegler had drinks with a Soviet team physician who admitted that they were using hormones. Said Dr. Ziegler, "I felt the Russians were going to use sports as the biggest international publicity trick going. . .and strength sports especially. They saw it as a political advantage 100 percent."

Dr. Ziegler went to the Ciba Pharmaceutical Company (now Ciba-Geigy), and together they worked out a program to develop an anabolic steroid to give weight lifters, the first to try it out, at the York (Pennsylvania) Barbell Club. The problem was that the weight lifters loved the drugs and weren't satisfied to stay on the recommended dosages. Said Dr. Ziegler, "They figured if one pill was good, three or four would be better, and they were eating them like candy." The news of anabolic steroids spread through the athletic community more like wildfire than candy, and soon drugs and stories of drugs became the chief topic of conversation at training camps and the subject of articles in all of the sports magazines.

So sadly, Dr. Ziegler's work, that he had viewed as American can-do science at its best, providing Americans with the tools to win, became distorted, misunderstood, and abused. Dr. Ziegler learned early and seeing the dangers signaled by anabolic steroids run wild, he ceased his advocacy of them, but it was too late. The magic growth genie wouldn't go back in the bottle.

THE PHYSICAL EFFECTS OF DRUGS ON ATHLETES

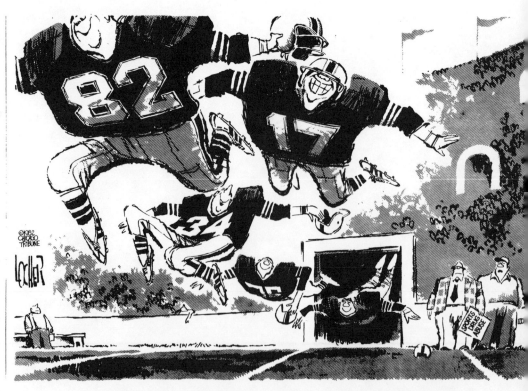

"I THINK THEY'RE HIGH FOR THIS GAME IN MORE WAYS THAN ONE!"

Copyright ©1982 by The Chicago Tribune. Reprinted with permission.

8
ERGOGENIC AIDS IN SPORTS —MYTH OR FACT

The merciless rigor of modern competitive sport, especially at the international level, the glory of victory, and the growing social and economical reward of sporting success (in no way any longer related to reality) increasingly forces athletes to improve their performance by any means available.

from *Manual on Doping* by the
Medical Commission of the International
Olympic Committee, 1972

ATHLETES TEND TO BE GULLIBLE AND WILLING TO TRY ANYTHING that might aid their athletic prowess. All it would take is the suggestion of a coach, trainer, or physician, peers, or fellow athletes, or even casual friends, for an athlete to be tempted into trying some kind of artificial aid. These aids are known as *ergogenic aids* and are any substance or method believed to aid or improve athletic performance. Generally there are three classes of ergogenic aids. In the general scope they may be artificial aids, anabolic steroids, and stimulants. North America, by nature, is a pill-popping society. Dr. Percy of the Arizona Health Sciences Center states in an article he wrote on ergogenic aids, "There is no scientific evidence to date, to my knowledge, that demonstrates that competitive training will cause a depletion of certain critical vitamins, nor that extra vitamins will improve upon performance." Vitamins are one example of artificial ergogenic aids. For the record, I feel that dietary aids have value, which I feel has been evidenced by a number of studies. In a study of the 1976 Olympics, Clement found some of the competitive athletes to have suboptimal intake of dietary protein. He performed blood

97

tests indicating that athletes might benefit from protein and mineral supplementation to maintain a normal hemoglobin level.

GENSING is a harmless root vegetable first discovered by American missionaries in the eighteenth century in China and has been used as an ergogenic aid by some as part of a dietary fad. However, in some cases manufacturers add phenylbutazone or aspirin to give the person taking gensing a feeling of well being.

Sometimes athletes use DIURETICS and sweatsuits to make weight for competition. This, combined with restricted fluid intake, is very dangerous because it can lead to electrolyte and fluid imbalances. Some individuals using anabolic steroids might take diuretics to rid their body of the retained fluids that accompany the drugs. *Your body is not a balloon. You cannot without extreme danger to your health pump yourself up with water and then lose the fluid with diuretics.* Some researchers have proposed that diuretics be placed on the banned drugs list for international competitions. A large number of the competitors tested in recent competitions have shown high concentrations of diuretics in their urine tests. There had been many times when I had to make weight during my competitive wrestling and power-lifting days, but I would just wear a heavy sweat suit and restrict my fluid intake. Sweating is a natural process; taking a drug to rid the body of needed fluids is a very dangerous habit.

I will attempt to cover many of the ergogenic aids used today by athletes. A complete list might be impossible because there are always new methods and drugs being created. People will try anything.

Dr. Lynne Pirie, D.O., physician-athlete and champion bodybuilder, had these comments on the abuse of diuretics by athletes:

> Early last spring Heinz Sallmayer, the 1980 IFBB Lightweight Mr. Universe, died of a heart attack while preparing for a professional competition. Sallmayer was hardly a candidate for a heart attack. An autopsy revealed a minor congenital heart malformation. But the cause of death was excessive use of diuretics, which led to heart arrhythmia (irregular heartbeat) and the heart attack.
>
> A few weeks later Andreas Cahling reported that an 18-year-old male Swedish bodybuilder also suffered a fatal heart seizure

following a competition in Stockholm. Again, massive dehydration from using potent diuretics was pegged as the cause of death.

...The loss of the electrolyte potassium from the system can precipitate arrhymia.

Electrolyte profiles of athletes in other sports who have abused potent diuretics to make weight for competition show seriously low amounts of sodium, potassium, calcium and chloride in the blood. The acidity of the blood has also been decreased, resulting in alkalosis, a condition of increased alkalinity of the blood and tissues.

These imbalances are reflected in fatigue, thirst, irritability, muscular cramping, gastrointestinal upsets and irregular heartbeat—all of which the average bodybuilder dismisses as part of the price he or she has to pay to achieve peak muscularity. This attitude seems very inappropriate for someone who desires the appearance of a healthy bodybuilder, however.

Diuretics can quickly deplete the circulation blood volume to such a low level that there will be no significant blood supply to the kidneys. Tests on dehydrated athletes have demonstrated impaired renal function that could possibly be permanent. Kidneys do not regenerate like the skin and hair. This decreased blood volume is a direct result of dehydration and/or the use of potent diuretics, which significantly reduce the kidneys' ability to reabsorb salt.

BLOOD PACKING. Bjorn Ekblom of Stockholm's Institute of Gymnastics in Sweden reported on a method to give athletes more oxygen, which increases endurance. Ekblom removed some of the athlete's blood (about 1,200 cc.) over a period spanning four days. This was taken at three separate times, and the blood was then placed in cold storage.

By removing this amount of blood, equal to about a quart, the athlete's oxygen-carrying capacity was lowered in their muscles. This also lowered their individual endurance by 30 percent. Now the body was forced to replace the lost blood. Dr. Ekblom then separated the red blood cells from the frozen samples, and then injected them back into the original donors, causing a rapid red cell increase in the athlete's circulatory system. There was a 25 percent increase noted in endurance, by measuring the running times. This type of boost did not last for more than fourteen days because the body quickly rids itself of the excess red blood cells. After about fourteen days, the runners returned to pre-blood-packing endurance levels.

To increase the amount of red blood cells in the athlete by this method would be of little use to the type of athlete who requires short bursts of energy (power lifters) but might prove useful if the weight trainer was attempting a maximum amount of repetitions at a quicker speed. This is possible due to the increased amount of oxygen placed in the blood.

Gledhill said that it takes five to six weeks to replace the 1,000 ml of blood that may be extracted during blood doping. Further, he reported that there is a substantial loss of red blood cells when the blood is stored. In reality he feels it takes even longer to replace the blood. Extreme caution must be exercised with blood doping because hazardous circumstances could occur when retransfusing the blood back into the athlete. Some of the problems that could occur are infection, potential coagulation defects (clotting) from increased viscosity (the ability of fluid to flow smoothly), and the chance of mismatched transfusion when more than one athlete is involved. I feel the dangers outweight the benefits, if any.

HYPNOSIS. Psychological factors play a very large role in competitive endeavors. I feel that the athlete's state of mind is 75 percent of winning. Desire is a vital characteristic to becoming a champion in any sport. If not for this powerful desire and drive, the athlete would not have ever reached the higher level of competition. Whether it be a pep talk from the coach, or even a conversation between the athlete and his peers, the *psych* is a major factor in the performance of the individual. Hypnosis, and the placing of a psychologist on the medical team, now plays an important role in national and international teams. There is tremendous precompetition tension that might be eased by a trained medical person. The right words, expressed in the proper manner, would be a great aid.

"One startling report which came out in the lay press after the 1976 Olympics was that the West Germans had used RECTAL INJECTIONS OF AIR in their swimming team, in an attempt to improve swimmers' performance by increasing their buoyancy. You are aware, of course, that there are four basic strokes in swimming and it would appear that the West Germans have now added a fifth stroke—the floater or Zeppelin stroke. One might truly say that their athletes have attempted to join the jet set." (E.C. Percy, *Medicine and Science in Sports*)

ALCOHOL was once thought to aid work performance but has now proven to detract from true work potentials. A series of testing procedures using a Johansson ergograph, which consists of an apparatus where the subject pulls weight with both hands, found definite drops in activity after a small initial boost. Herxheimer found alcohol to have bad effects on the performances of subjects running short distances and swimmers. Another researcher found a decrease in oxygen consumption with the ingestion of alcohol, where others found no change. There are conflicting studies as to whether alcohol can be used as an energy source for muscular contraction. Most researchers, on the whole, feel that alcohol is a detriment to performance, as can be seen with a simple driving test.

Many think alcohol will warm them during a football game. Alcohol acts as a mild dilator on the vascular system effecting the peripheral blood vessels (the small vessels near the surface of the skin). This results in a small drop in blood pressure. This vasodilation occurs as a result of the depressive action on the vasoconstrictor centers in the medulla. Higher brain centers, such as the hypothalamus, may mediate this action. These cells are normally in a state of vessel vasoconstriction. Alcohol dulls the cells, which emit constrictive impulses. With this stimulus gone, the vessels become relaxed and dilated. Now that these vessels are relaxed, they enlarge, allowing more blood to flow at the surface of the skin that is in contact with the outside environment. Heat is then lost from the body when the external environment is cooler than body temperature, leading to an increase in loss of body heat. So, the next time you take a drink during competition in the cold weather, remember you will be decreasing your body temperature.

MARIJUANA. Some athletes smoke prior to competition to relax themselves. The short-term effects of marijuana usually are a combination of the drug itself and the athlete's state of mind, personality, and environment. The person experiences slower reaction time and loses the steadiness of hand. This could be disastrous for skilled competitive sports that rely on reflexes. You may think you are doing great but in reality may be clumsy and slow. This drug can also distort time and visual perception. Taking this drug the night before a competition may cause you to sleep easier, but you may not feel well rested in the morning, sort of a post-hangover. I would not suggest indulging anywhere near a competition. Do it after it is all over, if you must. Smoke is still an irritant and may cut down your wind and hurt your cardiovascular potential.

AMPHETAMINES. Some common amphetamines are benzedrine and dexedrine. Some of the effects this class of drugs have are: (1) rise in blood pressure, (2) constriction of blood vessels, (3) increase in heart rate, (4) mydriasis (pupil dilation), (5) dilation of the bronchi, (6) intestinal muscle relaxation, (7) higher blood sugar, (8) increased muscle tone, (9) shorter blood-coagulation time, and (10) stimulation of the adrenal glands. Some athletes use amphetamines to control their weight. Initially they depress appetite, but after a while this effect is lost. These drugs have been and are used by athletes, but their value as an ergogenic aid is debatable. The majority of studies performed lead to negative results. During testing for the presence of these drugs during past Olympics, it was found that some of the losers had the drug present in their blood, while virtually none of the winners had any drug present. The way amphetamines work is by stimulating the release of epinephrine and norepinephrine from the adrenal glands and the nervous system, respectively. This increases muscle tension and heart rate and blood pressure, which makes the individual feel more awake. This elevated mood does not allow the athlete to evaluate his performance realistically. For example, one football player who had taken some "ups" before a game thought he had played great. The reality of the situation was that he was thrown out of the game for unnecessary roughness. This occurred because he would come upon the play too late, due to a slower reaction time.

Your body has natural defense mechanisms. With these drugs you might push yourself further than it would be safe, leading to circulatory collapse, due to an unnatural heat build up. *This can kill you. The heart is working harder than it has to. There have been a number of deaths by competitive cyclists and in other endurance sports. These drugs are addictive and can kill.* As Dave Meggyesy said in *Blood and Guts,* "The violent and brutal player that television viewers marvel over on Saturdays and Sundays is often a synthetic product."

A study done in 1968 and 1969 noted that National Football League team purchases of amphetamines averaged 60 to 70 mg./man/game. This did not include drugs obtained (legitimately or otherwise) by individual players. It appears that all this use of amphetamines began after World War II. Dr. L.A. Johnson's 1972 doctoral dissertation on amphetamine use in professional football looked into this subject. Dr. Johnson found the use greater on defensive than on offensive teams, the line more than the backfield, and the older more than the younger. One quarterback said the drug made "everything slow down while I read the defense."

In a 2¹/₂ year study, known as "The Sunday Syndrome," researchers evaluating NFL teams noticed that before the game there was a sudden emergence of uncharacteristic obscenity, violent diarrhea, vomiting, temper tantrums, and repetitious pacing back and forth.

The "Sunday Syndrome" reasearch published in the October 1981 *Federation Proceedings* went on to state:

> According to Al Davis of the Oakland Raiders, amphetamine was used by the special teams to counteract fear. High doses of amphetamine engender nearly psychotic paranoid rage. Comparable doses are used by the "pillhead" and intravenous "speed freaks." Reminiscent of animal behavior becoming stereotypic and of "speed art" being made up of detailed patterns endlessly drawn over and over, linemen who had taken very high doses of amphetamine had difficulty adjusting their play; one game film showed a veteran defensive end on high levels of amphetamine going inside on every play, disregarding the linebacker's signals. The opposing offense consistently aimed their running attack at the region he could be counted on to leave, and no amount of shouting by the defensive line coach during the game could change the defensive end's behavior; he said he was always playing a sweep to the other side. One might speculate that his brain had been driven to a limit cycle by the drug.
>
> The network of amphetamine distribution to football players has shifted over the last decade from open bottles of thousands of pills, to little white envelopes distributed by trainers, to prescriptions written in private by team physicians, to the present, when the sophisticated player uses a physician in town willing to prescribe for him, and the less knowledgeable rookie hits the streets for "black beauties."

However, in December 1982, the Symposium on Sports Medicine painted a slightly different picture. John Harvey, Jr., M.D., felt that the amphetamine abuses of the 1960s and 1970s is much less of a problem now.

> This decrease can be attributed to a growing awareness by youth that "speed kills," and to the liability concerns of professional teams and their physicians who have been sued by athletes injured while playing under the influence of these drugs. Use of amphetamines had been the major drug-related problem in athletics, so its decline is encouraging. . . .
>
> Obscuring an athlete's physiologic fatigue level may allow him to exceed his limits and precipitate a sudden collapse, elimi- .

nating him from the event. Football players on amphetamines seem to be able to ignore pain from injuries, thus allowing further play and thus even more damage. Such drugs can also make an athlete more aggressive, resulting in unnecessary brutality and rough play in contact sports, causing even more injuries. High doses may induce a paranoid, prepsychotic state or a paranoid schizophrenic syndrome, both of these apparently dose-related.

Jockeys and wrestlers have taken advantage of the anorexic effects of amphetamine-type drugs to lose weight in preparation for specific tournaments.

On the other end of the spectrum, the beta-adrenergic receptor antagonist PROPRANOLOL (a drug that slows down the heart) is sometimes used by ski jumpers to prevent palpitations that develop in anticipation of the run. Furthermore, alcohol, librium, valium, and serax have been known to be used by trap shooters, golfers, and archers to steady their hands and promote sleep before competition.

COCAINE abuse has run rampant in the 1980s. It is the "in" drug of the stars, athletic and movie alike. The epidemic had ruined enough lives, so on July 25, 1983, Football Commissioner Pete Rozelle chose to suspend four National Football League players for involvement with cocaine.

U.S. News and World Report of August 1983 carried the following account of the actions.

> The penalties, to run through four games in the coming season, will mean losses of $25,850 for Greg Stemrick of the New Orleans Saints, $33,350 for E.J. Junior of the St. Louis Cardinals, $34,600 for Pete Johnson of the Cincinnati Bengals and $37,600 for the Bengals' Ross Browner.
> Only weeks before Rozelle's action, baseball pitcher Steve Howe of the Los Angeles Dodgers was docked a month's pay— $54,000—after being treated a second time for cocaine dependency.
> One reason officials are cracking down: They fear that players with cocaine habits might try to pay off their debts to drug dealers by fixing games or providing inside information on injuries. "There is a potential threat to the integrity of the game," said NFL spokesman Jim Heffernan.

Mark Mulvoy of *Sports Illustrated* came to know the crisis first hand. He spent three months practically living with Don Reese when Reese approached SI for help. He put Reese into hospitals to get detoxified. "His life was in serious jeopardy when he came to us, in June of 1982, and resulted in probably the most important drug story in athletics up till that time," said Mulvoy.

> It begins at the top, with leagues getting millions of dollars for certain shows and what the viewers want to see—275-pound guys knocking each other down. The public seems to want drugged-up brutes crashing into each other—which loses the true essence of football. It is my wish that athletes could compete as themselves and not as some drug-induced robots. The sad thing is that the National Football League doesn't give a darn; they are just afraid of getting arrested.

Cocaine is a very powerful stimulant and affects the circulatory rates and the central nervous system. It increases muscular tension as well as having a direct sympathomimetic effect. Cocaine comes from the coca leaf and is used frequently by South American Indians. This gives these individuals the ability for remarkable feats of endurance. The drug tends to postpone the onset of fatigue. However, this drug is a dangerous habit-addictive drug. Athletes, and anyone for that matter, should avoid contact with this drug.

ALKALIES are buffers to help neutralize the accumulation of acids in the bloodstream during exercise and muscular exertion. It has been seen in some studies that sodium bicarbonate might allow greater oxygen depth or capacity, but there were no significant improvements in muscular performance.

Although the following theory has provided conflicting reports, Dennig and his coworkers found an increase in endurance with the following alkai intake:

sodium bicarbonate . . . . 3.5 gm.

sodium citrate . . . . 5.0 gm.

potassium citrate . . . . 1.5 gm.

These prescribed doses are taken two days before a contest and two after, taken once daily after a meal. One would continue the dose for the two days after competition to avoid an acidotic reaction. If the athletes were to take this for a longer period of time, it might hinder his performance.

CAFFEINE acts on the heart, blood vessels, and the nervous system.

The contractile power of the heart is increased, and dilation of the coronary artery, with simultaneous general vasoconstriction, takes place. Tea, along with the caffeine effects found in coffee, have been found to be beneficial in prolonged exertion studies. Cola from cola nuts had an even stronger effect on work performance than caffeine in one study comparing both of them. A cup of coffee usually contains 97–195 mg. of caffeine. I would not suggest this because it can become addictive.

GELATIN AND GLYCINE are rich in amino-acetic acid and is considered an incomplete protein. The amino-acetic acid comprises 25 percent of the weight of gelatin and glycine. Creatine and glycine are chemically related, and creatine is very important in muscular contraction. It is for this relationship that glycine and later on, gelatin have been used therapeutically to aid and improve muscular action. Several studies have pointed to the positive effects glycine has had on work performances in terms of decreased fatigue and work output increases, sometimes as high as 240 percent. But the results have been conflicting, aside from psychological factors (placebo effect). It is pretty much a fact, though, that adding gelatin to a diet will not improve strength.

FRUIT JUICE is a fine dietary supplement and has good vitamin and mineral contents, as well as possibly alkalizing the blood to aid work capacity. The increases in performance by some researchers were attributed to the supposed increase in blood alkalinity. However, as is the case with most ergogenic aids, there are conflicting reports as to the results of their use and benefits. Again, psychological factors may play a role. I am for this aid. Anyway, juice is hard to beat after a tough workout. I particularly like V-8 Juice, Motts apple juice, or the various citrus juices (Tropicana and Minute Maid are two trustworthy citrus juice companies).

PHOSPHATES are very important compounds that are necessary in order to furnish energy for muscular contraction. These phosphorous compounds also act as a buffer in the blood. Researchers have noted increases in ergogenic tests with the administration of sodium phosphate, in the form of Recresal. A dose of 3 gms. can provide feelings of euphoria and well-being, but too much will cause insomnia. Some researchers also found phosphates to be good laxatives and to aid in recovering from fatigue more quickly. However, there are some studies that show little or no benefit with the use of phosphates. On the whole, there is no definite proof that phosphate ingestion will lead to improved athletic ability.

LECITHIN contains phosphoric and fatty acids and belongs to the phosphatides, so it can be considered a fine source of phosphorus. It is considered to play a role in the oxidation and emulsification of neutral fats. The results as to its true benefits are conflicting.

OXYGEN is considered a limiting and crucial factor in an individual capacity and recovering from physical exertion. Therefore, some researchers believe that giving oxygen before and after athletic endeavors will enhance performance. They have also found that preliminary oxygen inhalation lowered lactic acid accumulation, as well as aiding the metabolic system for an additional fifteen minutes. Here again, there are conflicting studies as to the virtues of oxygen inhalation immediately prior to a competition.

SUGAR is the fuel for muscular exertion and contraction. During exertion of short duration, sugar is mostly a psychological aid more so than a physiological one. If an athlete takes too much, he might get nauseated or experience gastric disorders.

CARBOHYDRATE-LOADING. "For years," said Paul Slovic, "discussions about the influence of diet upon athletic performance tended to emphasize the benefits of protein and vitamins. However, few if any of the enthusiastic claims for these substances have been confirmed by scientific tests. Thus, it was rather surprising when highly respected Swedish physiologists described a diet whose proven effects on endurance surpassed even the wildest claims of health-food hucksters."

Slovic, a scientist with the Oregon Research Institute in Eugene, had just completed a study which told exactly how many minutes this diet could shave from a marathon runner's time. The Swedish diet was called "glycogen super-compensation" by scientific types and "carbohydrate-loading" by laymen. It had been popular among long distance runners since the later 1960s.

The Swedes had learned that (1) depleting muscle glycogen, (2) keeping the level down with a low-carbohydrate/high-protein diet, then (3) shifting the balance to high-carbohydrate intake did wonders for runners' energy. Muscle glycogen levels soared 100 percent above normal. This meant individuals could hold fatigue at bay for longer than usual periods.

In long races, where runners often run down like clocks in the later miles, this diet quickly won converts. The usual regimen was a "depletion" run one week before the race, then three high-protein days, then three high-carbohydrate days.

Swedish physiologists Karlsson and Saltin applied this routine in a test with ten distance runners. They ran two races each—30 kilometers (18.7 miles) three weeks apart. Before one race, they ate normally. Before the other, they "loaded." Times under loaded conditions were 7.7 minutes faster than with normal diets.

This group was small, though, and Paul Slovic wanted results on a bigger scale. So he questioned runners at the 1974 Trail's End marathon, and 181 of them responded. Of these, 98 were nonloaders, 27 partial loaders (increased carbohydrate intake but didn't follow the usual depletion sequence), and 56 were full-loaders.

"On the average," Slovic wrote, "the glycogen-loaders finished considerably faster than nonloaders (2:57 v. 3:23). However, the loaders also trained harder, had more experience with marathoning and were somewhat faster in the mile. These factors, rather than diet, may have determined their superior performance.

Slovic used complex statistical methods to take these factors into account, coming up with formulas that accurately predicted each runner's potential in the race. On this basis, the loaders enjoyed a 6–$11\frac{1}{2}$ minute advantage over nonloaders. Carbohydrate-loading apparently had improved marathon times by that much.

Slovic said, "Despite market differences between the design of this study and that of Karlsson and Saltin, the 6–$11\frac{1}{2}$ minute improvement is close to their 7.7-minute effect over 30 kilometers. Another similarity between the two studies is that diet has made little or no difference over the first half of the run, but was associated with marked changes in performance over the last quarter of the course." Loaders, as a group, were able to hold their pace while non-loaders slowed markedly.

Those are the advantages of carbohydrate-loading. The article which appears in the appendix, by Dr. Ben Londeree, an exercise physiologist at the University of Missouri, lists the techniques. But what about the limitations?

The most obvious one is that it only works in events lasting thirty to sixty minutes or more. Also, little is known about its effects outside of running, though it would seem to be useful in bicycling, cross-country skiing, race walking and similar endurance sports.

Another problem with the standard routine (three days low-carbohydrate, three days high) has been to survive the first three days. Athletes feel miserable during that period. They're tired and irritable from low blood sugar. Now physiologists are telling them they can forget the bad days.

Dr. Bob Fitts, a U.S. road running champion: "The final level of muscle glycogen super-compensation reached is not affected by the low-carbohydrate phase of the diet. The main purpose of this phase is to lengthen the amount of time between the depletion run and the race....I avoid the potential dangers of this phase by taking my long run on Tuesday, followed by a high-carbohydrate diet Tuesday night through Friday, with the race on Saturday morning."

One of America's original proponents of glycogen loading later moderated his opinion based on evidence that the loading regimen was not as effective as had been believed.

DMSO (DIMETHYL SULFOXIDE) is a new drug being used by athletes because of its amazing ability to penetrate the skin and through cell tissue, but a lot more research needs to be done, and objective research is difficult to do—as the accompanying quote from Dr. John Harvey shows.

> DMSO (Dimethyl Sulfoxide) is widely available as an over-the-counter preparation in pharmacies throughout this country, and it is widely used by athletes of all ages because of its alleged anti-inflammatory properties. Athletes rub it on an injured area in the belief that the inflammation (and therefore the pain and discomfort) will be relieved sooner than by the traditional conservative methods, such as rest and heat. The pungent odor of the breath within minutes of its being applied to the skin makes double-blind placebo-controlled studies difficult. However, one recent study compared the effectiveness against elbow tendinitis of the standard 70 percent solution with a 5 percent DMSO placebo, and no benefit could be ascertained.
>
> The problem with DMSO is that its human toxicity has not been fully explored. Its early use in humans as a treatment for arthritis was stopped when the FDA withdrew the drug from clinical use because of reports of eye toxicity in animals. It has since been reapproved only for instillation into the bladder in the treatment of interstitial cystitis. The principal worry about the compound is that it is both an excellent solvent and an extremely effective skin penetrant. It will therefore carry into the

body any substance contaminating the solution being used. As the industrial grade of DMSO is presumably the one being used by the athlete, its standard of purity does not approach that which would be required of a manufacturer if the chemical were a drug approved for human use. Its use should be discouraged until human research indicates that it is both safe and effective.

from "Overuse Syndrome in Young Athletes,"
by John Harvey Jr., M.D.
Pediatric Clinics of North America
(December 1982)

ULTRAVIOLET RAYS have little value, save psychological, if the individual receives an adequate amount of Vitamin D.

Last, and probably most important, is **HGH, HUMAN GROWTH HORMONE.** HGH is extracted from the pituitary glands of cadavers and is, therefore, a very rare substance indeed. A recent scientific breakthrough has led to synthesizing HGH in a laboratory. Its principal use was treating children with growth hormone deficiency, and with such a short supply, it used to infuriate me that so much HGH went to normal athletes rather than to these children who needed HGH to lead a normal life.

Some problems associated with HGH include: antibody formation against HGH, a sort of allergic reaction to a foreign substance in the body; hepatitis; hypoglycemia and diabetes, with the chance of diabetic coma in susceptible individuals, and acromegaly, or what I call the Frankenstein Syndrome (see the appendix on HGH), the most devastating reaction of all.

Since HGH has been reported in the lay press to quickly build muscle on athletes, and since its cost is likely to drop dramatically in the near future, there is no doubt that HGH will soon become the "in" drug of the near future. But the dangers are overwhelming.

As long as the aids do not injure the individual or are in any way a health danger, I would consider them ethical. Where health and the lives of the athletes can be adversely affected, the line should be drawn. Ergogenic aids may work directly on the muscle fibers; they may counteract normal fatigue products, such as lactic acid; they may delay the nervous system's reaction that causes the feeling of fatigue; they may increase the capacity of the circulatory system and heart, thereby increasing the transport efficiency of materials in the bloodstream, such as fuel (glucose), wastes, and oxygen; they may cause an increase in respiratory capacity, even if only a temporary one; and by counteracting the inhibitory effects of the nervous system, and they may allow the muscles to develop great force potentials.

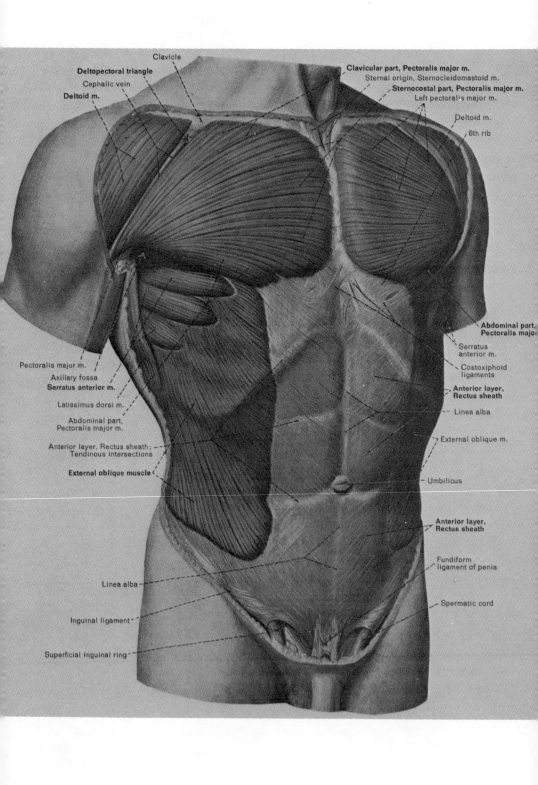

Clavicle

Deltopectoral triangle

Cephalic vein

Deltoid m.

Clavicular part, Pectoralis major m.
Sternal origin, Sternocleidomastoid m.
Sternocostal part, Pectoralis major m.
Left pectoralis major m.

Deltoid m.

6th rib

Abdominal part, Pectoralis major

Serratus anterior m.

Costoxiphoid ligaments

Anterior layer, Rectus sheath

Linea alba

External oblique m.

Umbilicus

Anterior layer, Rectus sheath

Fundiform ligament of penis

Spermatic cord

Pectoralis major m.

Axillary fossa

Serratus anterior m.

Latissimus dorsi m.

Abdominal part, Pectoralis major m.

Anterior layer, Rectus sheath; Tendinous intersections

External oblique muscle

Linea alba

Inguinal ligament

Superficial inguinal ring

Reprinted with permisson from Anatomy: A Regional Atlas of the Human Body, by Carmine D. Clemente, (Urban & Schwarzenberg, Publishers).

9
HOW STEROIDS DESTROY THE BODY

THE ENDOCRINE GLANDS—THE INTERNAL CONTROL SYSTEM

THERE ARE VARIOUS BODY SYSTEMS THAT WORK TOGETHER TO MAKE the unit function. Some have specific controls, while others have varied and general responsibilities. The endocrine glands are largely independent of each other both functionally and anatomically. The glands share an action that is as vital as the nervous system.

The endocrine glands secrete hormones directly into the blood stream for action. *Exocrine glands* (for example, the sweat and salivary glands) secrete directly onto the surface of the body or via a duct into the body. The *endocrine glands* secrete blood-borne entities into the bloodstream and are very specific and can effect action on areas and organs very distant to themselves. This does not include acetylcholine (the substances passed between nerve ends) and carbon dioxide, even though they are both chemical regulators.

Hormones generally alter cellular activity, decreasing or increasing an ongoing process, rather than starting a new process.

Hormones can:

1. alter the permeability of organelle and cell membranes to particular substances;
2. change the rates of reactions;
3. inactivate or activate an enzyme system;

113

4. influence the genes themselves;
5. change the speed of a reaction or a series of reactions by varying the amounts of one or more reactants;
6. cause an increase or decrease in enzyme production, as well as causing the production of additional enzymes.

The *target organ* is the tissue the hormone acts upon. The target organ may be just a few cells in the whole organ, and the actions are specific. The action may take from a few minutes to hours to take effect. An example of specificity is how antidiuretic hormone affects only the cells of collecting tubules in the kidney and not the loop of Henle (these two sections are very close to one another). However, some of the hormonal action may be general, such as the action of the thyroid hormone increasing the metabolic rate of all cells.

Even though hormones are secreted continually from their respective origin sites, the secretion rates vary with the needs of the body. In order to retain the low, continual level of hormones in the blood and system, hormones are constantly produced, secreted, inactivated, and excreted.

THE ENDOCRINE GLANDS

Adrenal gland (adrenal cortex and adrenal medulla)
Thyroid gland
Placenta
Kidney
Thymus
Pineal gland
Gonads (testis and ovary)
Pituitary gland (hypophysis)
Intermediate lobe
Anterior lobe (adenohypophysis)
Posterior lobe (neurohypophysis)
Parathyroid glands
Liver
Gastrointestinal tract

SOURCE	HORMONE	PRINCIPAL EFFECTS
Anterior pituitary	Growth hormone	Stress hormone (indirectly stimulates growth)
	Thyrotropic hormone	Stimulates the thyroid
	Adrenocorticotropic .... hormone (ACTH)	Stimulates the adrenal cortex
	Follicle-stimulating......... hormone (FSH)	Stimulates growth of ovarian follicles and of seminiferous tubules of the testes
	Luteinizing hormone (LH) ..	Stimulates conversion of follicles into corpora lutea; stimulates secretion of sex hormones by ovaries and testes
	Prolactin	Stimulates milk secretion by mammary glands
	Melanocyte-stimulating..... hormone	Controls cutaneous pigmentation in lower vertebrates
Posterior pituitary .... (storage organ for hormones apparently produced by hypothalamus)	Oxytocin	Stimulates contraction of uterine muscles: stimulates release of milk by mammary glands
	Vasopressin	Stimulates increased water reabsorption by kidneys; stimulates constriction of blood vessels (and other smooth muscle)
Intermediate lobe	Melanocyte-stimulating..... melantropin MSH, intermedin	Expands melanophores (changes skin color): no known function in humans
Adrenal cortex	Glucocorticoids (cortisol) ...	Inhibits incorporation of amino acids into protein in muscles; stimulates formation of glucose (largely from noncarbohydrate sources) and storage of glycogen
	Mineralocorticoids......... (aldosterone, deoxycorticosterone, etc.)	Regulates sodium-potassium metabolism
	Adrenal sex hormones......	Stimulates male secondary sexual characteristics, particularly those of the male
Hypothalamus	Releasing factors	Regulates hormone secretion by anterior pituitary
	Oxytocin, vasopressin......	See Posterior pituitary
Adrenal medulla..........	Adrenalin	Stimulates series of reactions commonly termed "fight or flight"
	Noradrenalin.............	Stimulates reactions similar to those produced by adrenalin, but causes more vasoconstriction and is less effective in conversion of glycogen into glucose

Pyloric mucosa of stomach	Gastrin...................	Stimulates secretion of gastric juice and HCl
Mucosa of duodenum	Secretin	Stimulates secretion of pancreatic juice
	Cholecystokinin	Stimulates release of bile and pancreatic digestive enzymes
	Enterogastrone	Inhibits secretion of gastric juice
Damaged tissues..........	Histamine	Increases capillary permeability
Pancreas	Insulin	Stimulates glycogen and lipid formation and storage; stimulates carbohydrate oxidation; inhibits formation of new glucose
	Glucagon................	Stimulates conversion of glycogen into glucose and the formation of new glucose
Kidney plus blood	Angiotensin II............ (Renin converted in lungs to Angiotensin I)	Stimulates vasoconstriction, and aldosterone synthesis, causing rise in blood pressure
Testes	Testosterone	Stimulates development and maintenance of male secondary sexual characteristics and behavior
Ovaries	17B Estradiol (estrogen)	Stimulates development and maintenance of female secondary sexual characteristics and behavior
	Progesterone.............	Stimulates female secondary sexual characteristics and behavior and maintains pregnancy
Thyroid	Thyroxin, triiodothyronine .	Stimulates oxidative metabolism, and is needed for normal growth and development and helps maintain the basal metabolic rate
	Calcitonin	Prevents excessive rise in blood calcium
Parathyroids	Parathormone.............	Regulates calcium-phosphate metabolism
Thymus	Thymosin	Stimulates immunologic competence in lymphoid tissues
Pineal...................	Melatonin	May help regulate pituitary, perhaps by regulating hypothalamic releasing centers

EFFECTS OF TESTOSTERONE AND ANDROGENS IN MALES

Testosterone and androgens have the following effects in men:
1. Exert an effect on sexual characteristics. At puberty: larynx enlargement; vocal cords become heavier to give a deeper

voice; increase in body hair; shoulders become broader; muscles grow heavier; oily secretion of skin (which may lead to acne).
2. Stimulate the growth of their target organs.
3. Promote protein anabolism (building).
4. Reduction in protein catabolism (breakdown).
5. Increase in the size of seminiferous tubules and testes.
6. Stimulate spermatogenesis (production of sperm).
7. Necessary for the development and maintenance of accessory sex organs, including enlargement and secretory functions and increase in external genitalia and tubule structures. Without androgens these structures would atrophy and cease to function.
8. Metabolic effects on muscle, bone and skin.
9. Closure of epiphyses in long bones (growth potential).
10. Associated with the mental pattern of aggressiveness and sex drive (libido).

These are all very carefully calibrated physiological developments that are upset with drug abuse.

Testosterone and other androgens or hormones bring about their changes by altering the permeability of cell membranes that control how nutrients and material enter and leave the cell; by stimulating or suppressing specific genes or characteristics, thereby decreasing or increasing their production; and by affecting specific enzyme systems within cells, which exert control over the rates of internal biochemical reactions within the cell.

The final actions and effects of hormones on a cell, and thus on the entire human organism, are the previous physical condition, sex, and age of the body or cell. Furthermore, these factors are also influenced by the predisposed state of balance and presence of other substances already present, such as other hormones, nutrients, and drugs.

All of these above-mentioned elements work together for maximum "normal," or homeostatic, function. This is monitored overall by a feedback system. Steroid abuse can cause minor or even permanent disruptions, of which even small quantities could lead to cell death or deterioration.

According to the tenth edition of *Harrison's Principles of Internal Medicine:*

> *Cancer* is the term to characterize abnormal growth of cells, which may result in the invasion of normal tissues or the spread to distant organs, termed *Metastasis.* The degree of malignancy

of a cancer is based upon the propensity of the cells for invasion and distant spread. A metastasis is a neoplastic lesion arising from another cancer, with which it is no longer in continuity. Regardless of mechanism, separation of malignant cells from the primary cancer is an essential part of the neoplastic process. The basic concept that metastases arrive directly from the constituent cells of primary cancer originates from observations of histologic similarities between the two. The mode of transport of cells from the primary to the presumptive secondary lesions is inferred from the many observations of cancer cells infiltrating tissues and invading blood vessels and lymphatic channels and the recognition of circulating cancer cells in the blood of patients with cancer.

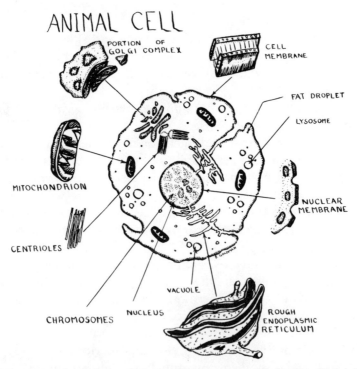

Our body tissues are made up of many individual units called *cells*, which help our body to assimilate chemically the nutrients we eat. The cellular processes of metabolism, catabolism (breakdown) and anabolism (building), control our body growth and function.

The cellular membrane controls what substances enter and leave the cell unit and is the first line of defense for the cell structure. The *rough endoplasmic reticulum* transports various items like a subway system. The *golgi apparatus* acts as a collecting system for secretory products. *Lysosomes* contain enzymes that break down proteins. They are involved in cell death (autolysis). The *mitochondria* serve as the powerhouse for the cell and are the primary energy sources of aerobic (oxygen using) metabolism. The *nucleus* is where the *chromosomes* lay, which are responsible for the genetic information transferred in reproduction. The *DNA* in the chromosomes controls the cell's activity.

EXAMPLES OF HUMORAL SUBSTANCES OR
SYNDROMES ASSOCIATED WITH NEOPLASMS

1. Hormones
2. Hormone precursors
3. Fetal proteins (e.g., carcinoembryonic antigen, alpha fetal protein)
4. Enzymes (e.g., alkaline phosphatase, thymidine kinase)
5. Central nervous system degenerative conditions
6. Myopathies
7. Myasthenic syndromes
8. Dermatologic syndromes (e.g., dermatomyositis, acanthosis nigricans, pachyderma)
9. Digital clubbing and arthropaties
10. Hematologic diseases (e.g., aplastic anemias, thrombophlebitis)
11. Fever

HORMONES (ECTOPIC) REPORTED TO BE
PRODUCED BY CANCERS

1. ACTH and PROACTH
2. Lipotropin
3. Chorionic gonadotropin
4. Alpha chain
5. Vasopressin
6. Hypoglycemia-producing factor
7. Somatomedins
8. Parathyroid hormone
9. Prostaglandins
10. Osteoclast-activating factor
11. Erythropoietin
12. Hypophosphatemia-producing factor
13. Growth hormone
14. Prolactin
15. Gastrin
16. Secretin
17. Glucagon
18. Corticotropin-releasing hormone
19. Growth hormone-releasing hormone
20. Somatostatin
21. Chorionic somatotropin

—Williams' *Textbook of Endocrinology*

CANCER

Male and female hormones are present in both women and men, but in different ratios. When these ratios are disturbed, there is an increased risk of cancer.

Further, in research done by Dobriner, Rhoads, and their coworkers (1947), it was found that in neoplastic disease, adrenocortical hormone production and metabolism were disturbed. It should be noted that steroid balance may well act as an autodefensive, antitumoral device. In other words, by upsetting the normal balance in the body, the body's ability to combat cancer is lessened or lost.

There are five possible causal relationships between cancer and hormones:
1. they may initiate the neoplastic change (cancer);
2. they may give origin to neoplasia-inciting metabolites;
3. they act in conjunction with other agents as co-factors or promoters;
4. they cause the tissues themselves to produce carcinogens (cancer cells);
5. they may provide for growth of tissues upon which other mechanism act.

CANCER'S WARNING SIGNS:

1. *a change in bowel or bladder habits;*
2. *a sore that does not heal;*
3. *unusual bleeding or discharge;*
4. *thickening or lump in breast or elsewhere (males included);*
5. *indigestion or difficulty in swallowing;*
6. *obvious change in a wart or mole;*
7. *a nagging cough or hoarseness.*

There are certain areas of the body in which cancer tends to lodge. These include the breasts, the prostate gland, and various glands in the endocrine system.

There are many different types of cancers, and many are dependent on the metabolic activity of specific hormones. These cancers are known as hormone-dependent tumors. It has been found in a number of studies that even small traces of hormones can cause wild, uncontrolled neoplastic growth that can be fatal.

It also appears that an imbalance of hormones causes cellular mutations and changes within the metabolic system. Normal homeostatic balance might have prevented this from happening.

Now let's pause for a word from Ciba Pharmaceutical, the company that manufactured Dianabol. This was published long before any athlete even knew what a steroid was:

A theory that carcinogenic hydrocarbons might come from steroids that occur naturally was formulated [by Cook Dodds and Kennaway]. At an International Conference of Physicians and Scientists, the results of which appeared in "Ciba Foundation Colloquia on Endocrinology, Steroid hormones and tumor growth," it was stated that, "there is a considerable body of evidence to be presented at this conference that steroids are directly implicated in the cancer problem."

CANCER OF THE PROSTATE

The prostate gland weighs only a few grams at birth, and due to the influence of androgens, it reaches its adult size of about twenty grams by age 20. Its size remains stable for about twenty-five years and in the fifth decade of life a second growth spurt begins in many men. This increase in size (hypertrophy) or Hyperplasia (increase in cell number) of the gland can cause urinary and/or rectal obstruction.

During a 1983 medical symposium, Dr. Charles Huggins, Nobel laureate for his work in prostatic cancer, directed the topic to prostatic disorders. He, along with world renowned scientist Dr. Liao, noted that 12 percent of all deaths by males of cancer is prostatic cancer and that a majority of males by the age of sixty or seventy years of age have a hyperplasia of the prostate gland. This does not denote cancer, but certain prostatic cancers are androgen dependent, and it is interesting to speculate on what the effects massive doses of androgens will have on the prostate glands of these individuals. They may end up with premature hyperplasias and hypertrophy of the prostate gland in their thirties and forties instead of their seventies. I would venture to say we might note more tragic instances of prostatic cancer in younger individuals.

Cancer of the prostate is the second most common malignancy in men (in those over fifty-five years old, it is the most common cause of cancer death after carcinomas of the lung and colon). Sixty-six thousand new cases and 21,500 lives were claimed by the disease in 1980. Although this disease is rare before age 50, steroid abuse could change this fatal distribution. You could have this disorder and be asymptomatic. Common symptoms are dysuria (pain on urination), difficulty in voiding, increased urinary frequency, complete urinary retention, back and hip pain, and hematuria (blood in the urine).

This is why the rectal exam by the physician is so important. This gland can be easily palpated. Cancer of the gland presents characteristically as hard, nodular, and irregular texture of the gland. Diagnosis can be confirmed by:

(1) computerized tomography (CT SCAN), (2) needle biopsy (taking a piece for microscopic examination) (3) elevated serum acid phosphatase, which is common in those individuals with spread (metastases) of the cancer to bone.

This cancer spreads from the gland right up the bones of the spinal column. This is because the veins there have no valves, so there is no stopping the spread. These cancers are androgen dependent, so the treatment is to remove the source of androgen, which means removing the testicles and give female hormones. Not a pleasant way to live one's adult life, guys!

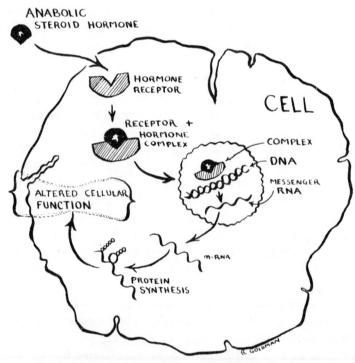

Steroid Hormones and Cell Growth

Steroids work by a hormonal-genetic interaction. When anabolic steroids are taken, they enter the cell and combine with the *hormone receptor*. The hormone-receptor complex then enters the *nucleus*, where specific genes are activated to alter protein production. This new message is carried by the *messenger RNA*, which leads to altered protein synthesis and cellular function.

THE LIVER

One area of the body that is often linked with steroid use is the liver. The liver is one of the most important organs in the body. It is a vital organ and the detoxifying area of the body. A large number of anabolics are liver conjugated (which means they are broken down and metabolized in the liver). The liver has many functions:

1. Regulation of glucose in the blood.
2. Storage of glycogen (complex glucose) and metabolism of carbohydrates.
3. Deamination—the removal of amino (NH_2) groups, This is to enable the body to gain energy from the amino acids in proteins.
4. Transamination—the interconversion of one amino acid to another kind (trans—as in transfer and amination—as in amino) used in the synthesis and degradation of amino acids.
5. It converts nitrogenous wastes into urea, so that the urea can be filtered by the kidney and excreted.
6. Vitamins A, D, E, and K are stored here.
7. Bile is synthesized to aid fat absorption.
8. The interconversion of various nutrients.
9. It is capable of resynthesizing glycogen (the stored form of glucose from some of the lactic acid (a waste product of exercise in the muscle) produced by the muscles.
10. Excretes bile pigments.
11. Destruction of old red blood cells.
12. It is the body's main line of defense against poisons.

LIVER PROBLEMS WARNING CHART

1. Look for atrophy (shrinkage) or enlargement of lobes of organ.
2. Change in texture, such as increases in hardness, softness, or nodularity.
3. Tenderness to palpatation.
4. Tenderness to ballottement (pushing to and fro)
5. Jaundice (yellow discoloration of skin and mucus membranes when they are stained by bile pigments) occurs when serum bilirubin exceeds 2 mg./dl. Jaundice most noticeable in conjunctiva of eyes. This condition may be accompanied by xan-

thoma (deposition of fat globules around eyes) and pruritus (itching).

6. Darkened urine (do not confuse with color incurred by high doses of vitamin B).
7. Abdominal pain of the visceral type; pain increased by coughing or movement and usually located in the right upper quadrant.
8. Palmar Erythema—(red palm) and spider angiomas—(brown spider-like blemish on skin) may reflect acute or chronic liver disease.
9. Finger clubbing (swelling of flesh at base of the nail bed on the fingers).
10. Change in mental state or neurologic function.

BILE

Bile pigment is mainly derived from the aging and destruction of red blood cells, from the turnover of non-hemoglobin and heme compounds, and from the metabolism of heme in the formation of new red blood cells. Anabolic steroids have resulted in elevated levels of conjugated bilirubin, hinting that some liver dysfunction might be resulting from intrahepatic cholestasis (the blockage of bile flow) or due to hepatic biliary obstruction.

Elevated levels of bile, or hyperbilirubinemia, have been reported with the use of 17-alkylated steroids. James E. Wright, Ph.D., a well known and respected steroid researcher, has organized a fine series of charts denoting the effects of anabolic steroids on liver function parameters (see appendix).

ANDROGEN-INDUCED HEPATOMAS (LIVER CANCER)

Hepatoma or Hepatocellular primary liver cell cancer accounts for 80-90 percent of all liver cancers. Clinically this disorder presents with hepatomegaly (increase in the size of the liver) and with pain or tenderness, usually in the upper right abdominal quadrant. The physician should attempt to palpate a tender mass in the liver. Anemia and elevated alkaline phosphatase levels are common laboratory findings. This may be confirmed by

1. Ultrasound.
2. CT SCAN.
3. Gallium 67 scan.

4. Alpha-fetoprotein (AFP) in the serum (70% of patients have high AFP levels between 500 ng./ml. and 5 mg./ml.).
5. Liver biopsy.

There have been a number of cases reported in the literature that strongly link anabolic steroid administration and liver cancer. At the time many of the cases were reported very few individuals were taking these drugs in comparison to the large population of men and women that are now taking huge amounts of these drugs. With this increased population pool, the chance of more individuals with a genetic susceptablity to liver cancer may manifest.

PELIOSIS HEPATIS

Peliosis hepatis is a pathological condition of the liver which is characterized by widespread and often cystic hepatic sinusoidal dilation. Blood pools or blood lakes are noted in the liver.

> The Greek word "peliosis" means extravasation of blood, or purpura, and was first used by Schoenlank in 1916 to describe a pathologic condition consisting of blood-filled cysts of the liver. Zak introduced the term to the English literature in 1950 in a description of a patient who also had a papillary adenocarcinoma of the kidney. Twenty-nine other cases were reviewed by Zak, and all but three were associated with tuberculosis. Subsequently, additional, sporadic cases have been regarded as coincidental postmortem curiosity, and has attracted little clinical attention. In cattle, it is recognized as a lesion that is associated with St. George disease, a severe wasting disorder of unknown cause....
>
> Although the pathogenesis is not known, sporadic reports have suggested a relation to anabolic-androgenic steroids. In 1952 Burger described a patient with peliosis hepatis who received "testosterone," but Gordon first suggested the association in two patients who received norethandrolone. Only isolated case reports have appeared subsequently. Although a number of different drugs have been administered to most patients, and the role of serious underlying disease has not yet been defined, seven of eight consecutively diagnosed cases at the University of Chicago Hospitals received some form of androgenic-anabolic steroid therapy, which strongly suggests that these hormones are directly related to the development of peliosis hepatis. Furthermore, in cases where androgens have not been administered, death is apparently unrelated to this lepatic lesion. In contrast, patients who develop peliosis hepatis in association with anabolic steroids appear to have a much more serious clinical form,

since death could be directly attributed to peliosis in four cases in this report and at least two in the literature.

Annals of Internal Medicine
81: 610-618, 1974

Dr. Nadell & Kosek examined this disorder very closely in a paper they published in 1977. In this exquisite review of the literature they comment,

That androgenic anabolic steroid administration may cause peliosis hepatis now seems very likely. There has been an abrupt increase in reports of peliosis recently, and most are of patients receiving anabolic steroid therapy. The disappearance of peliosis has been observed when treatment with the drug was withdrawn after biopsy diagnosis of the lesion (patient 9 and seen in the cases of Bagheri and Boyer and Poulsen and Winkler), and the lesion has been experimentally produced in rats by the oral administration of oxymethlolone (unpublished data, 1975). Also, the steroid-associated peliosis is dangerous. In the present review of 42 cases of peliosis, 14 of the 27 patients who had received androgenic anabolic steroid therapy died of liver failure and/or intraperitoneal hemorrhage resulting from peliosis hepatis, whereas peliosis hepatis was an incidental observation in the 17 nonsteroid-treated patients. Therefore, hepatic failure and massive hemorrhage must be accepted as risks of such steroid administration.

The mechanism by which these drugs induce peliosis is unknown. Although they may produce cholestasis and impaired sodium sulfobromophthalein excretion, they do not produce much histological or serum enzymatic evidence of hepatocellular injury and they seem rather to directly affect biliary secretion and canaliculi. This is not the case in peliosis, which is infrequently associated with cholestasis, at least it is not the case until liver failure is advanced.

Drug-induced injury to hepatocytes, with shrinkage or atrophy of liver cell plates, might result in abnormal dilation of sinusoids but would reduce the total liver size, whereas the livers in peliosis have usually been at least twice the normal size. Furthermore, the absence of hepatocellular regenerative signs in these cases makes primary hepatocellular injury seem less likely.

Archives of Pathological Medicine,
August 1977

The association of anabolic steroids and peliosis hepatis should not preclude their use in the treatment of serious illness such as aplastic anemia. However here are the early warning signs:

1. Abdominal pain

2. Liver (hepatic) enlargement.
3. Severe dysfunction of body.
4. Elevated liver enzymes.

Since this is a potentially fatal disorder that has been remedied by withholding steroid medication, it is wise to exercise caution.

KIDNEY DISORDERS

WILM'S TUMOR

I guess you can say I have a very close relationship with Wilm's Tumor, also known as nephroblastoma. This tumor of the kidney, the most common malignancy of the urinary tract in children and very rare among adults, is the reason this book was written. About a decade ago there was a great man who taught me how to exercise and lift weights. I wrote about him in chapter 1, "Death of an Athlete." He was one of those rare adults who died of this cancer. Then several years following his death, a report from the Harvard School of Medicine was published documenting another champion athlete who succumbed to this disorder. Both men were fine athletes and both men took anabolic steroids.

In half the cases, the condition is diagnosed before the age of four (90 percent before eight). Hematuria (blood in the urine), pain, fever, hypertension, and a palpable mass are diagnostic signs of this tumor. Flank, lumbar, or abdominal pain may also be early clues to the impending problem.

We don't know for sure if anabolic steroids were the cause of these deaths, but the prognosis for adults getting this cancer are normally very poor. So I am keeping a close eye on the literature for further correlations.

HEART DISEASE

Heart disease is the leading killer in this country, claiming over 100,000 people in 1983. This is almost triple the deaths due to cancer the same year. Before going into the dangers of steroids and other drugs on this vital body system I would like to discuss its makeup and composition.

Beating 10,000 times a day and moving 4,300 gallons of oxygen-rich blood through the circulatory system daily, this four-chambered miracle pump keeps us alive. We have 60,000 miles of blood vessels that must be supplied by the contractions of the heart muscle. A normal adult has about eight pints of blood, constantly recirculated through the body. The right side of the heart receives blood after it has delivered nutrients and oxygen to the body tissues, and then moves it on to the lungs. The second part of the two-part pumping system of the heart receives cleansed blood after it has been oxygenated by the lungs and has had the poisons (carbon dioxide) removed along with other blood gas wastes. This oxygenated blood is then pushed through the circulatory system until it eventually returns via the right side of the heart.

The normal heart rate of sixty to eighty beats per minute is controlled and activated by the sinoatrial node (SA node), which is also known as the "pacemaker" of the heart. This electrical impulse center is the heart-beat regulator. This is similar to the conduction impulses that pass through a copper wire, except now the conducting wire is the heart muscle.

The heart sounds (the lub-dubb sound) heard when you listen to a heart beat, are the sudden closing of valves and distinct vibrations of the blood, arteries and heart. The first heart sound is the closure of the atrioventricular valve. The second sound is due largely to the closure of the semilunar valves, and the heart vibrations in the chest wall and the heart, along with the relaxation of the ventrical. If heart murmurs are heard, this could be due to defects in the valves or other cardiovascular changes.

HYPERTENSION

Hypertension is known as the silent killer because in 90 percent of the cases the cause is unknown, and there is no real cure. Loss of body weight and dietary care (no more salt in the diet) seem to help. According to the American Heart Association, hypertension is the leading cause of death and disease in this country. One in six adults have some elevated blood pressure. Some of the dangers resulting from high blood pressure are coronary artery disease, stroke, kidney failure, and congestive heart failure. Hypertension has been detected in children as young as four years old.

The use of anabolic steroids causes an elevation of blood pressure due to the retained fluid in the body. It works like this. There are a number of substances in the body fluids such as sodium, potassium, chlorine, etc., and a specific amount of water to balance the amount of these elements in the body. Steroids cause the body to retain nitrogen. There is a specific ratio between the amount of nitrogen to water in the body. Since the body now is holding in more nitrogen, it must now also retain more water to balance this out. This condition results in edema. The extra fluid in the body elevates the blood pressure. The blood vessels are like flexible pipes which are used to accommodate a certain amount of fluid under a certain pressure. Now all of a sudden they have a lot more fluid to pump with the same machinery. The system is now overloaded, and elevation of blood pressure is noted. Hypertension is a deadly disease, and even a young athlete can develop hypertension and heart disease.

THE HEART IN PERIL

Anabolics have been known to increase atherosclerosis and damage many other areas of the cardiovascular system.

> Continually accumulating clinical and laboratory data indicate that dose and duration of use of oral anabolic and contraceptive steroids are the predominant factors influencing the development of hepatic lesions....
>
> Oral steroids have been increasingly implicated in the development of liver tumors....Conceivable, the use of anabolic hormones may lead to atherosclerosis, hypertension, and disorders of blood clotting—the three major causes of heart attacks and strokes. The biochemical and physiological events and reactions which can ultimately lead to these effects have been observed in humans administered the drugs under clinical conditions as well as produced experimentally in various laboratory animals.
>
> James Wright, Ph.D.
> *Anabolic Steroids and Sports*, volume II

Larry Pacifico, nine-time world power-lifting champion, found out the hard way. He almost died from advanced atherosclerosis at thirty-five years of age.

> One day in the fall of 1981 I was in the recovery room of a hospital following elbow surgery, and I had this terrible squeezing in my chest....The next morning they catheterized my arteries, and I learned that two arteries were approximately 70 percent blocked and one was almost completely closed—99.9 percent. I was immediately scheduled for a triple bypass, but

they decided to try angioplasty. It worked, but the whole experience had changed my life. I'm convinced my steroid use contributed to my coronary artery disease. I'm certain of it, and so is my doctor. I should have realized it was happening, because every time I went on a cycle of heavy steroid use I'd develop high blood pressure and my pulse rate would increase. Steroids aren't a part of my life now, but I'd be lying if I said I didn't miss them. And you know what? I may even take them again because I may not be able to *keep* myself from taking them.

Larry Pacifico*
Sports Illustrated
August 1983

Anabolic steroids remain in the bloodstream for extended periods of time. The body responds to this stress with the sympathetic ("fight or flight") portion of the autonomic nervous system. This increased activity of the sympathetic system initiates the release of adrenalin (epinephrine) and noradrenalin (norepinephrine), which are substances that affect the smooth muscle of blood vessel walls, causing them to constrict. This squeezing of the blood vessels increases body blood pressure.

Now the liver, which metabolizes anabolic drugs that are ingested, releases the breakdown products of these hormones, which cause increased retention of sodium and water. This, then, increases body fluids and blood volume, giving the heart even more to pump.

The resultant elevated blood pressure can lead to kidney and heart failure or even to stroke (a blood vessel bursting in the brain). In addition, the high blood pressure can augment the atherosclerotic process by damaging the linings of the inner walls of arteries.

These drugs have been noted to elevate both cholesterol and triglyceride levels in the blood stream. This is further supported by the fact that steroids lower HDL (high density lipoprotein) levels. HDLs protect the blood-vessel walls by removing excess cholesterol not being utilized and carry it to the liver to be converted into other products. Dangerously low HDL levels have been recorded in steroid-abusing athletes, which greatly increases their risk for heart attack.

HDLs (high density lipoproteins) are substantially effected by anabolic steroid use with the average in men being 40-50 mg./dl. and women 55 mg./dl. The Framingham study goes on to point out that

---

*Pacifico was interviewed here by Terry Todd. In subsequent interviews, he claimed that only a portion of what he said was quoted and felt that it might have been taken out of context, since he had a strong genetic predisposition to cardiovascular disease.

"for every 5 milligrams per deciliter of blood your HDL falls below the average value, your risk of heart attack increases by roughly 25 percent."

Dr. James Wright (*Anabolic Steroids in Sports*) has noted values as low as 5-10 mg./dl. in some of his patient athletes using moderate dosages of steroids.

Dr. Anthony Maddalo brought to light some interesting work published in the 1973 issue of *Medical Counterpoint*. In an article by K.A. Oster M.D. and L. Kesler M.D. they found that homogenizing milk causes xyanthene oxidase, one of the enzymes in milk to be coated in small liposomes in the fat molecule. Whereas normally it would be digested in the stomach, it now is coated within the protective coating of the liposome and can be absorbed in the intestine into the chyle in chylomicra to the lymph system into the blood. Now xyanthene oxidase has been shown to cause small lesions in arterial walls by attacking plasminogen, which is one of the cell membrane constituents in arterial walls, to cause a lesion. The body's natural defense is to lay down cholesterol or plaque to heal that lesion, and that's possibly one of the contributing mechanisms for atherosclerosis. What they have also found is that among the things that increase the activity of xyanthene oxidase are male sex hormones, histamines, and vitamin D_2 and D_3.

Now with exogenous or synthetic male hormone ingestion, you increase red-cell mass and histamine content in the blood. This ties in very closely with the reports of athletes taking anasoic steroids and increased atherosclerosis. Further studies should explore whether athletes on steroids have increased levels of xyanthene oxidase.

WATCH YOUR TENDONS

The tendons in your body are like supportive rubber bands. They connect the bone to muscle and add strength and support to body movement. If this very important body system is injured, serious problems will result. For instance, if your Achilles tendon snaps or ruptures, you would not be able to run or even walk on that leg. The pain associated with joint and tendon injury is intense and has stopped many a champion from winning, competing or even training. Without properly functioning connective tissue, many movements are seriously hampered.

Many times an individual abusing his body with steroids will up his poundage (the amount of weight normally used in an exercise). As George Turner has said in *Muscle Builder*,

> What he has done is bypass the work stages. He has failed to work on in-between poundages. That sudden dramatic strength increase is a heady trip all right, but the tendons that have to support all that muscle power fail to keep pace. Limited blood supply prevents it. Tendinitis sets in, and now he has got problems.

Bill Penner, in *Iron Man*, adds, "Former high hurdler and now physical education researcher, Gary Power, says that continued use can cause connective tissues—ligaments and tendons—to lose their elasticity. Instead of stretching they tear and pull after about three years of steroid use.

These opinions have been supported by a number of human and animal studies. In some therapeutic steroid studies, where glucocorticoids were used as anti-inflammatory steroids, there was an increase in tendon ruptures attributed to steroid use. These steroids also seemed to have an inhibitory effect on the healing process of the connective tissue. This has been evidenced by a number of fine studies where test animals were administered the drug in different doses. Many of today's athletes receive injections of anti-inflammatory steroids as popular therapy for tenosynovitis (tendinitis). How many times have you heard a peer athlete say, "I just got a shot of cortisone for the pain in my shoulder." Even though the anti-inflammatory steroids are believed to stabilize lysosomal membranes (lysosomes are packets in the cell containing digestive enzymes), thereby reducing collagen (the sticky stuff that holds cells together), these drugs may also inhibit the production of new collagen, as well as promote the removal of previously formed collagen. In other words, the steroids may weaken the structure by inhibiting the formation of collagen, which is the substance that holds the tendons and ligaments together. Even though repeated injections of drugs such as cortisone may allow an athlete to return to competition faster, they can lead to tendon rupture, which will put him out for good!

Terry Todd (former world powerlifting champion) discussed the danger to body tendon structures in *Sports Illustrated* (August 1983).

> One of the ways the old no-free-lunch lesson was learned by athletes who began to use testosterone was that as a group they began to suffer a great many more muscle and tendon injuries.

Before its widespread use such injuries were rare among strength athletes, whereas now they are alarmingly frequent. Among lifters the two areas that tend to rupture are the biceps tendon and the quadriceps, the muscle on the front of the thigh. Since the widespread use of testosterone began, scores of men have either had the unpleasant experience of watching their biceps muscle roll up their arm like a windowshade after the tendon at the point of insertion into the bone of the forearm gave way, or of collapsing to the platform after one or both of their quadriceps or patellar tendons ruptured. But although the increase in these injuries is not a matter of dispute, the reason, or reasons, for that increase aren't completely understood.

Some weight men argue that the injuries can all be attributed to the heavier poundages being lifted now. Others contend that because of the increased testosterone level something biochemical must happen to the muscle or tendon that makes it more brittle and likely to tear. Still others, and I lean toward their view, suggest that it can be explained by the aggressiveness produced by the testosterone, aggressiveness that causes the lifters to train hard when they should take it easy. This argument holds that the body normally tells an athlete when to back off, but the testosterone imperative to train hard and dominate the weights overrides these messages, with the result being injury.

SHOCK

ANAPHYLACTIC SHOCK

An extremely dangerous problem is when an allergic-condition reaction occurs when taking certain drugs. When you take steroids, you are taking a drug that is a synthetic foreign substance in the body. The body can react to the steroid or the vehicle it is carried in. The cardiac output and the arterial pressure drop drastically. Immediately after the antigen (the steroid) has entered the body, a massive antigen-antibody reaction takes place throughout the body. This is the body's defense mechanism against any invading agent it feels will cause harm. You might be taking a drug for many years, and then all of a sudden your body and protective antibody system will become allergic to it. This type of reaction is detrimental to the circulatory system in several ways. If the antigen-antibody reaction is to take place in direct contact with the vascular walls or cardiac musculature, these tissues can be damaged directly. In addition, when cells are damaged anywhere in the human body by this antigen-antibody reaction to a foreign substance, there are the release of some highly toxic substances into the bloodstream. These substances, one of which is histamine (or a histamine-like substance), have very strong vasodilator effects. When this happens, the venous dilation causes an increase in vascular capacity. Further, there is a great reduction in arterial pressure due to the dilation of the arterioles. The arterioles are the smallest arteries with a vascular wall. They are continuous with the capillary network. This whole effect causes a great reduction in venous return. The shock that follows is so severe that the individual dies within minutes.

Shortly after the drug is ingested, the person might become agitated and flushed and feel uneasy. It is possible to experience palpitations, tachycardia, paresthesias (numbness, pricking or burning feeling in the abnormal level), difficulty breathing, ear throbbing, or pruritis (itching). *If you suffer anaphylactic shock after ingesting steroids and do not receive emergency medical care, you will be one dead athlete within minutes.*

SEPTIC SHOCK

This disorder used to be known as "blood poisoning." This is a very dangerous infection that is carried by the blood to many areas of the body. There can be extensive damage. This type of shock is of great concern to medical people because it is one of the leading (shock-type) killers in the hospital. With so many athletes self-administering steroids, the danger of septic shock is magnified. You can get this devastating bacterial infection from contamination of either the drug or syringe. There is an elevated white blood cell count (the antibody system reacting to the foreign bacteria) and muscular weakness. Symptoms may appear eight to twelve hours after the ingestion of the drug. This can definitely prove fatal if left unattended.

Both of the above-mentioned conditions may occur when athletes self-administer injections without proper medical supervision. The inside of a gym bag or locker is chuck full of bacteria and fungi. You might say death lurks in the locker room, especially if an athlete has a private pharmacy next to his jock strap.

A good example of this behavior pattern was discussed in the August 1983 issue of the *Physician and Sportsmedicine*. Dr. K.D. Fitch, Australian Olympic team physician in the 1972 Munich Olympics and 1980 Moscow Games, relays the experience one of his colleagues had at the powerlifting championship at which no drug tests were performed.

> A championship weight lifter had been taking large doses of oral and parenteral anabolic steroids during the last seven pre-competitive weeks. Not surprisingly, he was at approximately 105% of allowable body weight. He reduced his weight the last 24 hours by restricting fluid and taking 320 mg. of furosemide (eight tablets). He planned to rehydrate by intravenous infusion (2.5 liters of 0.9 sodium chloride) during the 90 minutes between weigh-in and the start of competition. However, after five unsuccessful attempts to venipuncture his own arms in a men's room he abandoned this plan and drank fluid together with potassium, quinine sulfate, and sodium chloride tablets and Paroven (a vasodilator) capsules to minimize cramps.
>
> Before his first lift, he took 150 mg. of ephedrine sulfate (more was to be taken during the competition). After failing with his first squat, he then watched his challenger successfully negotiate the same weight. Perhaps as a consequence of his steroid-induced aggression and impaired decision-making ability due to overdosage with a sympathomimetic agent, compounded by dehydration and electrolyte imbalance, he called for additional weight and planned a much faster descent.
>
> As he attempted to halt his far too rapid descent, his left quadriceps tore completely at the lower tendomuscular junction. With the spotters watching helplessly, his right ankle inverted, resulting in a third-degree sprain. The unchecked heavy bar caused massive soft-tissue bruising of the dorsal trunk, with his hemoglobin falling to 9gm/100ml. Surgery was performed that day to repair these injuries and was required subsequently because of persistent left patella problems.

The risk of infection and even septic shock during the above-mentioned episode was immense. A tiny puncture site from a needle could initiate a very dangerous infection. During the Civil War, more soldiers died from infections than actual surgical procedures.

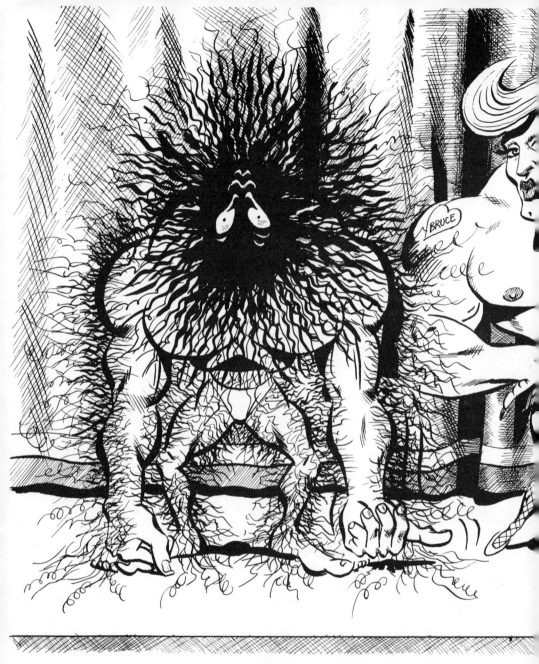

10
WITHDRAWAL SYMPTOMS

Using this stuff [steroids] makes you neurotic. I entered four pro shows this year and I started with it, and haven't been off it for a long time because of the constant competitions and shows...one after the

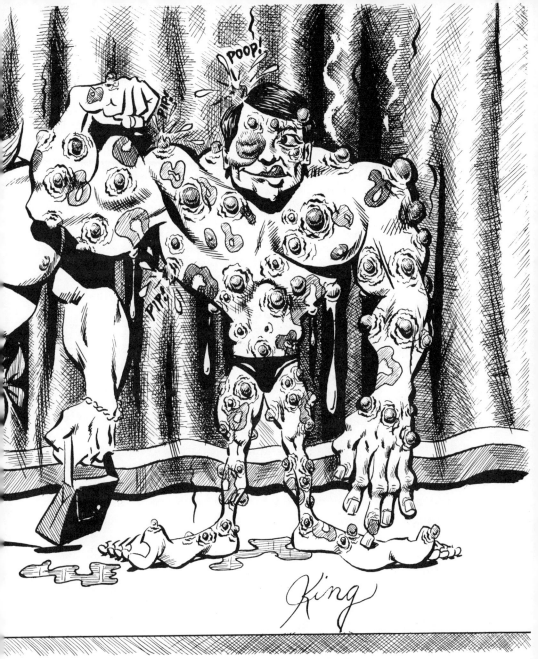

Drawing by Myron King, entitled "Steroids—No Side Effects."

other. I've been on it for a good part of the year. Anyone who goes on the stuff . . . your attitude changes, you get nasty . . . get real mad easy. I'm coming off now and I am very upset, depressed. My body feels *lousy and my workouts are terrible. I lost a lot of drive. I lost my psych to work out hard and train. When you really clean up your system, you get really paranoid. . .you feel like you're shrinking, you get very upset. This is what I am going through right now. It's a dramatic mental change. People notice and say, "you don't look so good." I don't want to have to go back on the stuff, I want to clean out my system. Some of those guys really go overboard. The kids are going nuts. . .young kids on the junk. No one is putting a gun to my head, but I am being forced indirectly because everyone else is taking it. To tell you the truth, I'm gonna experiment without it in the next year's pro shows. . . .I really want to stop. . .bad.*

Pro competitor, bodybuilder

OPEN DOOR TO DRUG ADDICTION

AS WITH ANY DRUG, THERE ARE DRAWBACKS, EVEN AFTER THE USE OF them has ceased. An alcoholic suffers tremors, a cigarette smoker nicotine fits, speed freaks the shakes, and heroin junkies total withdrawal accompanied by blind madness to get more. Anabolic steroids are not without withdrawal effects. These hormones are body stimulators, and many times may coerce certain body organs to be whipped into action when they should normally be dormant. What happens when you stop? What are the psychological implications?. . .psychological changes? I interviewed a number of athletes on their subjective experiences when coming down off these hormone drugs. To sum up their experiences in one word, I would have to pick—depression.

All of a sudden the hormone flow stops, and with it goes all the synthetic energy and power. The artificial steroids have cut off the natural body supply by inhibiting normal secretions. Normal body testosterone has dropped below normal to such an extent that even feminizing effects have been documented to occur. The body nitrogen level drops drastically so that the edema, water weight gained, is lost rapidly, so quickly that all gains disappear within weeks, to an even lower level than prior to drug ingestion. You see your body shrinking and growing weaker before your eyes. . .the gains just fading away, the muscle poundage just peeling away. Depression sets in as those around you comment that you do not look too good. "Are you sick?" they may ask.

Dr. John Ziegler, quoted in *Sports Illustrated*, found the athlete's addiction leads to increased dosages:

Everyone got more "studdy." The side effects were strong. Finally, in the late '50s, we got Dianabol, and it was about then that I read of the work that had been done in Germany on isometric contraction. It was in 1960 that I decided to try the steroids and the isometric contractions on a few of the top U.S. lifters, but I wish to God now I'd never done it. I'd like to go back and take that whole chapter out of my life.

Steroids were such a big secret at first, and that added to the hunger the lifters and football players had to get hold of them. I honestly believe that if I'd told people back then that rat manure would make them strong, they'd have eaten rat manure. What I failed to realize until it was too late was that most of the lifters had such obsessive personalities. To them, if two tablets were good, four would be better.

Terry Todd, in this same article, goes on to explore the strong clamps these drugs can place on stubborn competitors:

Athletes tend to take ever larger dosages over longer periods of time. Thus the apparent increasing need of the body *for* steroids and the growing psychological dependence *on* steroids join hands to encircle the ambitious athletes. . . .

One former athlete who understands this cycle is Dr. Craig Whitehead, a leading bodybuilder in the mid-1960s, who used steroids while competing. An ophthalmologist who now practices acupuncture in San Francisco, Whitehead for several years directed the drug rehabilitation unit of the Haight-Ashbury clinic. He is still involved in that field, and recently he said, "The dependence on steroids many people develop is classic. It's similar to that developed by people on so-called recreational drugs."

West German hammer thrower Uwe Beyer, who won the European championships in 1971 and broke the world record that same year, became so dependent on anabolic steroids during his training for the Montreal Olympics that he said that after he stopped taking the pills, "I was listless, depressed and despaired of winning anything. . . . I suffered withdrawal symptoms like a drug addict."

The personality traits exhibited with steroid abuse have been demonstrated in numerous animal experiments. Female monkeys have been noted to repeatedly mount each other in an attempt to copulate after testosterone injections. These changes have also been demonstrated in electroencephalographic research on humans. The human reactions are similar to amphetamine abuse—those being rage, uncontrollable aggression, and almost schizophrenic behavior. The mood swings of high highs, and really low lows plague the athlete.

The *Journal of Clinical Psychiatry* (April 1980) noted a case of anabolic-steroid abuse and acute schizophrenic episodes in a seventeen-year-old athlete.

> It is well documented and widely known that corticosteroids, estrogens, and progesterones have among their side effects various mental disturbances, which can mimic the schizophrenias and the manic-depressive psychoses. Relatively classic examples would include the agitated psychoses of Cushing's Disease, the schizophreniform psychosis of lupus cerebritis, and the "iatrogenic" depressive illness found with the use of contraceptives. To date, the anabolic, ergogenic steroids, such as methandienone, have not been associated with severe mental illness, although their structure and function might suggest some similarity to the corticosteroids.

The young weight-lifter's acute schizophrenic episode was linked to his ingestion of Dianabol:

> During his hospitalization, he informed the physician that he had been using anabolic steroids in 1977 and 1978 while weight-lifting to "gain weight." These were obtained on the black market and were used without medical supervision. He noted that 6 months after initiating this self-medication he began to feel uncomfortable, slept poorly and began having thought confusion, ruminations, paranoid ideation, and audible thoughts.
>
> . . . [further], we feel that with the widespread use of illicit anabolic steroids by athletes, and their unwillingness to offer this information to consulting physicians, the possibility of such an exogenous etiology for severe psychic disturbances going unnoticed is very high.

There is also the increased risk of suicidal thoughts and acts of uncontrolled violence. I have personally witnessed this rage and the depression that follows. I had to physically restrain a personal friend who thought he was going to keep a "hot date" with an open window, fifteen stories up.

A cautious eye toward the future was noted by my colleague, Dr. C.E. Finch, Ph.D., director of the Andrus Gerontology center at the University of Southern California. He has performed extensive research on laboratory-induced hormone levels on rodents. He says, "We have found that elevated levels of steroids can cause irreversible brain damage and target-cell damage in the brain. Our studies are with rodents, but it raises the question about future human studies in a pertinent way. We speculate that the abuse of steroids could cause neuronal [brain cell] death in humans because the evidence is very strong in laboratory animal studies." This is new brain research that is just beginning to surface in medical literature.

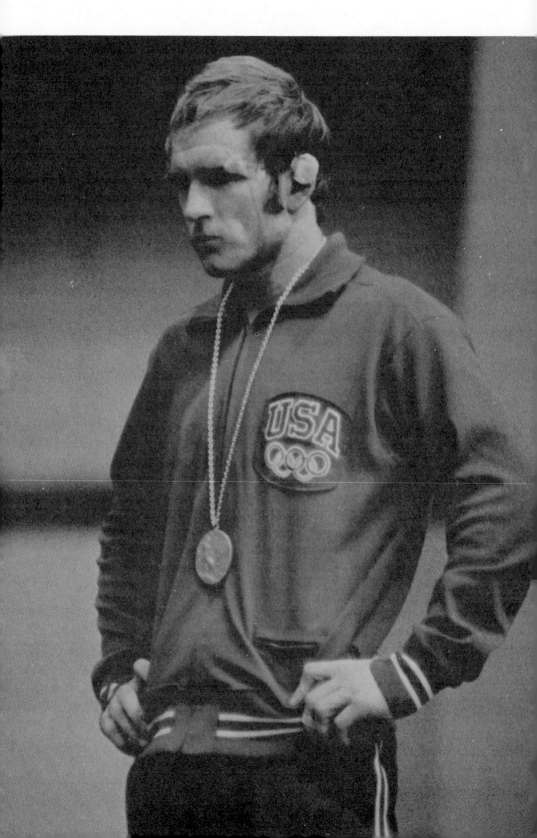

Dan Gable, 1972 Olympic Gold Medal Wrestling Champion and wrestling coach of the 1984 U.S. Olympic team says, "Anyone who is a serious contender for an Olympic championship would be foolish to gamble his career for drugs."

11
WHAT'S THE CURE?

The unfortunate and glaringly inconsistent aspect of steroid and general drug abuse in sport today is that it violates the very code of athletic participation in that we are supposed to be involved in sports to exercise the body with at least the hope and promise of some spinoff physical benefits. Indiscriminate drug use opposes this concept in the most villainous way.

Robert Kennedy, Publisher
Muscle Mag. International

WHAT CAN BE DONE? MY OWN DEALINGS HAVE LED TO A LOT OF FRUStration. At first, I attempted to bring hard-core, bland, medically referenced data into articles published in common-carrier sport magazines. These found their way into the locker-room trash cans.

Then, through the coaxing of Denie, the sport photo-journalist and magazine editor who gave me my start, I developed a more embellished and vivid writing style, something to the tune of:

> Many of the athletes you now see pictured in this magazine will be dead within 10-15 years. Their deaths will not be painless or due to old age. The abusive use of anabolic steroids will make their passing an ugly sight, as cancer rips through their bodies, unmercifully eating them up alive. Once great mountains of muscle and health, they will be reduced to flaccid skin and bone in the horror soon to come.
>
> It is remarkable how athletes that possess such training, discipline, and the will to improve health are now carrying hypodermic needles and synthetic drugs in their gym bags instead of fresh fruit.

> The dosages of steroids now being shoved down throats might very well lead to a hospital bed with tubes and needles stuck in every opening, every breath seething with pain, wasting away.

Whew! And that was only my first article published five years ago. To be honest, that was mild compared with those that followed. The purpose was to paint a mental picture for the readers. Young athletes can only relate to pain; death is too foreign. Denie and I tried in desperation to reach these young minds and reverse the ominous trend we saw growing, engulfing, strangling the sport world we so love.

The series of articles that followed may at times have been over-embellished with excessive adjectives, but the basic theories have all come to pass as true. We were ridiculed for our fears and confronted with, "We don't see anyone dying or getting sick!" Those voices have long since been replaced with reported cases of liver and kidney failure and fatalities.

However, this approach did little to curb the tidal wave of drug abuse engulfing all of sport. In this chapter, I leave you with some solutions and thoughts of experts in the sports-medicine field.

I interviewed hundreds of athletes, coaches, officials, trainers, sports-medicine physicians and scientists, news reporters and media people in an attempt to formulate a viable, systematic approach to dealing with drug abuse in sports. Some individuals had unique and interesting ideas, and I hope this sounding board can be used as a guide for would-be steroid users as a warning. It will take the cooperation of all the above and political and sociological changes to make it work, but if we all work together in earnest, perhaps we can map out a plan that is fair and feasible.

I am not concerned with pointing a finger and saying, "So and so uses drugs." What is important is making the social changes needed so that drug abuse can come under control, and the right of fair competition and the health of every country's young athletes is protected.

World heavyweight powerlifting champion *Terry Todd* had this to say in *Sports Illustrated* (August 1983):

> So I took Dianabol intermittently from 1963 through early 1967, at which time I retired from competition. My best guess is

that during that period I took approximately 1,200 pills, which would be 6,000 milligrams. When I tell young athletes these days of my dosage levels they look at me as if I were describing how margarine used to look during the Second World War, before the yellow coloring was added. Exactly how high the levels have gone is a matter of conjecture, but I have both testimony and published reports indicating that on occasion athletes have taken in less than two weeks the 6,000 milligrams that I, weighing more than 300 pounds, took in four years.

Terry's wife, *Jan Todd*, head of the International Powerlifting Federation for Women and a world record-holder in women's powerlifting, reinforces this feeling further in an article in *USA Today*:

> Part of the difficulty is that they are so easy to get. Although a prescription drug, steroids are not classed as controlled substances—which makes the job of those who buy and sell them on the black market much simpler.
>
> All controlled substances are carefully monitored from the time they are manufactured until they are sold by a pharmacist. They range from class 1 (heroin) through class 5 (paregoric). Their sale requires much more thorough recordkeeping than does the sale of simple "legend" drugs such as those in the steroid group.
>
> According to Gene Vykukal, president of Southwestern Drug Corp., if the Food and Drug Administration reclassified anabolic steroids as controlled substances, it would not only be more difficult for unethical drug wholesalers or pharmacists to deal in these drugs, it would allow the Drug Enforcement Agency to more vigorously prosecute those who profit from them.
>
> If the appropriate government agencies act now to designate anabolic steroids as controlled substances, perhaps the fiasco in Caracas will not have been in vain.

In the same article, it was reported that The Athletics Congress' women's committee had voted to have drug testing at the national championships, but this proposal was ruled out because of expense. This prompted Lorna Griffin, the top American women's shot-putter in 1982 to say that she might have to quit competing soon because she could not keep up with athletes using steroids.

Jennifer Weyland, women's middleweight world powerlifting champion, who has bench pressed 282 pounds at a body weight of 156 pounds, had this to say:

> It seems to me the one person that is being overlooked is the

athlete. They are most affected by the rules and have the small-est voice in political say so and rule making. Under the current conditions, the drug-testing system is not foolproof enough for me to feel comfortable with. Many times, the officials who have the final say were not even athletes themselves. Without the ath-letes, there is no sport. The whole situation is almost like the handgun law. The people that arms are safe with, such as the businessman or homeowner, won't have access to guns, while the criminal does.

She went on to bring up an important point—that officials should come to a reasonable list of substances and not test every medication under the sun. Cold tablets if one has a cold, an anti-diarrheal agent to stop the runs, or a mild analgesic such as aspirin should not cas-trate an athlete competitively. I personally feel we must draw a rea-sonable line as far as the list of banned substances. A cup of coffee or a can of cola should not be sufficient to blow away years of training.

Cheryl Jones, mother of three, housewife, gym owner, and female world powerlifting champion in the 97-pound class, who has squat-ted 282 pounds and has deadlifted 297 pounds, noted:

> When you see lifters going up two or three weight classes, with their lifts going up 100 points in a year, it's very frustrating, especially when you win and people attribute it to drugs when you're clean. One time I had taken a cough syrup for a cold, which had codeine in it, so I had to bow out of one test so that I would not forfeit my position for future world competitions. Then it was alluded to in one magazine that I didn't take the test because of steroids. You can't lift to your full potential if you have a stomach cramp, headache, diarrhea, or menstrual dis-comfort.

Finally, one more woman powerlifter, *Maris Anne Sternberg*, 198-pound world powerlifting champion, who has squatted with 450 pounds on her back, says:

> People should work to the best of their own personal ability and not concern themselves with the habits of others. To further support this concept that "vitamins and nutritional aids are also chemical substances," there has to be a limit to chemical bans. I don't like the idea of tests because some people may get around it, but if a test is required for me to lift, then I will take it.
>
> Further, it's frustrating to see the medical people in other coun-tries spending loads of money on how to help their athletes with drugs and how to get around the tests, while here we spend our

money on how to catch the athletes. Why not spend the money to help our athletes find a way to use these drugs healthfully instead of making criminals out of the competitors?

David P. Webster, vice-president, Commonwealth Games Weightlifting Federation, has seen these rulings come into power despite strong initial opposition by the bulk of athletic society in Europe. He is the main driving force to bring equal and drug-free competition back to the level of true sport. "I believe that the best method to stop the problem is to inflict very severe penalties, as is done in Scotland most successfully. I am appalled that the authorities in America have knuckled down to the pressures being put upon them. The threat of legal action is not new; it is one which we have had to face, and while very apprehensive, we have won through in the end. Sports organizations are entitled to make their own rules, and people must abide by these rules regarding this matter. And in spite of what is said in America, the tests are very satisfactory and highly sophisticated."

Jack Kelly, a competitor on four Olympic teams in rowing and still a national masters champion hopes, "that the new equipment will be comprehensive and accurate and that the Eastern bloc countries have not devised chemical substances that will be undetectable. In those countries, athletes are closely followed by sports physicians and technicians, while here we often only see our athletes as they are being chosen for the Olympic squads." As first vice-president of the U.S. Olympic Committee, he noted, "The Russians have their top 100 swimmers training in Moscow at a year-round special camp, and with them they have 50 medical sports-technicians for a 1:2 ratio of specialists on a regular basis. I don't think many of these athletes know what is being given to them in the way of pills or shots. They are only told that they will be monitored and weaned of the drugs come testing time.

"Those athletes might be on drugs not even on the drug lists, I fear."

The problems of drug abuse spans many sports. I don't really think they are necessary to reach champion status. A good example is *Al Oerter,* who hails from Long Island, New York. Here is a former Olympian who has won the gold medal four times (1956, Melbourne; 1960, Rome; 1964, Tokyo; 1968, Mexico), and at the ripe old age of 44 came out of retirement to attempt a fifth gold medal at the 1980 Olympics in Moscow. Al was asked about steroids and other drugs in an interview in *Muscle Training Illustrated,*

I'm really not quite sure. In all honesty I don't know if they have any value or not. I know a number of athletes, and from what I ascertain, it's obvious that the greatest percentage of athletes are very much into the use of steroids, and the use of hormone programs to stabilize weight and increase strength...or assist them theoretically at least in being able to work harder.

To a certain extent, the hormone programs they're using today can be a detriment, particularly mentally. Because the precompetition testing programs are quite real and the officials are throwing out lots of athletes because their tests for drugs are coming up positive. Now, what does an athlete do when he believes that his capability is purely the result of the chemicals and drugs he is taking in? You take away that chemical and his confidence in his own capability disappears. How can he then compete with any sense of being able to do anything?

I am very ambivalent about it. It's very dangerous to begin with and I just don't subscribe to a lot of the things I hear.

U.S. Olympic Committee Executive Director Col. F. Donald Miller promised a crackdown after the Pan-Am Games scandal. "We have been making cheats and liars out of our athletes. We have got a drug problem. It's about time we've done something about it." *(Newsweek, Sept. 1983)*

William Simon, U.S. Olympic Committee president, is very emphatic about the situation. "Testing of banned substances will continue to take place, and athletes are going to recognize that they will be disqualified if found to be using them—period! We are going to enforce this stringently, not only in the U.S. at all the trials and domestic meets but also at international competition for every country in the world. Not only is it dangerous for these fine young athletes, but it is cheating!"

Sports Illustrated received this college athlete's lament, which points to a new way of looking at drugs and a new and more difficult milieu than before the 1970s.

When we went to the dining hall we were given a paper cup with a bunch of pills in it. Most were vitamin pills of one sort or another, but there were 30 milligrams of anabolic steroids in there, too. And they chewed our butts if we didn't take everything. Still, that was mild compared to what I saw back home in New Jersey recently. I was at a local gym and this little black kid comes up to me with a bottle of pills in his hand and asks me what they are. They were Dianabol tablets, and when I asked him where he'd gotten them, he said his football coach had told him to go to the doctor and get some pills and take them. We all knew about that doctor; you could go to his office and without giving your age or taking any kind of a test, you could get a prescription for steroids. All you needed was the money, at 14 years old?

One ex-bodybuilder spoke graphically of the side effects.

> I've got something wrong with my kidneys...really bad. The doctors don't know either. He sent me to a radiologist. When I was on the stuff, I got these back pains, sort of like it came from the kidney—a sharp pain which would go away. Then when I went off, the pain came back. A few months later, the pain came back as if I was on the stuff. At this time, I was getting it on the right side of the kidney in the back, then a month later the pain ran from the back of the right side all the way to the front, then it hit both sides. It felt like someone or something was inside the kidney...sort of like kidney stones. Like a burr inside being bounced around. The pain was unbearable. I was on Dianabol for 6 weeks in 1977, then 6 weeks in 1978. I was getting a shot a week [1 full cc. equals 100 mgs.]. When I went off, I was losing weight and could not maintain my weight, then I started to get very frustrated. You keep fooling yourself; "it won't happen to me." The pain is ridiculous. I threw the rest of the drug out. After I went off I was smaller than I was before I ever even started. Now I am scared as shit. They found protein in my urine a few months ago, but now they don't find anything wrong with my urine or blood. But the pain is still so bad I don't know what to do. I am waiting to hear about my X-rays. I've got something definitely wrong back there. The pain is sharp and unreal. It keeps coming back. I damaged it and it's trying to repair itself.

Bodybuilders have taken a large share of criticism for their involvement with steroids. But officially the International Federation of Body Builders could not be more forthright in warning bodybuilders about the dangers. The IFBB will begin testing at the 1985 World Bodybuilding Championships. Here's a statement from *Ben Weider*, IFBB international president.

> One of the big problems bodybuilders face is the use of shortcuts to obtain maximum muscular development. They read about other athletes in heavy athletics, such as weightlifting, shot-put, wrestling etc., using steroids, and they feel they can improve their chances of winning bodybuilding contests with the use of steroids.
> Bodybuilding is a way of life. We believe that bodybuilders should train through natural methods and eat natural foods to

obtain their results. The official position of the IFBB is that steroids are dangerous to health, and the side effects could cause horrendous harm. No amount of possible results could compensate for the dangers an athlete is putting himself in, when he uses steroids.

Steroids has its place in medicine and under the control of a medical doctor, they can be used for health improvement. However, in sport, steroids have no place and we are totally against them.

Ken Sprague, AAU vice-president, physique committee, former owner of Gold's Gym; in the last few years has been responsible for many of the positive changes in the sport of bodybuilding.

As manager of Gold's Gym, I have seen people take 100 times the recommended dosage of the common steroids used. And they are not just taking one steroid but 100 times the recommended dosage of several different steroids at the same time (synergistic effects). I have known people to go into shock and have to be rushed to the emergency room. One fellow dropped dead at home. He was a power lifter and trained regularly at the gym. He was from New York, Rochester, and he was only 28 years old.

I think we should mandate drug tests, but the problem is how far into the personal life of an individual do you go. I am sure if it could be shown how truly dangerous these drugs are, backed up with scientific evidence, I think the AAU would move towards some tighter regulations. Everybody knows everybody takes them. Like the wallpaper, they're there. There are also these other drugs they are bringing in from other countries, like a new one from Spain, that takes fat out from under the skin. The key is though that the tolerance to these drugs has been broken, and those athletes taking injectables where they can't even read the label...from Mexico and Spain, you name it. They get it in through a black market system. They are purchased and then sent from Germany, Italy, Spain, etc. They are sent through the mail illegally by parcel post. It's no secret that you can purchase Primobolin in Mexico for $1.35, and it sells in Pittsburgh for $20.00. Then there are a lot of doctors who prescribe the drugs. There is a physician I have filed suit against for pushing these drugs through an athlete at my gym. This guy would get all the Dianabol he wanted and give it out without even seeing the patient. Now you have monkey and horse steroids. If aspirin is okay, then morphine must be also. That's the danger that is occuring. If you told the bodybuilder that he would die, I don't know if he would stop. You have to outlaw the athletes that use them from competition. We must find a test that is not too expensive. It's a very touchy situation. You have guys backstage "pumping up," and you try to draw blood from them. That's rough? If it is done well in advance, it might work.

One time in the gym, a guy's heart stopped...they stuck in the big needle...and he was only 30. He went into shock after taking an injectable steroid. I saw another guy take 100 Dianabol tablets after breakfast (500 milligrams) and 50 Anavar tablets. He does this every day when he is training for a contest. Plus he takes injectables every day, but I am not sure of the quantity; also thyroid in heavy dosages. You can almost imagine that some athletes who take animal steroids begin to look like one, but I think this is mostly due to the fact that they looked a bit weird to begin with.

Sometimes these guys go on zero carbohydrates for two months before a contest, combined with the many drugs and thyroid extracts, and poor, unhealthy diets. I can't see that not killing somebody.

The use of these drugs is not restricted to bodybuilders though. There is a big scandal out in San Diego against a team physician who was giving the [steroids] out to the team as part of daily training.

Dr. Allan J. Ryan, editor-in-chief of *The Physician and Sportsmedicine*, has written some of the finest papers on possible solutions. He utilized the August 1983 issue to air the opinions of several experts.

Daniel Hanley, M.D., former chief physician to the U.S. Olympic teams between 1965 and 1976, seemed to feel that testing athletes once every four years will not control doping in sport and that lab-test programs have become too expensive. Further:

Selective testing of 20% of the athletes means that 80% of the competing athletes are not tested.

Always testing the first six athletes to finish fixes in the minds of all that doping and winning are connected, while the truth is just the opposite.

Dope testing has become a contest of pharmacy between the athlete and the tester. When a substance is banned and easily detected, athletes use other substances, usually more potent and potentially more harmful. For example, athletes now use adrenalin instead of ephedrine, testosterone instead of anabolic steroids, or growth hormone instead of both.

Another physician suggested:

That participation in Olympic Games and World Championships be restricted to persons at least 18 years of age, which would decrease the health risks involved in training children for top performance.

Dr. E. C. Percy feels the disadvantages of testing

> are outweighed by the fact that our athletes are using drugs that are not only illegal but can also have harmful side-effects. After all, we have been testing race horses since 1905 to protect them from drugs administered by their trainers and owners. Why not test our human athletes to protect them from the health hazards of drugs, when it is obvious that these intelligent performers are unwilling to accept the fact that these substances are dangerous?

The original tests for urine testing were developed by Professors Raymond Brooks and *Arnold Beckett* at St. Thomas' Hospital, University of London. These procedures analyze urine samples by radioimmunoassay and then by mass spectrometry and gas chromatography. Professor Beckett of Chelsea College and the International Olympic Committee medical commission takes a balanced view of it all. He says,

> What we must always remember is this. It is a never ending process. We can never eradicate drug use among athletes, but I think if we stay on our toes we can continue to develop procedures that will cause the athletes to use small amounts of drugs near the competitions, and this will promote fairness and health. That's our job. Consider the alternative.

George Verras, former director at Lenox Hill Hospital's Institute of Sports Medicine and Athletic Trauma, added: "I feel we need additional biochemical research. I think the research that has already been done indicates that the negative factors are there...we need more in-depth stuff. We need tighter international restraint [controls], especially between the European and American sport foundations..." *Dr. Thomas W. Allen*, masters powerlifter and specialist in pulmonary and internal medicine at the Chicago College of Osteopathic Medicine, reinforces this point by saying:

> The reason we have not told the athletes the whole truth is because we do not know all the ramifications yet, but there are still physicians and scientists who tell athletes steroids don't make a difference, while those using these drug preparations have found this not to be the case. We cannot lie to athletes on this basic point and then expect them to believe us on others. We must discuss all the effects, positive and negative physiologically, and

then the negative effects, ethically, about competing fairly. But if you're going to play the game, you must play by the rules of the game. . . . We will test and discipline those that break the rules of the game, period.

We can't use scare tactics because as with the use of cigarettes and alcohol, not everyone dies of heart disease or lung cancer or emphysema. [So too] athletes see others take drugs without any apparent ill effect. So the rules must be you can't use steroids and play in our ballgame, whether you believe us about the dangers or not—you can't use them and play. . . . If the athletes lose at trying to outsmart the testing officials, then they pay the price.

Philip Rosenthal, assistant director of the Institute of Sports Medicine and Athletic Trauma at Lenox Hill Hospital, New York:

> [What is needed is] education, starting at the elementary-school level, discussing drugs and their actions and adverse effects. You can't wait until college and the pro levels. This should begin for the student athlete and get away from the old hygiene classes where you are told alcohol, tobacco, and drugs are bad for you. There is great value in bringing in former pro athletes, who student athletes will identify with, when they say, "I paid the price." This education must be continued up through the ranks, while on the other front, testing at the international level should show them they won't get away with it. The National Basketball Association is going to take the stance as per newspaper reports that any player convicted of using cocaine will be expelled from the NBA. You need a fine line that is obeyed.

Dr. James A. Nicholas, founder of the Institute of Sports Medicine and Athletic Trauma in New York and a brilliant orthopedic surgeon and sports-medicine scientist, has aided me in the past with some of my publications. He was the keeper of Joe Namath's knees and treats the New York Jets and Giants, the Cosmos, the New York Knicks basketball team, and the Rangers hockey team. His personal experience with utilizing these drugs to treat the sick goes back to the 1950s. He was very interested in metabolic bone disease, particularly osteoporosis, and patient recovery response to trauma and surgery.

> We have noted pretibial edema and hirsutism in some patients on steroids and have found much of the weight gained by our athletes who were taking steroids to be fluid retention. They diuresed rapidly and lost fifteen pounds of fluid with cessation of the steroids. We are noting a backlash at this time to the

abuses that have occurred, with some athletes going natural again.

One major problem is that we now have a group of alternative medical-care systems. There are a number of nonmedical people who advocate medical treatments without the proper credentials and educational background. Self-appointed experts who proclaim certain facts in common-carrier publications should not be given free run without the proper credentials. Athletes must be made aware that the body is a biological machine that can respond in a lethal manner to toxic doses of self-medication and that they must be supervised by someone with the proper scientific background and not anecdotal experience.

Further, the brain is a computer, and there are compulsive traits developed by people in athletics as well as other areas of society, and I think legislation should be enacted to recognize these drugs as potentially lethal. These drugs should be reclassified by their toxicity at certain dose levels. There has to be disclosures of the true facts, not in newspapers but in the medical literature. Medicine spans the spectrum from birth to death, and one must realize that in scanning contemporary medical research pathology starts with birth, and one must realize when someone walks into a prescribing situation, you don't know what the person's liver is like, or prostate, and that testing procedures will not even give you the full story, so in many ways the evaluation is archaic in what these drugs are really doing to the body. By the time abnormal liver-function tests or an enlarged prostate is noted, the situation could be far gone.

Dr. Irving Dardik, chairman of the United States Olympic Committee Council on Sports Medicine, says,

> The first thing to do is to apply the rules and to enforce them while simultaneously developing a major educational program for all levels of athletics.
>
> The drug problem is in essence partly the fault of sports medicine as a whole. The tendency of the sports medicine science community is to act like the drug problem belongs to the athletes and that "we," the scientific community, have had very little to do with it. The major thing that needs to be accomplished is for the sports medicine community, physicians, and scientists to recognize their personal responsibility in this area. This deals with one principle to develop ideas, resources, and capabilities that we can apply when working with athletes to optimize performance. The athlete is "science in action," and science is a powerful adjunct tool to work with the athlete in his training program. We need to marshal our resources and bring our finest technology and scientists to work with our athletes. This would also open

up the channels of communication. The biggest problem with the drugs is that we stuck our head in the sand and we've mislead the athletes and have not told the truth. The athletes then tell the sports science community, "Don't preach to us from Mount Olympus. Where were you when we needed you? We'll do what we want." We must really publicize this information and what we can do for athletes. There have been many scientists publishing papers on what they can do for the athletes; the paper is published, and the author is gone from the scene.

We need people whom the athletes respect and can communicate with, not the preaching, disciplinarian type. The medical community also *alludes* to numerous panaceas and miracle breakthroughs that supposedly will help one win a gold medal but don't work in reality under true-to-life conditions. But the implications are not fully thought out.

Harold Zimman, public relations executive for the United States Olympic Committee, believes "There is a lack of education that is substantiated by research. Even with research it is a difficult situation. The surgeon general has more than adequately demonstrated the hazards of smoking, yet this has not stopped people. The IOC must allocate significant research funds toward finding the long-term negative effects of steroids on athletes."

Dr. David Lamb, former president of the American College of Sports Medicine, leans toward "randomized spot testing of athletes. It's a shame we have to go to a policing approach, but athletes are not cooperating with the rule systems."

Douglas Decker, researcher in xyanthene oxidase, associated with Dr. Dennis Levenson at the University of Chicago, has noted that "xyanthene oxidase is androgen dependent, and some of the effects androgens program the cellular mechanisms at birth and before. There also is an imprinting of androgen in the neonatal period, as well as the effects of androgens on brain differentiation in the intra-uterine period. Some enzymes are hormonally controlled and involve the integration of many facets at critical times, and levels of a number of hormones. When aphysiologic doses of anabolics are taken, it's analogous to taking a stick of dynamite to blow up a paper bag."

Pat Stewart, special agent in the narcotics division of the U.S. Department of Justice and a multi-title bodybuilding champion in his own right, feels that "steroids should be put under some controls or under a controlled-substances act. We have attempted to initiate some congressional hearings to establish this fact and explore the issue. There have been cases where an athlete has been detained by customs or by a state official for carrying large quantities of anabolics but being charged only with a misdemeanor. I feel these drugs should be reclassified and put under stricter control by wholesalers and retailers. It's getting to the point where even people who are not athletes are taking steroids to look better."

Sportswriters are no less concerned. Here is what *Henry Freeman*, sports editor-in-chief of *USA Today* had to say: "The pressure to win at any cost and keeping up with the sports Joneses is very strong. This is not a problem we got into simply, so the solution is not simple either."

Larry Fox, sports editor for the *New York Daily News*, noted the seeds of the problem:

> You have these high schools in Texas where parents will hold back students, red shirt high school and junior high school students, so that when the time comes for them to go to college, they are nineteen- or twenty-year-old freshmen, with the idea that they will have a jump on getting a scholarship. This is certainly inhibiting these kids' social and educational development. Drugs appear to be the next step.
>
> An example of this attitude appeared in *Sports Illustrated* when they wrote of H. Brown, the coach of the New York Knickerbockers basketball team. When he got his first high school coaching job, he took over a school with a poor winning record. The first thing he did as coach was cut all the seniors from the squad to give a message to the people that he meant business. To me that was a terrible thing and took high school sports out of context and sacrificing them [the seniors] so this coach could build a winning record and improve his career and go on to become a successful, highly paid pro coach. That's the kind of attitude, the "little league syndrome," of throwing eight-year-old kids into a must-win situation. That is what leads to drugs in sports.

Joe Carnicelli, executive sports editor for UPI, feels that

> an audiovisual educational program would work best. Show people exactly what happens to the body, what they should look like, and what they do look like after drug abuses with steroids. It's just like the driving clinics and the drunk drivers, where they show you a movie of someone being decapitated in a tragic car accident. The visual effects are more impressive than any writing you can do. Someone can speak to you of starving children, but until you actually see a picture of the kid it doesn't hit home. Shock value is very valuable; you don't forget a horrible picture

so fast. I remember the V.D. films in the army—they straightened me right out. If I remembered one thing from the army aside from tear gas, it's the V.D. films!

Walter Bingham, editor for *TIME* Magazine and a marathon runner of note said, "It's not in the spirit of the Olympics for people to win because of drug-induced edge." And *Matt Clark*, medicine editor of *Newsweek*, noted that "the casual disregard with which certain drugs are given to athletes is especially hazardous for young developing children." *Los Angeles Times* reporter *Randy Harvey* said that

> Anabolic steroids are much more dangerous when used without supervision and with as much as 90 percent of our world-class athletes using these types of preparations, something must be done to keep them from going to the black market, because that's where they have proven to be lethal.
>
> Most athletes don't make a lot of money and only have four to six years to make it to the top; so they feel pressured to take a short cut so that they can get there earlier and stay on top longer. Our athletes are not government subsidized as athletes in other countries are, so a long, starving road to the top is not very attractive. It's like the little league syndrome—parents bring their kids in to some physicians and say, "my son is 14 and he's only 5'4" and he's got no chance to be a pro basketball player. What can you give him?" The social and parental pressure to win is awesome.

Paul Hartlage, sports reporter for WISN-TV, added the comment that the public really does not know enough about steroids: "Cocaine has received much media attention, [but] steroids are actually more harmful due to the long-term effects. The media must bring this problem to the forefront. Just a ban won't stop them [athletes taking steroids]."

The Pan Am Games in the summer of 1983 brought out the problem for the first time to many people. *Mark Bloom*, editor of *The Runner* Magazine, made the point that the publicity might spur athletes to clean up before the 1984 Olympics, adding, "More frequent and organized worldwide testing is the way to go."

The entire question of *testing*—how to do it, what standards to use, and how to enforce penalties—were uppermost in the minds of several respondents. *Joe Weider*, publisher of *Muscle & Fitness* Magazine, would like to see an "iron-clad testing procedure that will prevent competitors from beating the test. Athletes should not be discriminated against because they are not as educated or don't have a personal pharmico-physiologist as a trainer. Otherwise, in the long run the con artists who know the racket will have the edge." This view was strongly supported by *Jim Manion*, international vice president of the International Federation of Body Builders and president of the National Physique Committee, the amateur arm of bodybuilding in this country, who felt that "with a legitimate, sure-fire test, the bodybuilder would go for it, but many are afraid. They feel that since the testing procedure was invented by an East German physician, they [the East Germans] already know how to beat the test. In addition, the extensive costs of testing make it prohibitive for promoters of contests to test everyone. Hopefully, a less expensive test will be designed to make it affordable to all."

Education was on the lips of many of our respondents. *Jack Bell*, who is in charge of the sports medicine program of the American Medical Association, leans toward a comprehensive education program starting at an early age. He goes on to say, "There should be incorporated into this program information on the very idea of sport and the over-emphasis of winning. We might try and instill the values of competing instead of just the value of winning."

Former *New York Times* reporter *Neil Amdur* (new editor of *World Tennis*) feels a multi-level approach is warranted.

> First we need a multi-level educational program directed from the International Olympic Committee to examine the hazards to the health of the athletes. Next would be to test at international competitions and not just the winning medalist but also randomly, along with random screening year round, which would also include countries not in the free world. Doping education should also begin at the grass-roots level as part of the health-education programs internationally. Athletes should be monitored as part of their training curriculum so that they are aware that their year-round training program is as important as the actual competitions.
>
> Included in the education programs should be a section of learning of doping control for all sports, at all levels. Wrestlers, for example, get caught up in their training and become dehydrated, and gymnasts develop anorexia. This is all part of the education of the aspects of conditioning and the excesses athletes will go to. There are some areas the International Olympic Committee has not been able to explore because it has allowed the individual international federations to handle the situation improperly, either because of lack of funds, or because they don't choose to look at it, or because the athletes are so involved in their sport and competing, they don't wish to do anything that would look unpleasant for the sport, so they ignore it.

John Jeansonne, sports reporter for *Newsday* and a personal friend, is looking for

> consistency and an expansion of knowledge about these and other chemical substances. At times there is a fine line between vitamins and drugs. When I was at the Pan Am Games, misinformation abounded, where people in positions of responsibility didn't quiet know what was going on. Early on, they tried to give the impression that these were testing procedures they never had before so that it appeared they were giving a really solid warning to those who were going to cheat, and the ones who were clean were saying, "At last, they're going to finally clean it up." But as the week went on, we found that the doctors saying this were either misinformed or indeed were trying to use this as a scare tactic. It was frustrating to discover that the test machines were essentially unchanged and the thinking there was still to get a way around the tests. This lost credibility for the physicians among the athletes, who now began to mistrust the doctors' view on other issues. "So if this doc lied about the test, why should I believe him when he tells me steroids will give me cancer or will kill me?" athletes thought.

Terry Todd offers yet another solution:

> My own feeling, for what it's worth, is that the ergogenic aids the athlete chooses to use are his or her own business, up to a point. If a person wants to take 2,000 mg. of anabolic steroids a day along with 3 cc. of testosterone and say to hell with the risk-to-benefit ratio, I think that person should have the right to do so, outside official competitions. But after seeing what I've seen over the past five years or so; after hearing Jan console so many young girls who call weeping to share with her the frustrations they feel as they face competition against women who have risked virilization and God knows what else to achieve the strength advantages conferred on them by the steroids; after seeing some of my friends wounded in body, in mind or both by steroid use; and after seeing many good people leave powerlifting because of their unwillingness to either take steroids or compete with the odds so against them, I think it's not unreasonable to tell those who wish to take steroids, "Look, use the drugs if you must, but don't stand in the way of reasonable drug testing in your sport. Either back off enough to be able to pass the IOC test at the big competitions or else stay out. Join another federation if you like, but you shouldn't expect the right to come in loaded against someone who's clean. If you wonder why, ask yourself why it would be unfair to begin a chess game with three queens to your opponent's one.

One of the problems with testing is that there is a rat race between two separate medical teams, one trying to devise a test to detect the drugs, while the other team attempts to mask the drugs or modify their chemical structures to make them undetectable.

High-level sport competition is all too familiar with the "testosterone loophole" or "masking effect." The competitor discontinues anabolic steroid intake while increasing intake of testosterone. This enables the athlete to retain the effect of anabolics and still pass some test procedures. However, pure testosterone is far more dangerous (re: cancer, liver damage, etc.) than the steroids.

Even more insane are "urine transfusions." Believe it or not, this is done by the athlete taking a strong diuretic which causes him/her to empty the bladder of urine. Then a catheter (a plastic tube) is passed through the penis/urethra into the bladder and the athlete receives a supply of "clean" urine from another individual on the other end of the tube. The West German female swimmers have even been known to be given air enemas to make them more bouyant (or jet propelled). This, however, could lead to a fatal air embolus.

These few examples are not doubt mild compared with those that will be used at future Olympic competitions. Perhaps the most comprehensive answer came from *Chicago Tribune* sports reporter *John Husar*, whose long, important statement I want to quote in full:

> You're talking about the reeducation of basic behavior patterns. Even though we didn't approve of these practices in the past and paid lip service to it, we still tolerated it. I wrote about steroids and weight lifting ten years ago with no effect. The hard point we have to face is that this is a form of corruption, and we are dealing with a corruption within our own culture. What I have learned as a sportswriter, if I've gained any wisdom, is that I like being close to the microcosm. I believe from an anthropological point of view you can tell an awful lot about people by watching how they play their games. We have seen a number of behavior patterns in our society since I've been watching games from the 1950s on. We have gone from an altruistic system to various cheating and corruptions, such as I saw in the Big 8 when I played there, the circumnavigating of rules, as well as in the Big 10, winning by cheating.
>
> We saw this, and we tolerated it. We saw the "Lombardism" creep in, the win-at-all-cost thing, the perversions in the little league. These behavior patterns were being permitted in our sports. This was a sign of the times—the corruption in our homes, our government, our working world, so, of course, we tolerated them in our games and our children's games. We have

seen all this, having gone through the protest years into another era. We are now in the "cleaning up" era, a period of cleansing. Look back at this period ten years from now, and you will see that we began to clean up in this period. That is the phase our pendulum happens to be at this point. You must identify the source of corruption within the culture and attack those sources and then be patient, knowing you are dealing with generations of programmed behavior.

For example, look back to the 1960s, where we saw people revolting and rejecting the ideals. There were reasons for these rejections, accumulated over several generations, and young people went around tearing down the establishment. These kids managed to go through high school and college during the protest years without getting proper educations—some with college degrees who could not write or communicate or who lacked the basic skills because they were pushed through schools that didn't know how to deal with the protests of the kids, the teachers, and such. So we ended up producing several generations of college-educated illiterates. All the standards were relaxed, and these people now have no concept of the classic literature or the proper background in their fields of study.

Now we have a new generation of students who are almost frightfully back to the fifties, they are so straight and conservative. They have reacted against the preceding generation, and they are aggressive achievers. But we still see a lot of "Me-ism" in the schools. These things occur in major cultural movements. It's not you or I sitting on a street corner saying, "Hey, I think I'm gonna cheat." We are motivated to cheat by the standards that are around us. That's where the problem is. We are children of a society and members of a culture. If it's okay to cheat on your taxes, then we do it. If it's not okay, we wouldn't. At one time it was unheard of not to pay a parking ticket. Who pays them now? *In sports we see the mirror. All the elements of culture seem to come together in the way we play our games.*

Strong stuff. John's statement hit home for me. I remember during the later 1960s, there were two factions—the jocks and the hippies. The "cool" guy on campus was the dope pusher, the most admired and respected individual around, and like the doped-up music idols women clawed over, it seemed as if the world had gone to the dogs.

So here were these dope heads blowing their brains out on LSD, and here I was, a jock with short hair and a conscientious student being looked upon as not being "with it." Now all the long-haired heads of the past are into vitamins, natural foods, and long-distance running with the little of their cerebral cortex that remains, and the cycle has repeated itself.

When, six years ago, I first began writing of the dangers of drugs and the injustice they were doing to sport, I was ridiculed as not being "with it" and a party pooper. The steroid pushers were again the heros...until just recently, when people have come to see the true destruction for what it is. Twenty years from now, when these young athletes taking steroids come down with prostatic cancer in their thirties and forties, it won't be me they'll be cursing as their trophies gather dust in a box in the basement.

I'm going to leave the last word of this chapter to a personal hero of mine—1972 Olympic gold medalist in wrestling and probably the winningest free-style wrestler in history, *Dan Gable*, who is the 1984 Olympic wrestling coach and is coach for the University of Iowa, probably the dominant wrestling power in the United States.

> I consider myself a very tolerant and flexible coach, but drug use I'm hard fast on. This doesn't mean I will throw an athlete out if I find he is on drugs. Hopefully I have laid the groundwork so that would not occur. By the time a kid reaches my level of coaching, at the collegiate and Olympic levels, he is pretty set in his ways. He needs to be indoctrinated at an early age about the disciplines of being an athlete and in the education of his particular sport. I sure don't need a wrestler coming to me with bad habits. Now with the advent of multiple testing, anyone who is a serious contender for an Olympic championship would be foolish to gamble his career for drugs.

I have no magic answers, but I feel very strongly that we forge our own destiny. I learned the hard way; you can talk your heart out and get blue in the face in an attempt to reach the obsessed athletic mind—to no avail.

However, we must make an attempt to protect people from themselves and self-destruction, no matter how futile the effort.

We can never stop crime, nor cure all disease; but law enforcement and medical personnel fight these battles. The lives of our finest product—our youth—are at stake, and I strongly feel we must make the effort to protect our own—even if the enemy is themselves.

One final note: Dr. Anthony Maddalo, a close friend and colleague and author of the self-screening examination that follows this chapter, sent me this story about a steroid-related death. I will let him tell the story in his own words:

A twenty-three-year-old bodybuilder, a magnificent physical specimen, who reminded me of Mike Mentzer...not, too tall, but remarkable muscle mass and definition. He had brown hair and mustache and was a fine-looking athlete. He had experimented with Deca-Durobolin, Anavar, and several other anabolic steroids in the past. At this particular occasion he had been taking Dianabol. In the first four weeks, he started developing a pruirtis [itching of the skin] and a mild jaundice [liver disease caused by problems with bilirubin and resulting in a yellowing of the skin]. At that time, he took benedryl [an antihistimine] for the itch. Two weeks after that he continued to take Dianabol and became frankly jaundiced and lethargic, at which time his parents brought him into the emergency room. He was totally uptunded and very combative at times. He was then admitted to the intensive care unit with acute hepato-renal [liver-kidney] failure. His creatine was over 7, his CPK was over 6,000, his liver enzymes were off the board, and he was in total electrolyte imbalance. He was treated as a normal hepatic shutdown, like a cirrhotic patient would be treated, but he was noted not to have any detectable infectious hepatitis.

On the fourth hospital day, he suffered a cardiac arrest and died. The autopsy showed severe hepatic necrosis [death of liver tissue], complete renal shutdown, and acute tubular necrosis. He also had severely degenerating testes with few fragmented sperm and very few Sertoli and Leydig cells. A great reduction in mass of both testes was noted. The histological [cellular exam] of testicular tissue showed him to be sterile. I wish I could have had all the people I try to treat for side effects in that room with me the night he came in. It was just terrible. I don't know if any of his friends are aware of his death. I sure hope they are—the reason why he died!

12

A SELF-SCREENING EXAMINATION FOR THE MALE ATHLETE TAKING ANABOLIC STEROIDS
by Anthony V. Maddalo M.D.

THE HUMAN BODY IS A COMPLEX SYSTEM OF CHECKS AND BAL-
ances, and drugs such as anabolic steroids can upset this balance and
cause seemingly unrelated signs and symptoms. Athletes frequently
experience discomforts while taking anabolic steroids, but because of
a lack of medical knowledge, they may not attribute these signs and
symptoms to the use of anabolic steroids. Furthermore, many athletes become confused when reading literature in this area because
some articles regarding the use of steroids ignore their side effects
while others dramatize their harmful effects. An alternative is to provide the athlete with enough information so that he may recognize
for himself the effects steroids are having on his body. The purpose
of this article is to present to the athlete the clinical signs and symptoms of some of the disorders caused by anabolic steroids.

If the athlete has one or more of the symptoms on the screening examination, he can refer to the appropriate paragraph indicated by
Roman numerals for an explanation of how these symptoms relate to
anabolic steroid use. However, the absence of these signs and symptoms does not preclude the possibility of an adverse effect which has
no clinically noticeable signs.

A SCREENING EXAMINATION FOR THE MALE ATHLETE TAKING ANABOLIC STEROIDS

Part I. External Exam

A. Skin

1. Color..............flushing (VIII), yellow tint (IV, VI)
2. Bruises ....more frequent with minor injuries (III, VI)
3. Eruptions ....usually on back (I)
4. Itching.............in general (II, VI), after hot bath (VIII)
5. Sweating...........greatly increased with anabolics (IV)
6. Stretch marks ....greater incidence than before anabolics (III)

B. Head

1. Face...............puffy or "moon" face (III)
2. Eyes...............yellow (VI), red, irritated (II), blurred vision (IV)
3. Mouth.............bleeding from underside of tongue (VI)
4. Nose ....unprovoked bleeds (V), take longer to stop (VI)

C. Chest

1. Gynecomastia ....female breast tissue over pectorals (VI)
2. Palpitations ....heart pounds heavily against chest (IV, V)

D. Abdomen

1. Mass ....left or right side (VI)
2. Flank pain ....may radiate to back or groin (II)
3. Upper abd. pain .....relieved by eating (II), after fatty meals (IV)

E. Genitals

1. Testes..............decreased in size (X)
2. Pain...............can be radiating from flank (II)

F. Extremities

1. Edema.............swelling, usually at ankles (III, V, VI)
2. Joints..............swelling, pain, stiffness, usually in the hands (II)
3. Trembling..........tremor or shaking, usually of hands (IV)

Part II. Internal Exam

A. General

1. Headaches ....in morning at back of head (II, IV, V)
2. Fatigue ....muscle weakness, tire easily (II, IV)

B. Cardiovascular

1. Blood Pressure....... 10 diastolic,   20 systolic at rest
(II, III, V)
2. Heart rate........... 7-10 beats/min. above normal (II, III, IV, V)

C. Nervous System

1. Hyperactivity........irritable, restless; insomnia (VII), psychotic (III)
2. Hypoactivity ....drowsy, apathetic (II), depressed (II, III, VII)
3. Lightheadedness .....dizzy (IV, V)

D. Gastrointestinal

1. Vomiting............blood or coffee ground material (II, VI)
2. Stools ....bright red (II), black tarry (II), clay color (IV, VI)
3. Hemorrhoids ....sometimes bleeding (VI)

E. Urogenital

1. Semen ....decrease in ejaculate volume (X)
2. Urination ....painful; small, frequent (IX)
3. Urine color.........brown (VI), red (II)
4. Urine "Bili-Labstix" Values*
   a. pH less than 5 ....acid urine (II)
   b. ketones + ...(IV)
   c. bilirubin + ...(IV, VI)
   d. blood + + + ...(II) or normal after stress

*"Bili-Labstix" are manufactured by Miles Laboratories and can be purchased without a prescription.

I. ACNE

The androgenic effect of anabolic steroids can cause an increase in oil production by the sebaceous glands of the skin (1). As a result, large painful follicles may develop anywhere on the body, with a greater distribution on the back (2). As these follicles enlarge and subsequently burst, the skin will be perforated many times which will make it vulnerable to bacterial infection. Onset of infection will require appropriate medical treatment and cessation of anabolic steroids.

II. HYPERCALCEMIA

Anabolic steroids have been show to inhibit calcium excretion and cause a subsequent increase in serum calcium (3). This increase can cause some of the common signs and symptoms of hypercalcemia. As calcium levels become elevated, the athlete may become weak and easily fatigues (3). Blood pressure will also rise and symptoms of hypertension may appear (4).

Severe hypercalcemia may lead to kidney stones (5), peptic ulcer (6), behavioral changes (7) and abnormal calcium deposits in the joints (8), eyes (9) and skin (10). Kidney stones are a serious problem because they can lead to permanent kidney damage (11). Symptoms may include severe flank pain radiating to the back or groin and blood in the urine. The danger period for kidney stone formation is not limited to the period of administration of anabolic steroids; in fact, the period just after anabolic drugs are stopped is when the highest concentration of calcium is passing through the kidneys. In addition, there is a greater incidence of kidney stone formation if the athlete is restricting his fluid intake, or is on a high protein diet. Both conditions promote kidney stone formation by creating acid urine.

A peptic ulcer may occur as a result of increased stomach acid secretion caused by high calcium levels. Peptic ulcers may be recognized by the passing of bloody or black, tarry stools, vomiting blood or coffee ground material or by a dull aching upper abdominal pain which is sometimes relieved by eating. As calcium levels increase, behavioral changes will be noticed either by the athlete or the people around him. He will become listless, drowsy, apathetic and depressed, and mental functions will be slow.

Although they are not very common, abnormal calcium deposits causing irritation and redness of the eyes, itching of the skin and swelling, numbness and pain around some joints have been attributed to hypercalcemia. The onset of any of the above symptoms requires increased fluid intake, cessation of anabolic drugs and prompt medical attention.

III. HYPERCORTISOLEMIA

Anabolic steroids have produced increased serum cortisol levels in men undergoing athletic training (12). This increase in cortisol is probably due to a decrease in the breakdown of cortisol by the liver. Because they have similar structures, anabolic steroids compete with cortisol for the pathway in the liver which deactivates both hormones (13). Moreover, 17α-alkylated anabolic steroids directly inhibit the main enzyme in this pathway, giving oral anabolics an added effect in the inhibition of cortisol metabolism.

Cortisol affects several systems of the human body. One of the effects is retention of salt and water by the kidneys, causing high blood pressure and edema. Cortisol also affects the central nervous system by creating behavior changes ranging from depression to psychotic behavior. In addition, metabolic changes in the subcutaneous fat and collagen tissues in the skin can result in abnormal fat deposits and a weakening or rupture of the dermis. These two conditions can cause a "moon" or puffy face and an increased incidence of stretch marks and bruises, respectively.

Although some of these individual signs and symptoms may be caused by conditions other than hypercortisolemia, as a group they are distinguishing characteristics of hypercortisolemia and should be brought to the attention of a physician.

IV. ALTERED CARBOHYDRATE METABOLISM

Anabolic steroids can have several effects on carbohydrate metabolism. In diabetic or pre-diabetic people, all anabolic steroids seem to decrease serum glucose levels, whereas only 17α-alkylated anabolic steroids have been shown to decrease serum glucose levels in the non-diabetic person (14, 15). The first effect is probably due to an increase in the body's sensitivity to insulin, making the initial amount of insulin more effective. If the initial glucose level is high, as in diabetes mellitus, the liver will not respond by deactivating insulin unless glucose levels approach normal. However, if glucose levels are normal, the liver will deactivate up to 40 percent of the circulating insulin in order to compensate for the increased sensitivity. This ability to deactivate insulin is altered by 17α-alkalyted steroids, and abnormally low glucose levels may be unavoidable. Although this degree of hypoglycemia does not usually become symptomatic, symptoms of hypoglycemia should be recognized by the athlete. If the early signs such as sweating, trembling, palpitations, headaches, lightheadedness, or blurred vision should occur after periods of fasting, a physician should be consulted.

As a result of a decreased serum glucose, the body must mobilize fat as a source of energy (16). This increased fat mobilization may produce one of the following conditions. If an anabolic steroid is used, there will be a rise in serum-free fatty acids (FFA) due to an alteration of liver functions (17). However, if liver functions are not altered, as with the 19-nortestosterones, the liver will convert FFA into cholesterol and ketones. An increase in serum cholesterol levels increases the incidence of gall stones, which cause upper abdominal discomfort after fatty meals, cholestatic jaundice, and clay-colored stools. Ketones can cause abdominal cramps and will be present in the urine. In both cases, the increase in fat mobilization will lead to "fatty liver", which is the formation of fat globules in the liver, causing liver damage.

V. HYPERTENSION

Anabolic steroids can cause high blood pressure. The exact mechanism is not clearly understood; it may be that hypercalcemia and hypercortisolemia play a significant role in raising blood pressure. Although most cases result in little more than slightly elevated readings, several cases have been reported in which athletes have passed out due to hypertension (1).

Recording the actual blood pressure with a sphygmomanometer (blood pressure cuff) is the most accurate method the athlete has to detect hypertension. Recording blood pressures is not difficult for the properly instructed individual, and with the commercial availability of sphygmomanometers, it is quite convenient. This gives the athlete a reliable monitoring system for his blood pressure. However, if this is not possible, the athlete should be alerted to certain physical signs and symptoms of hypertension. Severe hypertension can result in morning headaches, palpitations, unprovoked nose bleeds, blurred vision, lightheadedness, and fainting. If any of these symptoms occur, a resting blood pressure should be recorded and compared to a pre-drug reading. If there is an increase of ten or more units in diastolic (bottom) number or an increase in twenty or more in the systolic (top) number, all anabolic drugs should be stopped and a physician should be consulted. A hypertensive crisis can lead to kidney damage or stroke.

VI. LIVER DYSFUNCTION

Nearly all oral anabolic steroids contain a 17α-alkyl group which increases their intestinal absorption and prevents their inactivation by the liver (18). Originally , this structural modification seemed to be an improvement in oral anabolic therapy. However, because of the abundance of reports citing the hepatotoxic effects of 17α-alka-layted steroids (13, 19, 20, 21), they have virtually been abandoned as a mode of anabolic therapy. In the following section, hepatotoxic effects such as cholestatic jaundice, hepatoma, and peliosis hepatis will be discussed.

Cholestasis is the reduction of bile flow. Liver cells normally extract bile from the blood, concentrate it and send it to the gall bladder or intestine via small vessels in the liver. Oral anabolics have a toxic effect on these liver cells and inhibit their normal function (22). This causes an increase in bile in the blood and can cause yellow discoloration of the skin and eyes, itching, clay-colored stools, and a brown-colored urine that is positive for bilirubin. Continued toxic effects on these liver cells can lead to cell death and cirrhosis, which will impair normal liver functions.

One vital function of the liver is to produce some of the clotting factors of the blood. If they are not produced, prolonged nose bleeds, easy bruisability, and bleeding from the underside of the tongue may occur as signs of decreased clotting ability of the blood. Another vital function of the liver is the deactivation of estrogens from the adrenal gland. If this function is impaired, female breast development (gynecomastia) may occur (23). Furthermore, if liver functions are impaired for a long period of time, and cirrhosis becomes severe, congestion of the hepatic blood vessels will result. This obstruction of blood vessels can lead to an enlarged liver, enlarged spleen, edema, hemorrhoids, or vomiting of blood or coffee-ground material due to bleeding in the esophagus. This group of effects is known as portal hypertension.

Hepatoma, also known as hepatocellular carcinoma, may not be reflected in liver enzyme tests; however, the athlete will experience right abdominal pain and note a palpable mass in the same area. Most of the literature reports hepatoma in patients treated with oral anabolic steroids.

Peliosis hepatis is the formation of blood-filled cysts in the liver. These cysts result from dead liver cells blocking small veins in the liver, causing blood to pool behind the obstruction. These cysts may rupture and cause painful abdominal bleeding and possibly death; unfortunately, they usually cannot be detected by serum liver enzyme levels and must be diagnosed by a liver scan.

Bringing all these symptoms to the attention of a physician is critical. The symptoms described above are not early warning signs but rather signs of ongoing liver damage. Thus, cessation of anabolic steroids and immediate medical attention is necessary.

VII. BEHAVIORAL DISORDERS

Several types of behavioral changes have been attributed to anabolic steroid use. Anabolic steroids may cause an indirect increase in neurotransmitters in the central nervous system. This increase would have a stimulatory effect and could be responsible for the increased sexual drive, increased excitability, irritability, and insomnia seen during anabolic steroid therapy.

If there is an increased cortisol level, more drastic behavioral changes may be noticed. As mentioned in section III, the athlete may experience mood changes ranging from depression to psychotic behavior.

As mentioned in section II, hypercalcemia can also cause behavioral changes including listlessness, drowsiness, fatigue, and depression.

Of course, any combination of the above symptoms can occur and thus the underlying disease cannot be identified solely by the changes in the behavior. Any severe behavioral changes should be brought to the attention of a physician so that further workup may be done.

VIII. POLYCYTHEMIA

Secondary polycythemia is the overproduction of red blood cells without any apparent demand for them (24). One of the primary therapeutic uses of anabolic steroids is the treatment of certain anemias (25). Anabolic steroids cause the secretion of a hormone that in turn stimulates the bone marrow to produce more red blood cells. In normal individuals, this may result in red blood cell counts well above normal (26). Polycythemia may result in flushing of the skin and an itching sensation after a hot bath or shower. Long-term elevation of red blood cell counts may increase the severity of the side effects and necessitate the discontinuation of anabolic therapy. If itching or flushing does occur, an occasional complete blood count (CBC) should be done by a physician to monitor the number of red blood cells.

IX. PROSTATIC ENLARGEMENT

There is strong evidence to suggest that the androgenic effect of anabolic steroids can cause benign hypertrophy of the prostate gland (27). Although the evidence regarding cancer of the prostate is not as convincing (28), this possibility must also be considered when evaluating the adverse effects of anabolic steroids. Although investigators vary in the reported incidence of steroid-induced prostatic hypertrophy, there is speculation that the hypertrophic effect is dose related.

Enlargement of the prostate may cause several distinct signs. The individual may experience painful urinations, inability to maintain a steady stream of urine and a frequent urge to urinate resulting only in frequent and small urinations. Benign prostatic hypertrophy has been shown to be reversible when caused by anabolic steroids; however, this may not be the case in carcinoma of the prostate. Any symptoms of prostatic enlargement require cessation of anabolic drugs and medical attention.

X. TESTICULAR ATROPHY

Anabolic steroids block the release of two hormones form the pituitary gland that normally stimulate the testes (2, 29). Anabolic steroids' interference with the release of these two hormones will cause the testes to atrophy and become dormant. Subsequently, the testes will shrink in size, sperm production will be markedly surpressed, and the volume of semen per ejaculate may be decreased.

Although sperm counts may reach an infertile level, most athletes who take anabolic steroids either choose to ignore this fact or simply assume that sperm counts will return to normal. However, athletes should give serious consideration to the cases reported in which men on anabolic steroids did not return to pre-drug rates of sperm productions (2, 29).

References

1. Freed, D.C., A.J. Banks, D. Longson, D.M. Burley. Anabolic steroids in athletics: Crossover double-blind trial on weightlifters. Brit. Med. J., 1975, ii, p. 471.
2. Mauss, J., K. Borsch, et al. Effect of long term testosterone Oenanthate administration on male reproductive function. Acta Endocrin., 78 (1975), 373-384.
3. Maxwell, M.H. and C.R. Kleeman. Clinical Disorders of Fluid and Electrolyte Metabolism. McGraw-Hill Book Company, 1972.

4. Earll, J.M. et al. Hypercalcemia and Hypertension. Ann. Int. Med., 64(2), Feb. 1966, 378-380.
5. Williams, H.E. Nephrolithiasis. New Eng. J. Med. 290:33, 1974.
6. Smallwood, R.A. Effect of intravenous calcium administration on gastric secretion of acid and pepsin in man. Gut, 1967, 8, 592.
7. Petersen, P. Psychiatric Disorders in Primary Hyperparathyroidism. J. Clin. Endocr. 28:1491, 1968.
8. Holman, C.B. Roentgenologic Manifestations of Vitamin D Intoxication. Radiology 59 (6):805, Dec. 1952.
9. Walsh, F.B. and J.E. Howard. Conjunctival & Corneal Lesions in Hypercalcemia.
10. McMillan, D.E. and R.B. Freeman. The Milk Alkali Syndrome. Medicine (Balt.) 44:486 (1965).
11. Epstein, F.H., Calcium and the Kidney. Am. J. Med. 45:700 (1968).
12. Hervey, G.R. and I. Hutchinson. Anabolic effects of Methandienone in men undergoing athletic training. Lancet Oct. 2, 1976;699.
13. Johnsen, S.G. Maintenance of spermtogenesis induced by HMG treatment by means of continuous HGC treatment in hypogonadotrophic men. Acta Endocrin, 89:763 1978.
14. Landon, J., V. Wynn and E. Samols. The effect of anabolic steroids on blood sugar and plasma insulin levels in man. Metab. 12 (10):924 Oct. 1963.
15. Tainter, M.L. et al. Anabolic steroids in the management of the diabetic patient. N.Y. State J. Med. April 15, 1964, p. 1001.
16. Keele, C.A. and E. Neil. Samson Wrights Applied Physiology (twelfth ed.) Oxford University Press, 1971.
17. Srikanta, S.G. et al. Effect of a C17-alkylated steroid Methandrostenolone on plasma lipids of normal subjects. Am. J. Med. Sci. Aug. 1967. p. 201.
18. Hirschhauser, C., et al. Testosterone Undecanoate: A new orally active androgen. Acta Endocrin. 80 (1975):179-187.
19. Farrell, G.C. and D.E. Joshua. Androgen-induced Hepatoma. Lancet, Feb. 22, 1975 p. 430.
20. Johnsen, S.G. Long-term oral testosterone and liver function. Lancet Jan. 7, 1978 p. 50.
21. Westaby, D., et al. Liver damage from long-term methyl testosterone. Lancet Aug. 6, 1977 p. 261.
22. Schiff, L. et al. Diseases of the Liver (fourth ed.) J.B. Lippincott Company 1977.
23. Van Thiel, D.H. et al. Plasma estrone and prolactin concentrations are elevated in men with gynecomastia and spider angiomata. Gastroenterology 68 (4) April 1975 p. 934.
24. Erslev, A.J. Secondary Polycythemia. In Hematology by W.J. Williams, McGraw-Hill Book Company 1972 p. 544.
25. Hendler, E.D. et al. Controlled study of androgen therapy in anemia of patients on maintenance hemodialysis. New Eng. J. Med 291 (20):1046 Nov. 14, 1974.

26. Galetti, F. et al. Erythropoietic action of an oral non-17-alkylated anabolic steroid. Clin. Ter. 1979, Nov. 15:91 (3) 267-78.
27. Feyel-Cabanes. Combined effect of testosterone and estrogen on rat ventral prostates. Cancer research 38: (11 Pt. 2) 4126-34 Nov. 1978.
28. Walsh, P.C. et al. The binding of a potent synthetic androgen Methyltrienolone (R1881) to cytosol preparations of human prostate cancer. Trans. Am. Assoc. Genitourin. Surg. 69:78, 1978.
29. Steinberger, E., and K.D. Smith. Effect of chronic administration of testosterone enanthate on sperm production and plasma testosterone, FSH and LH leves. Fertil Steril. 28, 1977 p. 1320.

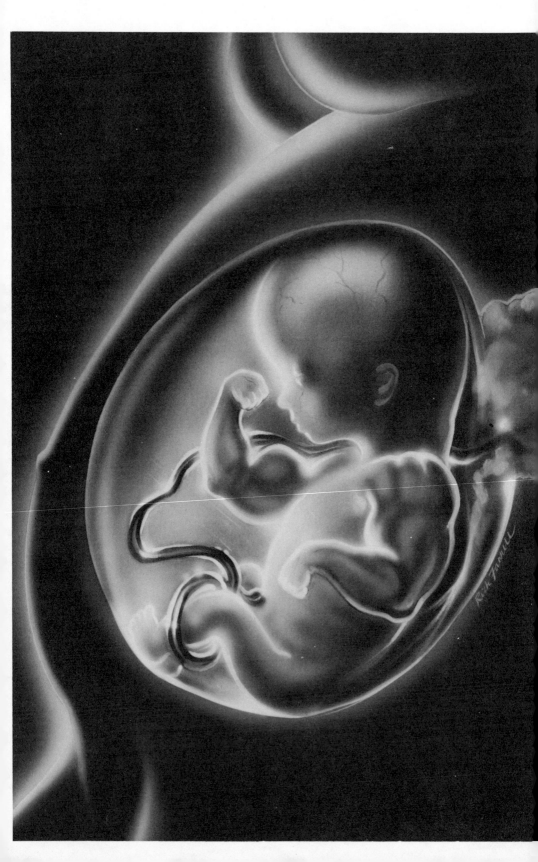

APPENDICES

1
POSITION STATEMENT ON THE USE AND ABUSE OF ANABOLIC-ANDROGENIC STEROIDS IN SPORTS

Based on a comprehensive survey of the world literature and a careful analysis of the claims made for and against the efficacy of anabolic-androgenic steroids in improving human physical performance, it is the position of the American College of Sports Medicine that:

1) The administration of anabolic-androgenic steroids to healthy humans below age 50 in medically approved therapeutic doses often does not of itself bring about any significant improvements in strength, aerobic endurance, lean body mass, or body weight.

2) There is no conclusive scientific evidence that extremely large doses of anabolic-androgenic steroids either aid or hinder athletic performance.

3) The prolonged use of oral anabolic-androgenic steroids (C_{17}-alkylated derivatives of testosterone) has resulted in liver disorders in some persons. Some of these disorders are apparently reversible with the cessation of drug usage, but others are not.

4) The administration of anabolic-androgenic steroids to male humans may result in a decrease in testicular size and function and a decrease in sperm production. Although these effects appear to be reversible when small doses of steroids are used for short periods of time, the reversibility of the effects of large doses over extended periods of time is unclear.

5) Serious and continuing effort should be made to educate male and female athletes, coaches, physical educators, physicians, trainers, and the general public regarding the inconsistent effects of anabolic-androgenic steroids on improvement of human physical performance and the potential dangers of taking certain forms of these substances, especially in large doses, for prolonged periods.

RESEARCH BACKGROUND FOR THE POSITION STATEMENT

This position stand has been developed from an extensive survey and analysis of the world literature in the fields of medicine, physiology, endocrinology, and physical education. Although the reactions of humans to the use of drugs, including hormones or drugs which simulate the actions of natural hormones, are individual and not entirely predictable, some conclusions can nevertheless be drawn with regard to what desirable and what undesirable effects may be achieved. Accordingly, whereas positive effects of drugs may sometimes arise because persons have been led to expect such changes ("placebo" effect) (8), repeated experiments of a similar nature often fail to support the initial positive effects and lead to the conclusion that any positive effect that does exist may not be substantial.

1) Administration of testosterone-like synthetic drugs which have anabolic (tissue building) and androgenic (development of male secondary sex characteristics) properties in amounts up to twice those normally prescribed for medical use have been associated with increased strength, lean body mass and/or body weight in some studies (6, 19, 20, 26, 27, 33, 34, 36) but not in others (9, 10, 12, 13, 21, 35, 36). One study (13) reported an increase in the amount of weight the steroid group could lift compared to controls but found no difference in isometric strength which suggests a placebo effect in the drug group, a learning effect or possibly a differential drug effect on isotonic compared to isometric strength. An initial report of enhanced aerobic endurance after administration of an anabolic-androgenic steroid (20) has not been confirmed (6, 9, 19, 21, 27). Because of the lack of adequate control groups in many studies it seems likely that some of the positive effects on strength that have been reported are due to "placebo" effects (3, 8), but a few apparently well-designed studies have also shown beneficial effects of steroid administration on muscular strength and lean body mass. Some of the discrepancies in results may also be due to differences in the type of drug administered, the method of drug administration, the nature of the exercise programs involved, the duration of the experiment, and individual differences in sensitivity to the administered drug. High protein dietary supplements do not insure the effectiveness of the steroids (13, 21, 36). Because of the many failures to show improved muscular strength, lean body mass, or body weight after therapeutic doses of androgenic-anabolic steroids it is obvious that for many individuals any benefits are likely to be small and not worth the health risks involved.

2) Testimonial evidence by individual athletes suggests that athletes often use much larger doses of steroids than those ordinarily prescribed by physicians and those evaluated in published research. Because of the health risks involved with the long-term use of high doses and requirements for informed consent it is unlikely that scientifically acceptable evidence will be forthcoming to evaluate the effectiveness of such large doses of drugs on athletic performance.

3) Alterations of normal liver function have been found in as many as 80 percent of one series of 69 patients treated with C_{17}-alkylated testosterone derivatives (oral androgenic-anabolic steroids) (29). Cholestasis has been observed histologically in the livers of persons taking these substances (31). These changes appear to be benign and reversible (30). Five reports (4, 7,

23, 31, 39) document the occurrence of peliosis hepatitis in 17 patients without evidence of significant liver disease who were treated with C_{17}-alkylated androgenic steroids. Seven of these patients died of liver failure. The first case of hepatocellular carcinoma associated with taking an anabolic-androgenic steroid was reported in 1965 (28). Since then at least 13 other patients taking C_{17}-alkylated androgenic steroids have developed hepatocellular carcinoma (5, 11, 14, 15, 16, 17, 18, 25). In some cases dosages as low as 10-15 mg/day taken for only three or four months have caused liver complications (13, 25).

4) Administration of therapeutic doses of anabolic-androgenic steroids in men often (15, 22), but not always (1, 10, 19), reduces the output of testosterone and gonadotropins and reduces spermatogenesis. Some steroids are less potent than others in causing these effects (1). Although these effects on the reproductive system appear to be reversible in animals, the long-term results of taking large doses by humans is unknown.

5) Precise information concerning the abuse of anabolic steroids by female athletes is unavailable. Nevertheless, there is no reason to believe females will not be tempted to adopt the use of these medicines. The use of anabolic steroids by females, particularly those who are either prepubertal or have not attained full growth, is especially dangerous. The undesired side effects include masculinization (2, 29, 30), disruption of normal growth pattern (30), voice changes (2, 30, 32), acne (2, 29, 30, 32), hirsutism (29, 30, 32), and enlargement of the clitoris (29). The long-term effects on reproductive function are unknown, but anabolic steroids may be harmful in this area. Their ability to interfere with the menstrual cycle has been well documented (29). For these reasons, all concerned with advising, training, coaching, and providing medical care for female athletes should exercise all persuasions available to prevent the use of anabolic steroids by female athletes.

REFERENCES

1. A.Aakvaag and S.B. Stromme, "The Effect of Mesterolone Administration to Normal Men on the Pituitary-Testicular Function." *Acta Endocrinol*, (1974)77:380-386.
2. D.M. Allen, M.H. Fine, T.F. Necheles, and W. Dameshek, "Oxymetholene Therapy in Aplastic Anemia," *Blood*, 32 (July 1968):83-89.
3. G. Ariel and W. Saville, "Anabolic Steroids: The Physiological Effects of Placebos," *Med. Sci. Sports*, 4 (1972):124-126.
4. S.A. Bagheri and J.L. Boyer, "Peliosis Hepatitis Associated with Androgenic-Anabolic Steroid Therapy," *Ann. Int. Med.*, 81 (1974):610-618.
5. M.S. Bernstein, R.L. Hunter and S. Yachrin, "Hepatoma and Peliosis Hepatitis Developing in a Patient with Fanconi's Anemia," *N. Engl. J.*

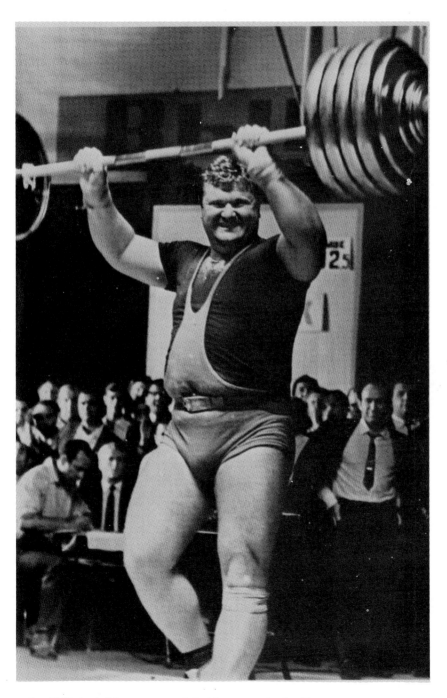

Leonid Zhabotinskii was preoccupied with perpetuating his Olympic crown into eternity. It lasted eight years (photo by Yuri Shalamov, from *Big Red Machine*, by Yuri Brokhov).

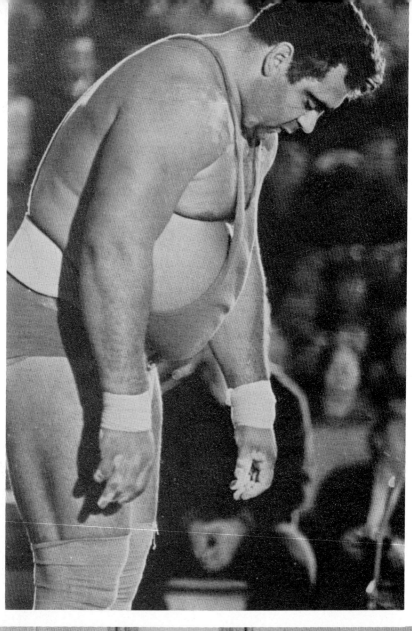

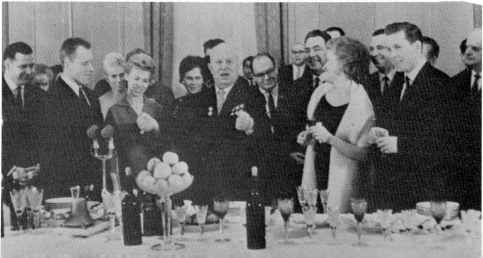

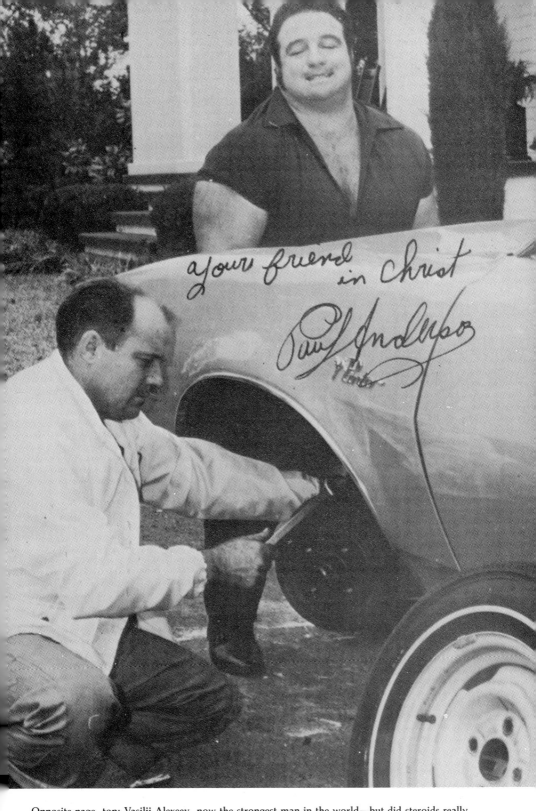

your friend in Christ

Paul Anderson

Opposite page, top: Vasilii Alexeev, now the strongest man in the world—but did steroids really help? Bottom: Nikita Khrushchev and Leonid Brezhnev with the Soviet Olympic Champions. "Beat the hell out of the capitalists!" (Yuri Shalamov, *Big Red Machine*.) Above: Paul Anderson, 1956 Olympic champion weight lifter and one of the strongest men in history: "I will give thumbs down to any athlete using steroids." (Photo courtesy of Mr. Anderson.)

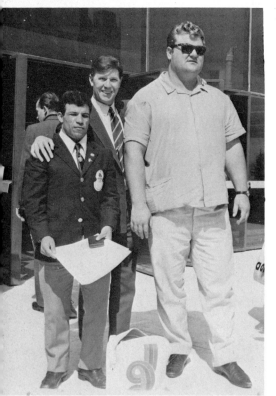
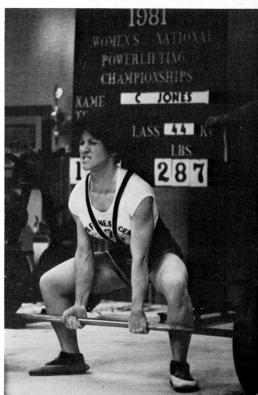
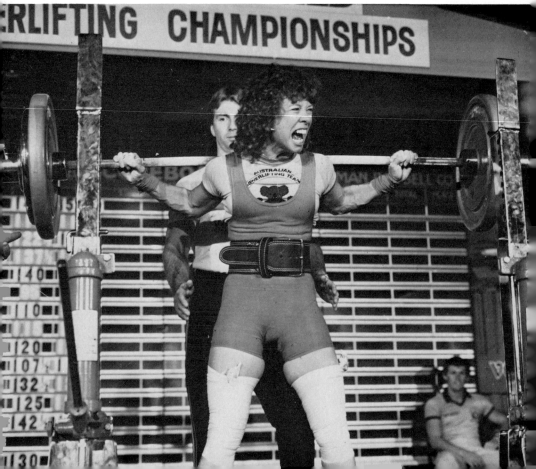

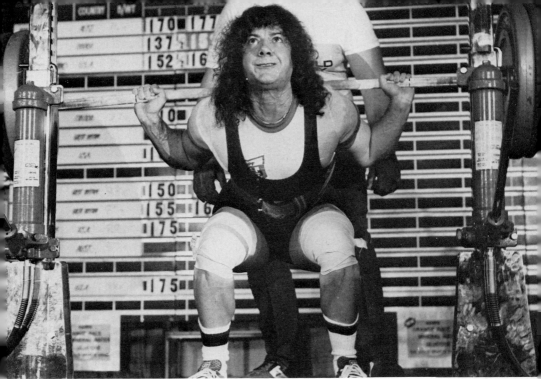

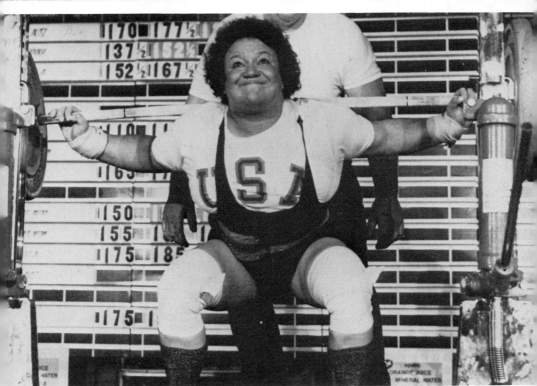

Opposite page, top left: David Webster, flanked here by two Soviet weight lifting champions (Nassiri and Zhabotinskii), has led the fight against doping in Europe and is a hardliner for drug testing for athletes. (Photo courtesy of Mr. Webster.) Top right: Cheryl Jones, women's world lifting champion in the 97-pound class. (Photo by Doris Barrilleaux.) Bottom: Sue Jordan, after completing her world record squat of 152 kg. at the women's world championships in May 1983 in Adelaide, Australia. (Photo by Jim Lewis.) Above, top to bottom: Women's world weight lifter Jennifer Weyland is shown squatting 396 lbs.; Maris Sternberg, 198-pound world powerlifting champion. (Both photos by Jim Lewis.)

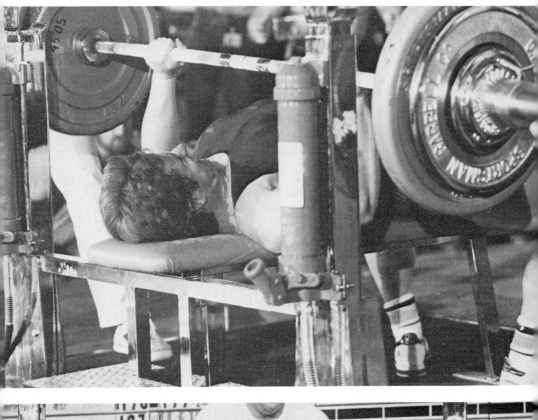

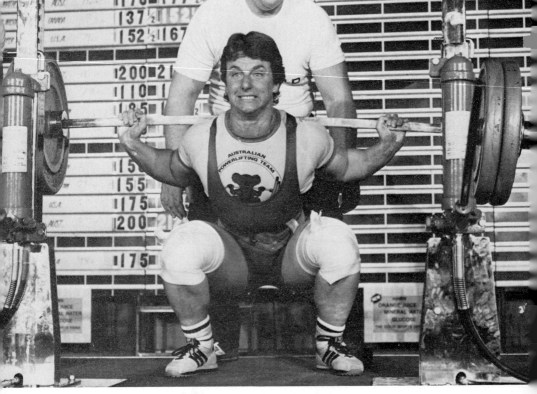

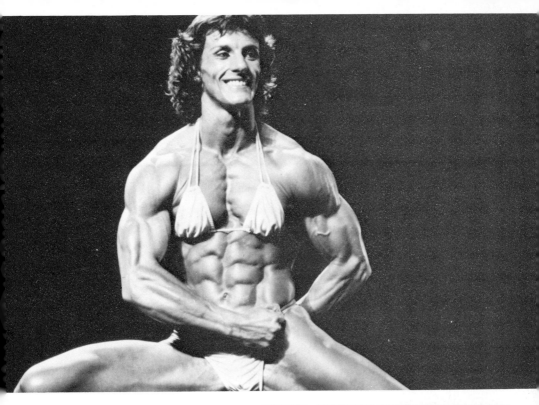

The incredible Bev Francis came close to
locking a world record bench press of 152.5 kg.
at the 1983 world championships in Australia,
but she did set the squat in the 82.5 kg. class
with an amazing 217.5 kg. lift, shown here.
(Photos by Jim Lewis.) The photos above show
clearly that Mrs. Francis has begun devoting
herself to physique contests. She trains four
hours a day and has never tested positive for
drugs in any competition. She is a woman
athlete in a class by herself. (Photos by Mike
Neveus, courtesy of *Flex* Magazine, copyright
1983.)

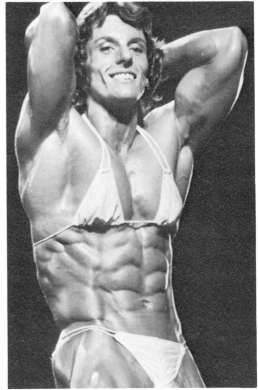

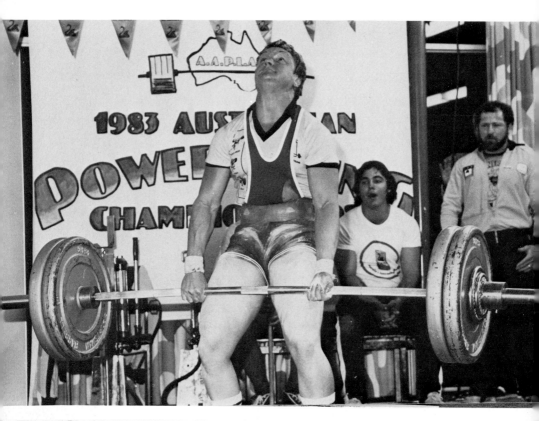

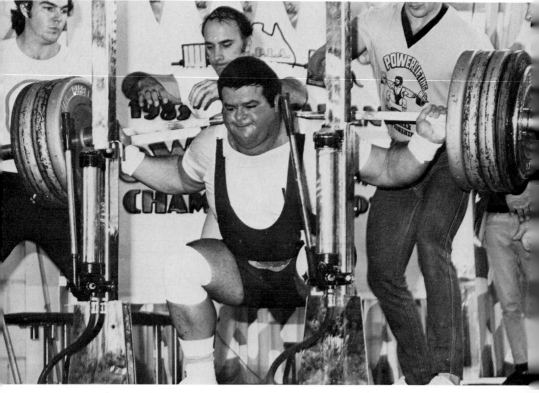

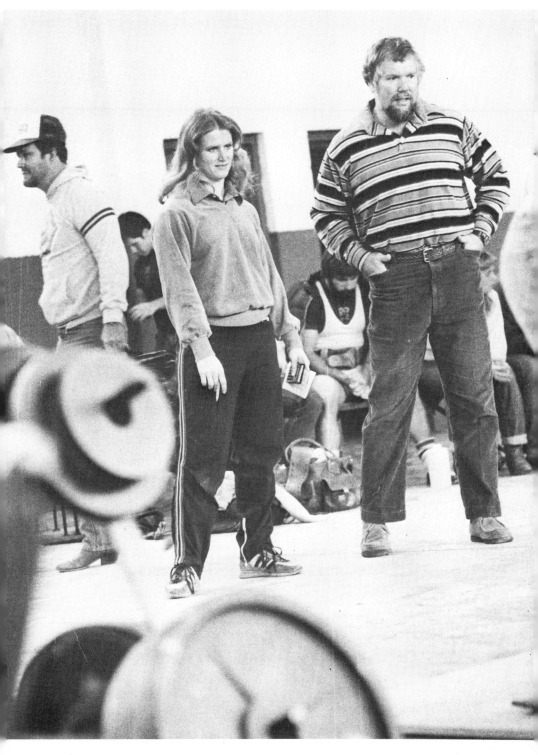

Opposite page, top and bottom: Linda Miller of Australia holds the unofficial world record deadlift of 212.5 kg. at a bodyweight of 75 kg. Australia's superheavyweight Ray Rigby is shown squatting 365 kg. Rigby's championship lifts go back to 1970, when he won the gold in Olympic lifting in the Commonwealth Games in Scotland. (Photos by Jim Lewis.) Above are Terry and Jan Todd, world powerlifting champions. (Photo courtesy of Sports Illustrated.)

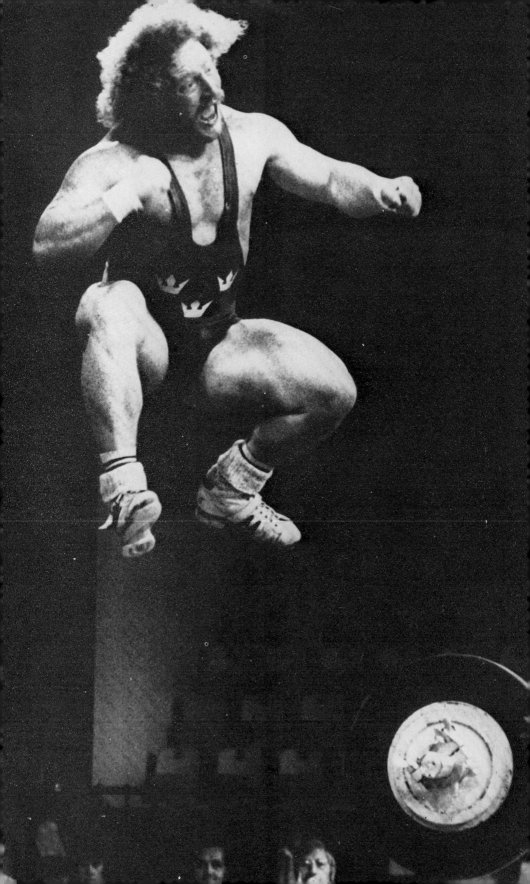

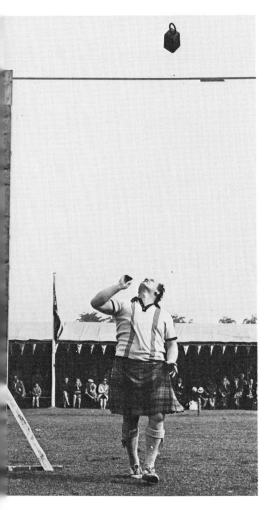
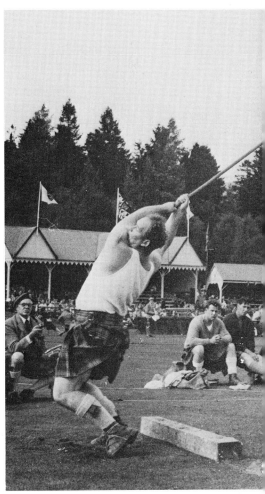

Opposite page: Sweden's Lennart Dahlgren exhibits the thrill of victory after placing first in the 110 kg. group B with a lift of 355 kg. at the Montreal Olympics, July 26, 1976. (Agence France-Presse photo.) Above photos show some of the native strength sports of Scotland. (Photos courtesy of David Webster.)

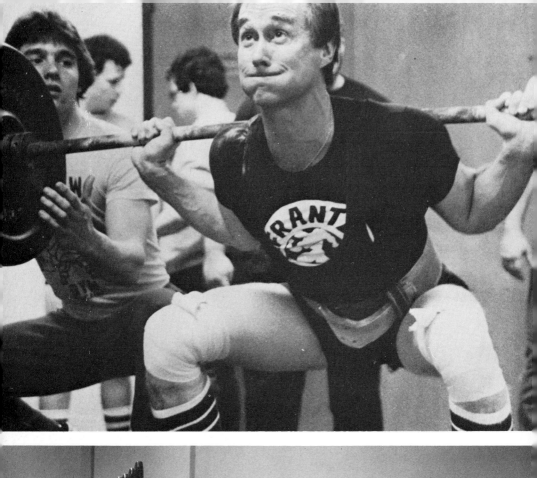

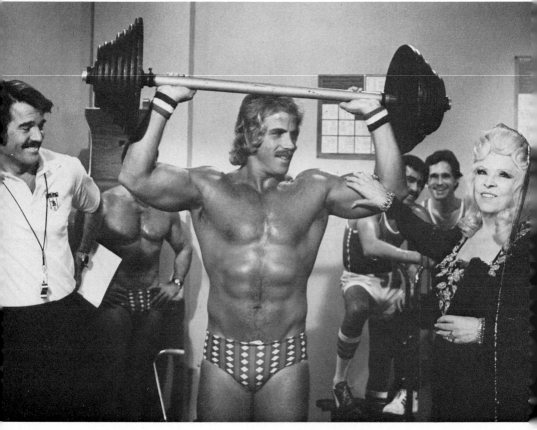

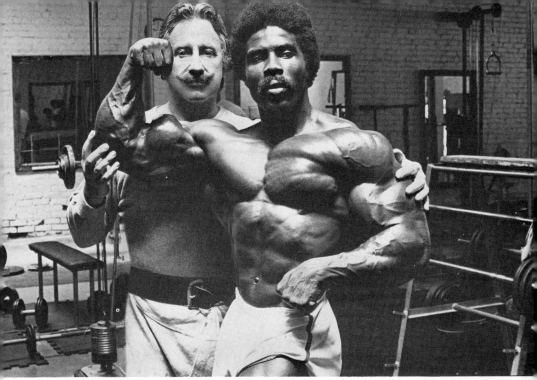

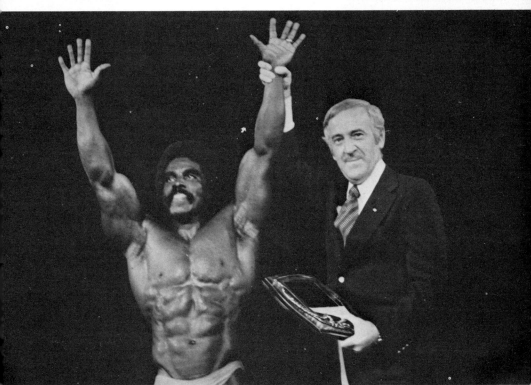

Opposite page, top to bottom: Dr. Thomas Allen, pulmonary medicine specialist and 45-year-old natural masters powerlifting champion is shown here squatting 385 lbs. with a bodyweight of only 148 lbs. (Photo by Maris Sternberg.) One of Mae West's "beautiful body" men in the motion picture *The Sextets*, Ric Draysin, almost died of steriod abuse. As it was, he lost a kidney and a great deal of body weight. Above, top to bottom: Joe Weider with Mr. Universe Robby Robinson, who found that steroids bloated his physique, giving him a puffy, uncut look. "I felt lousy on the drug and suffered dangerous jumps in my blood pressure." (Photo by Craig Deitz, courtesy of *Muscle & Fitness.*) Robinson is shown accepting the title from IFBB president Ben Weider. (Photo by Caruso.)

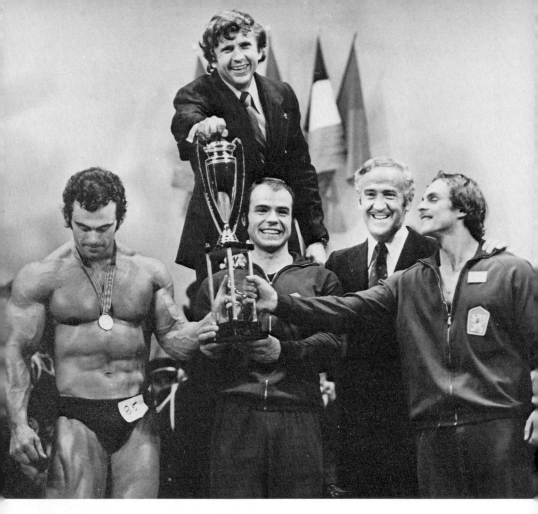
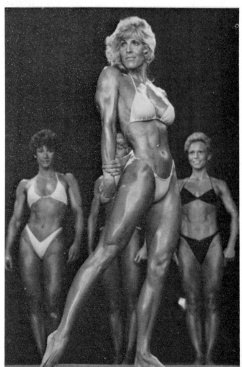
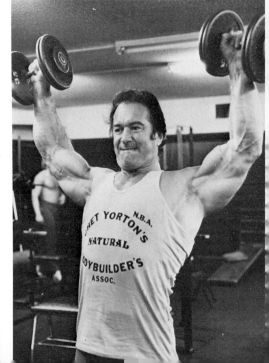

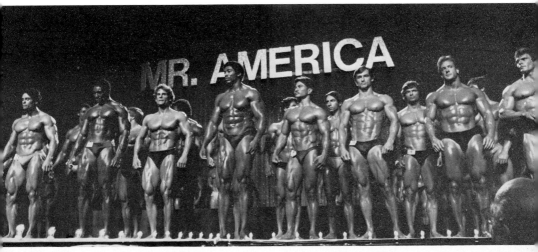

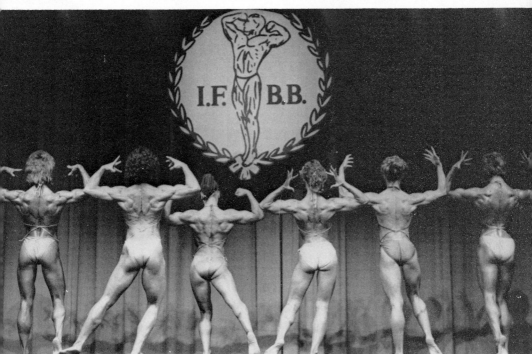

Opposite page, top: Ben Weider, shown here with the Czechoslovakian bodybuilding team, has ordered drug testing to begin at the 1985 Mr. Universe competition. If an athlete tests positive for steroids, he will be suspended for eighteen months; a second offense will result in a lifetime ban. Bottom left: champion bodybuilder Georgia Fudge is considering dropping out of competition rather than compete against she-men. (Photo by Doris Barrilleaux.) bottom right: Chet Yorton, former Mr. Universe, began promoting the first steroid-free bodybuilding competitions in 1978. "I want to provide athletes with the opportunity to compete without the 'drug monsters.' (Photo by Denie.) Above, many bodybuilders are pressured into anabolic steroid use for fear of losing that 2-5 percent edge. The new and exciting sport of women's bodybuilding should be protected from infiltration of steroid abuse. (Photos by Doris Barrilleaux.)

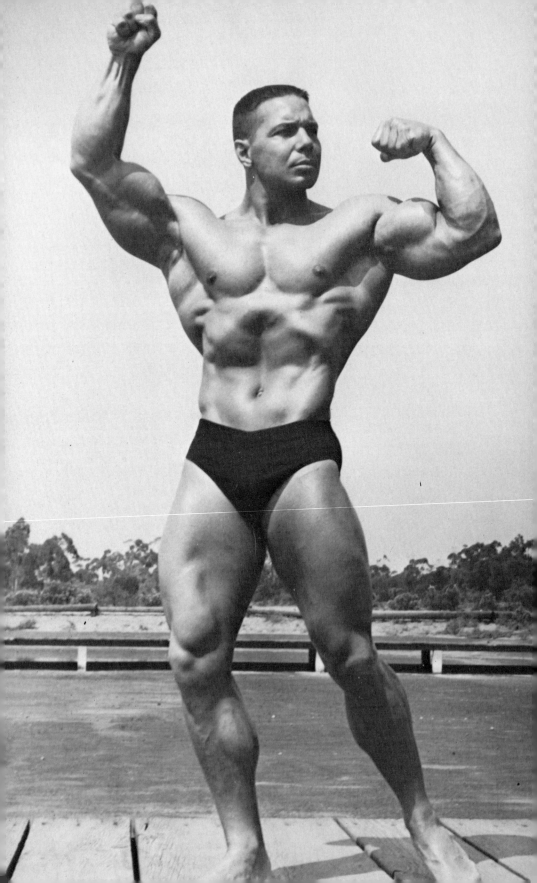

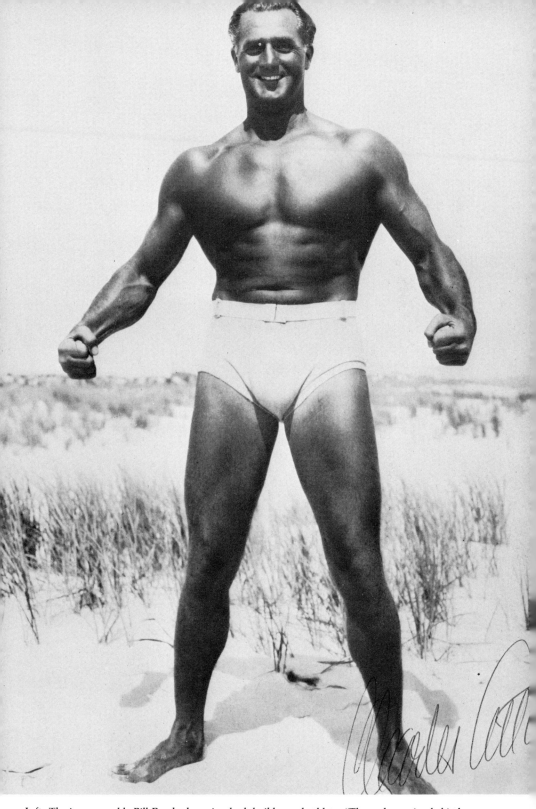

Left: The incomparable Bill Pearl, champion bodybuilder and athlete: "The real meaning behind weight training is the health aspect, and pumping in drugs and steroids into the system is just the opposite of what sport is about." (Photo by Leo Stern, courtesy of Weider Publications.) Above: Charles Atlas inspired the youth of yesteryear to build their bodies with the good nutrition and dynamic tension exercises. (Photo reproduced with permission from Charles Atlas, Ltd.)

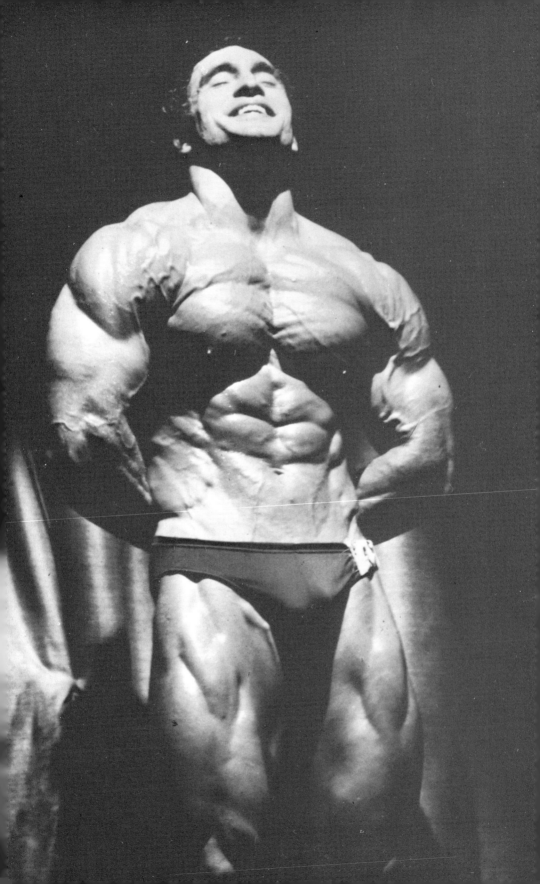

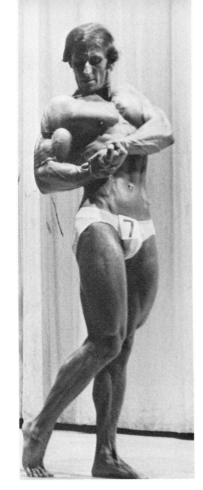

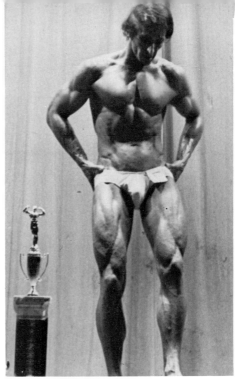

Left: Champion Enunlu in exhaltation. (Photo by Denie.) Above: This bodybuilder died the night before his competition due to steroid drug use and extreme diet habits. (Photos by Denie.) Below: Dennis Tinerino is shown donating blood sample for steroid testing before he went on to win the first American National Physique Championship. (Photo by Mark Lurie.)

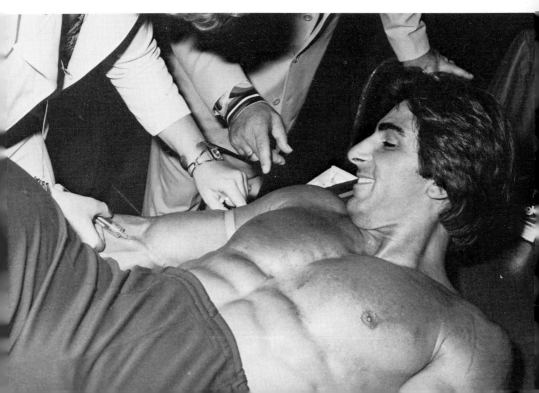

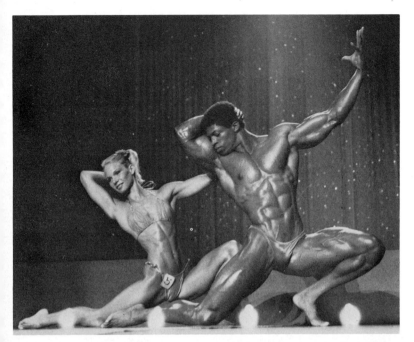

Left: The beauty and grace of bodybuilding is typified by champions Shelley Gruwell and John Brown. (Photo by Doris Barrilleaux.) Hard work and good coaching make winners—not drugs, but some high school athletes are informed by their coaches that steroids will help them make the team. Photo at right courtesy of DePaul Sports Information.

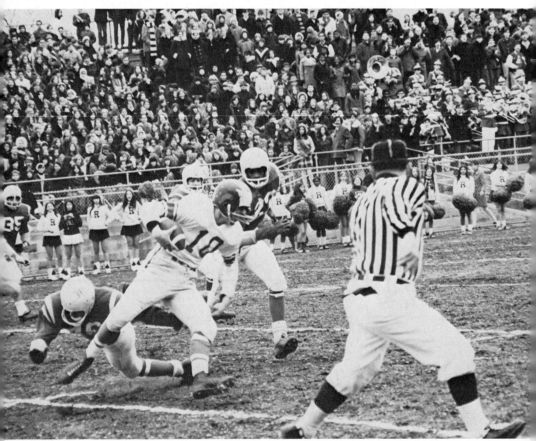

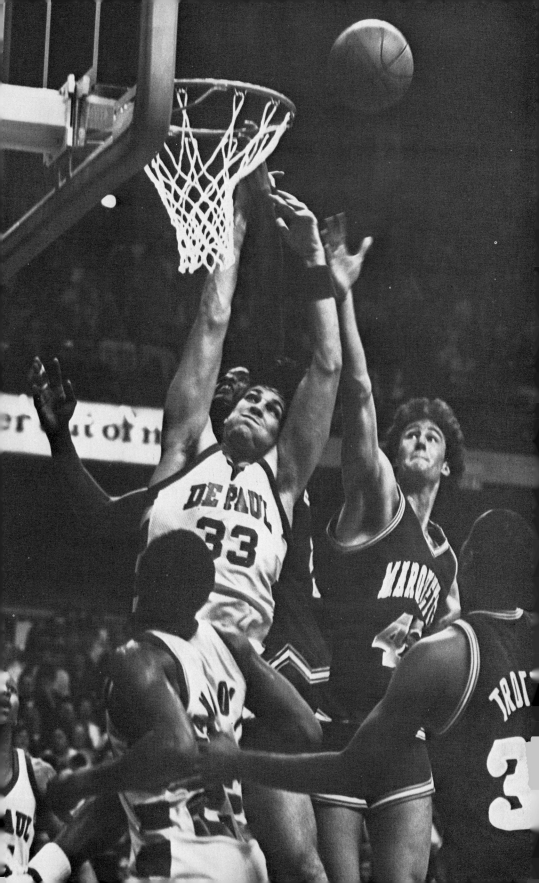

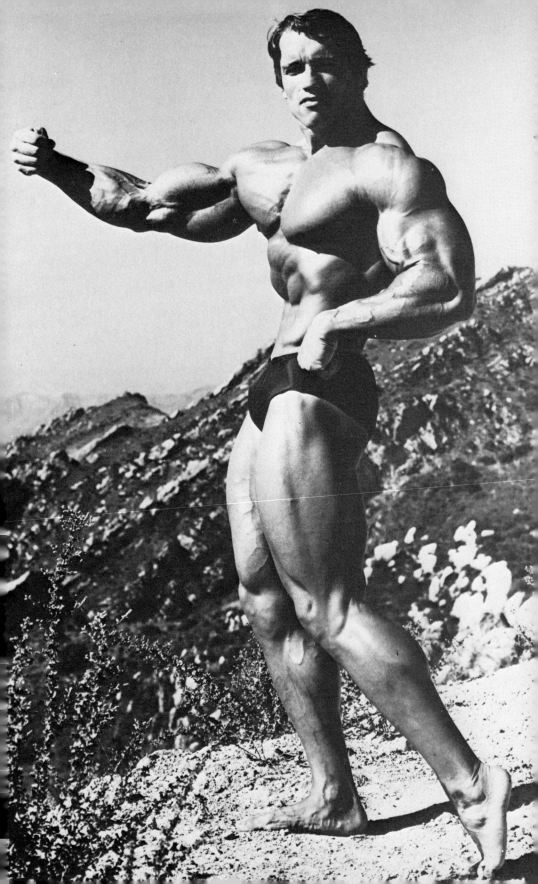

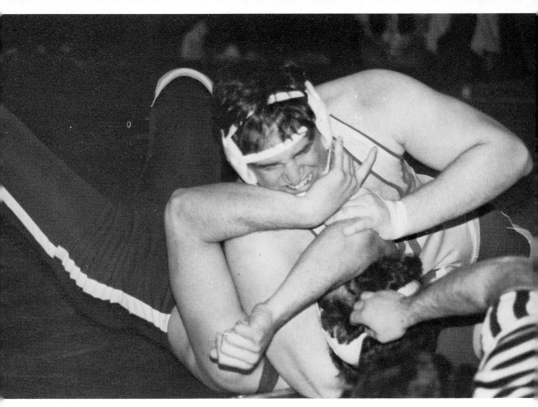

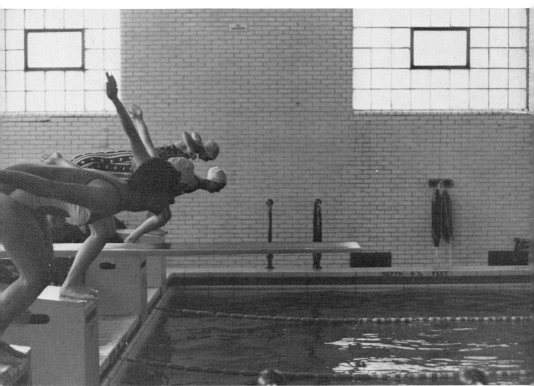

Left: The amazing Arnold Schwarzenegger, eight-times Mr. Olympia, says, "Steroids have never created a champion...Anyone who thinks he can defeat a John Grimek, Steve Reeves, Reg Park, Sergio Oliva or Franco Columbu just by taking a better drug is a fool. If it were up to me, I would eliminate steroids entirely from sports." (Photo by Art Zeller, courtesy of Joe Weider.) This pressure to win has forced even junior high school athletes into steroid use.

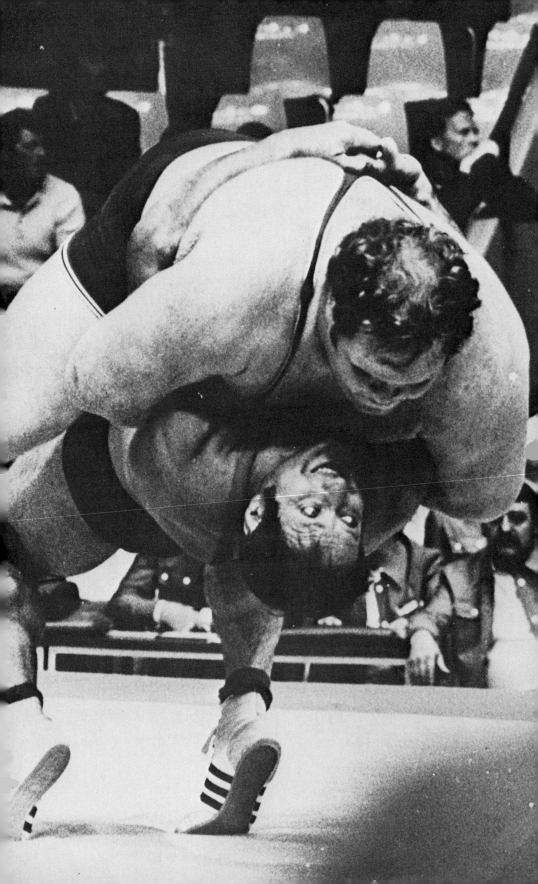

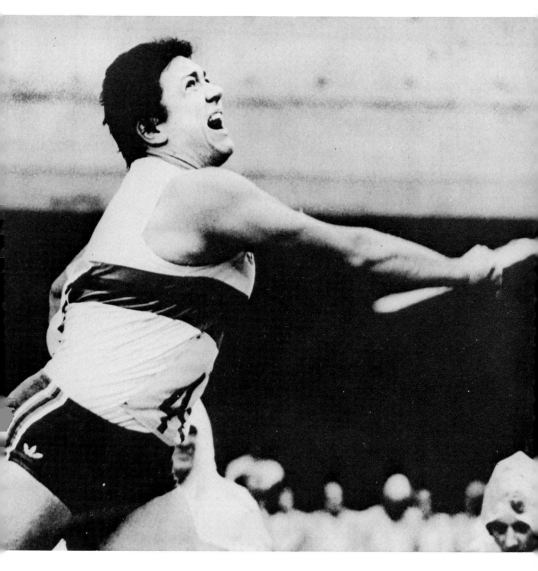

Left: Prize-winning picture by Ollie Seijbold of Sweden's *Dagens Nyheter* shows 400-pounder Chris Taylor of the United States being thrown by Germany's Wilfried Diedrich at the 1972 Munich Olympics. Above: Bulgaria's Ivanka Christova putting the shot 21.16 meters to win the gold at the Montreal Olympics, July 31, 1976. (AFP photo.)

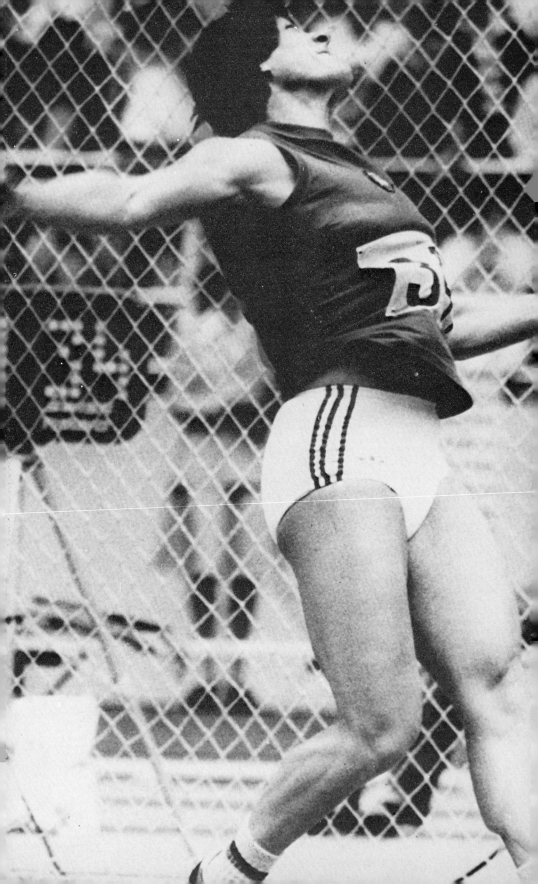

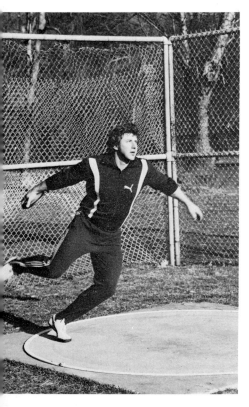
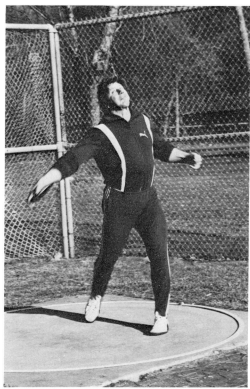
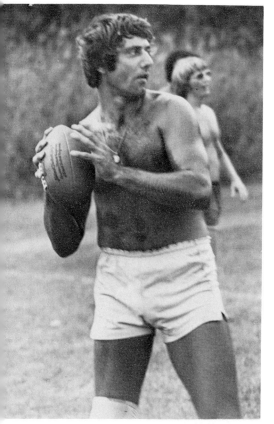

Top photos show the great Al Oerter, four-time gold medal Olympian in the discus: "Athletes who rely on drugs risk losing their confidence when testing eliminates their chemical edge. The hormone programs they're using today can be a detriment, particularly mentally." Left: Joe Namath believes that "the use of steroids is not only unethical but extremely dangerous." (Photos by Denie.) Soviet discus champion Faina Melnik surprisingly finished second at the Montreal Olympics in 1976 and then had her silver medal disqualified five hours later when judges ruled that she had taken three starts to throw on her fifth and best attempt.

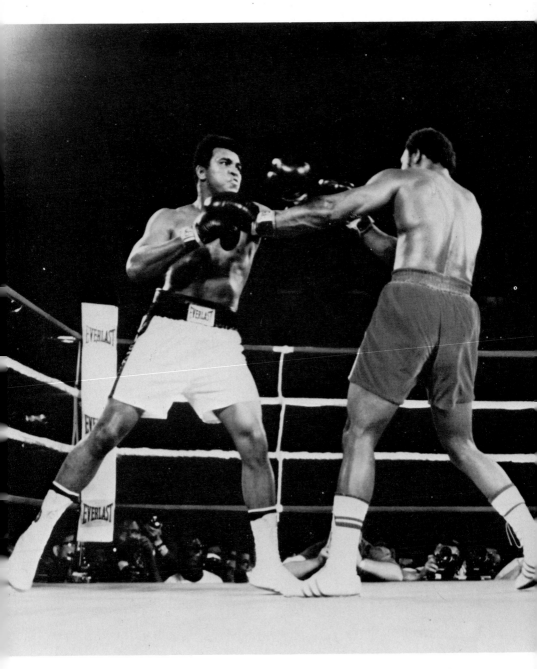

Champion Muhammad Ali, shown above in his victorious fight over George Foreman, has long been against drug abuse by athletes and has conveyed his thoughts to many young ghetto athletes who idolize him. (PR release photo.) Right: This exquisite drawing of the neck and thorax, showing the thyroid gland, is from C. Clemente's *Atlas of the Human Body*, courtesy of Urban and Schwarzenberg, West Germany

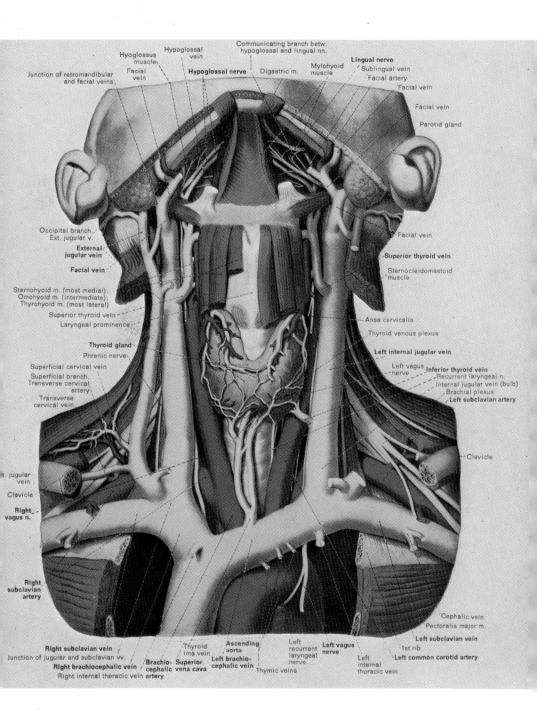

Communicating branch betw. hypoglossal and lingual nn.

Hypoglossus muscle

Hypoglossal vein

Hypoglossal nerve

Facial vein

Junction of retromandibular and facial veins

Digastric m.

Mylohyoid muscle

Lingual nerve

Sublingual vein

Facial artery

Facial vein

Facial vein

Parotid gland

Occipital branch, Ext. jugular v.

External jugular vein

Facial vein

Facial vein

Superior thyroid vein

Sternocleidomastoid muscle

Sternohyoid m. (most medial); Omohyoid m. (intermediate); Thyrohyoid m. (most lateral)

Superior thyroid vein

Laryngeal prominence

Thyroid gland

Phrenic nerve

Superficial cervical vein

Superficial branch, Transverse cervical artery

Transverse cervical vein

Ansa cervicalis

Thyroid venous plexus

Left internal jugular vein

Left vagus nerve

Inferior thyroid vein

Recurrent laryngeal n.

Internal jugular vein (bulb)

Brachial plexus

Left subclavian artery

Rt. jugular vein

Clavicle

Right vagus n.

Clavicle

Right subclavian artery

Cephalic vein

Pectoralis major m.

Left subclavian vein

Right subclavian vein

Junction of jugular and subclavian vv.

Right brachiocephalic vein

Right internal thoracic vein

Thyroid ima vein

Brachio-cephalic artery

Superior vena cava

Ascending aorta

Left brachio-cephalic vein

Thymic veins

Left recurrent laryngeal nerve

Left vagus nerve

1st rib

Left internal thoracic vein

Left common carotid artery

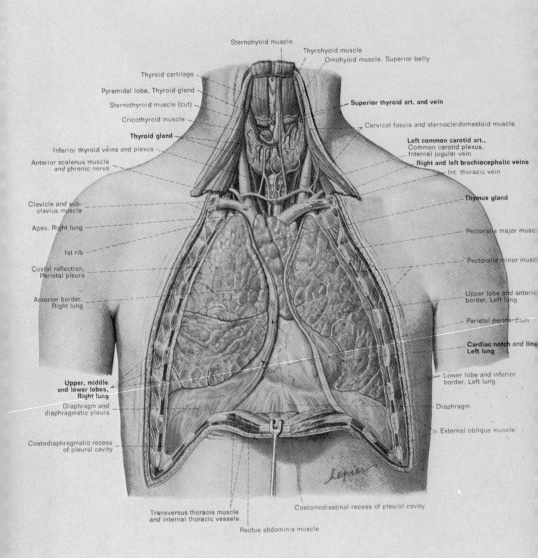

Sternohyoid muscle

Thyrohyoid muscle
Omohyoid muscle. Superior belly

Thyroid cartilage

Pyramidal lobe, Thyroid gland

Sternothyroid muscle (cut)

Cricothyroid muscle

Superior thyroid art. and vein

Cervical fascia *and* sternocleidomastoid muscle

Thyroid gland

Left common carotid art.,
Common carotid plexus.
Internal jugular vein

Inferior thyroid veins *and* plexus

Right and left brachiocephalic veins

Anterior scalenus muscle
and phrenic nerve

Int. thoracic vein

Clavicle *and* sub-
clavius muscle

Thymus gland

Apex, Right lung

Pectoralis major muscle

1st rib

Pectoralis minor muscle

Costal reflection,
Parietal pleura

Anterior border,
Right lung

Upper lobe *and* anterior
border, Left lung

Parietal pericardium

**Cardiac notch and lingula,
Left lung**

Upper, middle
**and lower lobes,
Right lung**

Lower lobe *and* inferior
border, Left lung

Diaphragm *and*
diaphragmatic pleura

Diaphragm

External oblique muscle

Costodiaphragmatic recess
of pleural cavity

Transversus thoracis muscle
and internal thoracic vessels

Costomediastinal recess of pleural cavity

Rectus abdominis muscle

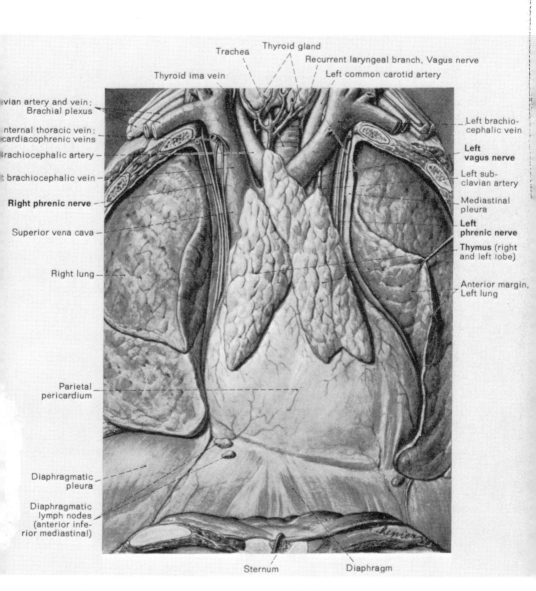

Trachea

Thyroid gland

Recurrent laryngeal branch, Vagus nerve

Thyroid ima vein

Left common carotid artery

vian artery and vein;
Brachial plexus

nternal thoracic vein;
cardiacophrenic veins

Brachiocephalic artery

brachiocephalic vein

Right phrenic nerve

Superior vena cava

Right lung

Parietal
pericardium

Diaphragmatic
pleura

Diaphragmatic
lymph nodes
(anterior infe-
rior mediastinal)

Left brachio-
cephalic vein

**Left
vagus nerve**

Left sub-
clavian artery

Mediastinal
pleura

**Left
phrenic nerve**

Thymus (right
and left lobe)

Anterior margin,
Left lung

Sternum

Diaphragm

The thymus gland is exhibited in this pair of drawings from C. Clemente's *Atlas of the Human Body*, courtesy of Urban & Schwarzenberg, West Germany.

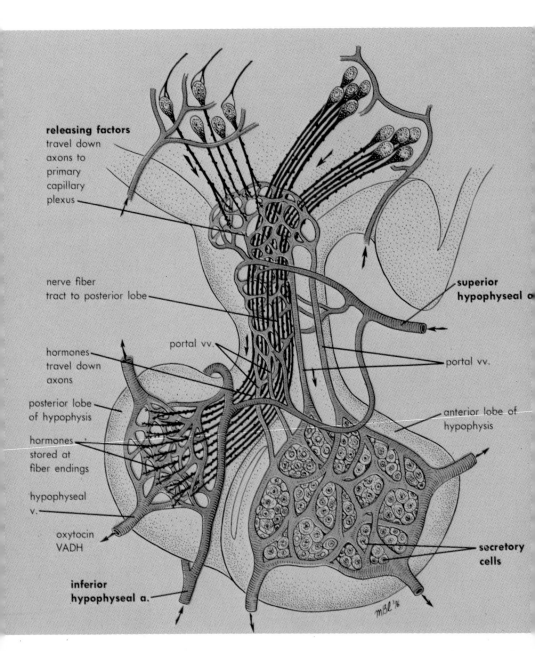

releasing factors travel down axons to primary capillary plexus

nerve fiber tract to posterior lobe

superior hypophyseal a

portal vv.

hormones travel down axons

portal vv.

posterior lobe of hypophysis

anterior lobe of hypophysis

hormones stored at fiber endings

hypophyseal v.

oxytocin VADH

secretory cells

inferior hypophyseal a.

Hypophysis of the pituitary gland, showing nerve and vascular supply. Drawing from *Essential Human Anatomy: A Text Atlas*, by J.E. Crouch, 1982, courtesy of the publisher, Lea & Febiger.

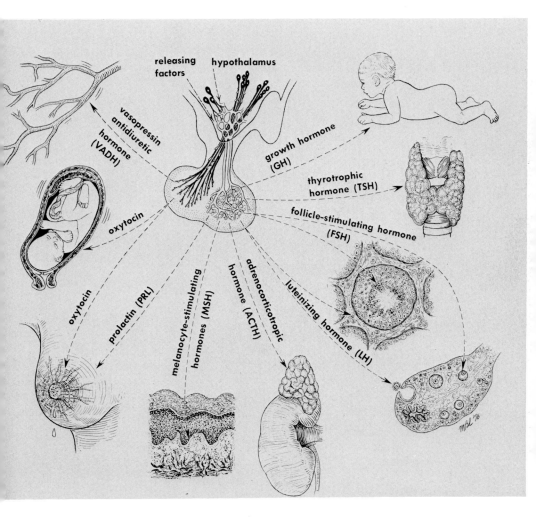

Hypophysis, showing its structural and functional relationships to the hypothalamus and to other endocrine glands and other tissues. (Drawing from *Essential Human Anatomy: A Text Atlas*, by J.E. Crouch, 1982, courtesy of the publisher, Lea & Febiger.)

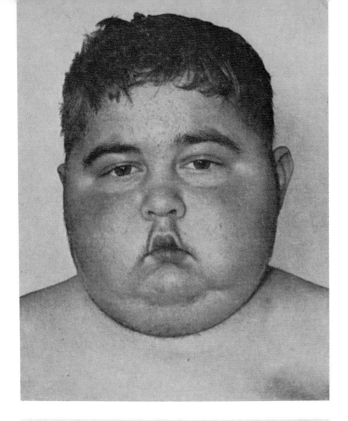

Left: The half-moon look of the typical Cushing's syndrome patient, from Jerzy Kosowicz' *Atlas of Endocrine Diseases* (Bowie, MD: Charles Press). Photo courtesy of Dr. Kosowicz. Below and right: Normal adult female breast anatomy. (From C. Clemente, *Atlas of the Human Body,* courtesy of Urban & Schwarzenberg, publisher.)

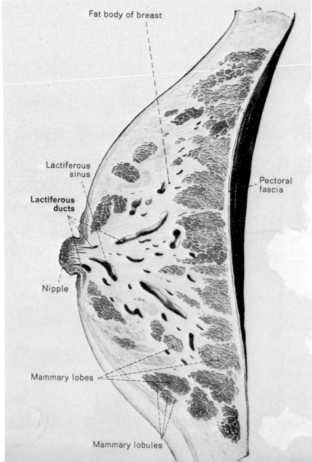

Fat body of breast

Lactiferous sinus

Lactiferous ducts

Nipple

Pectoral fascia

Mammary lobes

Mammary lobules

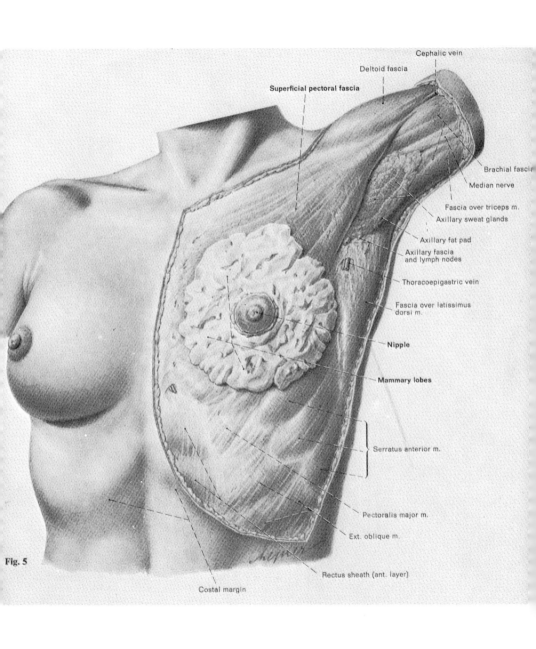

Cephalic vein

Deltoid fascia

Superficial pectoral fascia

Brachial fascia

Median nerve

Fascia over triceps m.

Axillary sweat glands

Axillary fat pad

Axillary fascia
and lymph nodes

Thoracoepigastric vein

Fascia over latissimus
dorsi m.

Nipple

Mammary lobes

Serratus anterior m.

Pectoralis major m.

Ext. oblique m.

Rectus sheath (ant. layer)

Costal margin

Fig. 5

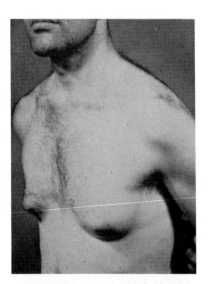

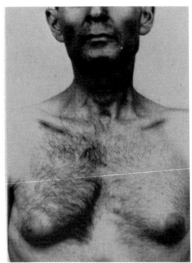

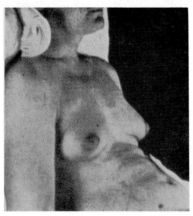

Following the disturbance of normal hormonal balance, men may develop female breast tissue known as gynocomastia. This occurs because both men and women have male and female hormones. Ingestion of anabolic steroids shuts off the male's own body androgen secretion so that when he comes off the drug, his ratio of female-to-male hormones is elevated, which can lead to this condition. (Photos on this page from *Atlas of Clinical Endocrinology* [2nd ed.], by Lisser and Escamilla, courtesy of Elizabeth S. Escamilla.) On right: Male pelvic area, showing relationship of pelvic visera (including prostate gland) to external genitalia. Both internal body hormone production and prostate size are seriously affected by anabolic steroids. (Drawings from Clemente, *Atlas of the Human Body,* courtesy of Urban & Schwarzenberg, publisher.)

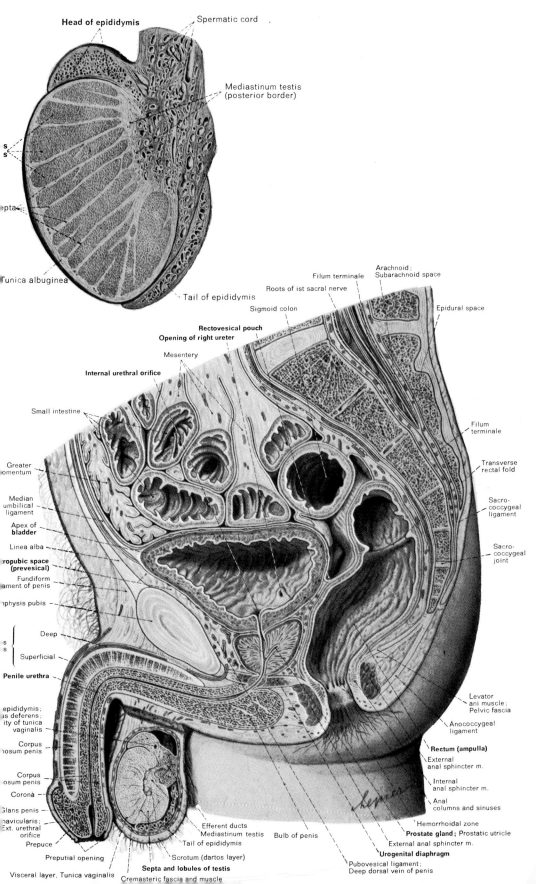

Head of epididymis

Spermatic cord

Mediastinum testis
(posterior border)

s
s

pta

Tunica albuginea

Tail of epididymis

Arachnoid;
Subarachnoid space

Filum terminale

Roots of 1st sacral nerve

Sigmoid colon

Epidural space

Rectovesical pouch

Opening of right ureter

Mesentery

Internal urethral orifice

Filum
terminale

Small intestine

Transverse
rectal fold

Greater
omentum

Sacro-
coccygeal
ligament

Median
umbilical
ligament

Apex of
bladder

Sacro-
coccygeal
joint

Linea alba

ropubic space
(prevesical)

Fundiform
ament of penis

physis pubis

Deep

Superficial

Levator
ani muscle;
Pelvic fascia

Penile urethra

Anococcygeal
ligament

epididymis;
is deferens;
ity of tunica
vaginalis

Corpus
hosum penis

Rectum (ampulla)

External
anal sphincter m.

Corpus
osum penis

Internal
anal sphincter m.

Corona

Anal
columns and sinuses

Glans penis

Hemorrhoidal zone

navicularis;
Ext. urethral
orifice

Efferent ducts

Prostate gland; Prostatic utricle

Mediastinum testis

Prepuce

Tail of epididymis

Bulb of penis

External anal sphincter m.

Urogenital diaphragm

Preputial opening

Scrotum (dartos layer)

Pubovesical ligament;
Deep dorsal vein of penis

Visceral layer, Tunica vaginalis

Septa and lobules of testis

Cremasteric fascia and muscle

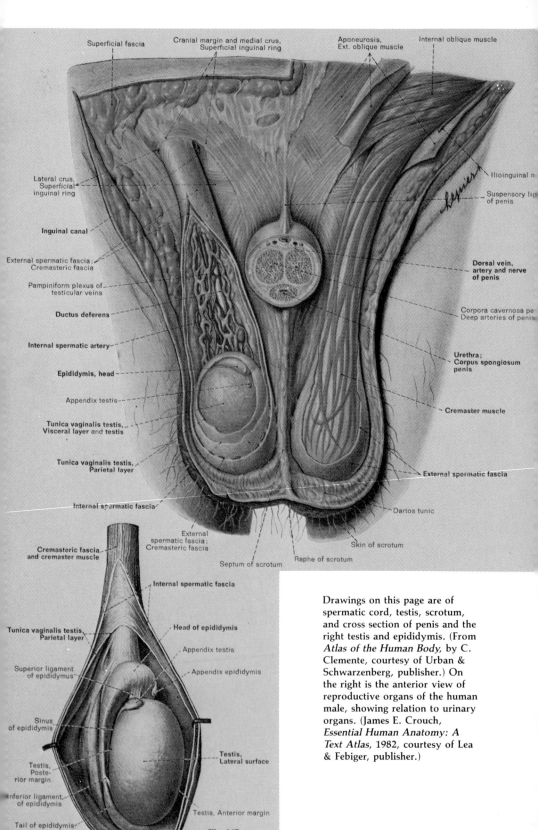

Superficial fascia

Cranial margin and medial crus, Superficial inguinal ring

Aponeurosis, Ext. oblique muscle

Internal oblique muscle

Lateral crus, Superficial inguinal ring

Ilioinguinal n

Suspensory lig of penis

Inguinal canal

External spermatic fascia; Cremasteric fascia

Dorsal vein, artery and nerve of penis

Pampiniform plexus of testicular veins

Ductus deferens

Corpora cavernosa pe Deep arteries of penis

Internal spermatic artery

Epididymis, head

Urethra; Corpus spongiosum penis

Appendix testis

Tunica vaginalis testis, Visceral layer and testis

Tunica vaginalis testis, Parietal layer

Cremaster muscle

Internal spermatic fascia

External spermatic fascia

External spermatic fascia; Cremasteric fascia

Dartos tunic

Septum of scrotum

Raphe of scrotum

Skin of scrotum

Cremasteric fascia and cremaster muscle

Internal spermatic fascia

Tunica vaginalis testis, Parietal layer

Head of epididymis

Appendix testis

Superior ligament of epididymus

Appendix epididymis

Sinus of epididymis

Testis, Posterior margin

Testis, Lateral surface

Inferior ligament of epididymis

Tail of epididymis

Testis, Anterior margin

Fig. 167

Drawings on this page are of spermatic cord, testis, scrotum, and cross section of penis and the right testis and epididymis. (From *Atlas of the Human Body*, by C. Clemente, courtesy of Urban & Schwarzenberg, publisher.) On the right is the anterior view of reproductive organs of the human male, showing relation to urinary organs. (James E. Crouch, *Essential Human Anatomy: A Text Atlas*, 1982, courtesy of Lea & Febiger, publisher.)

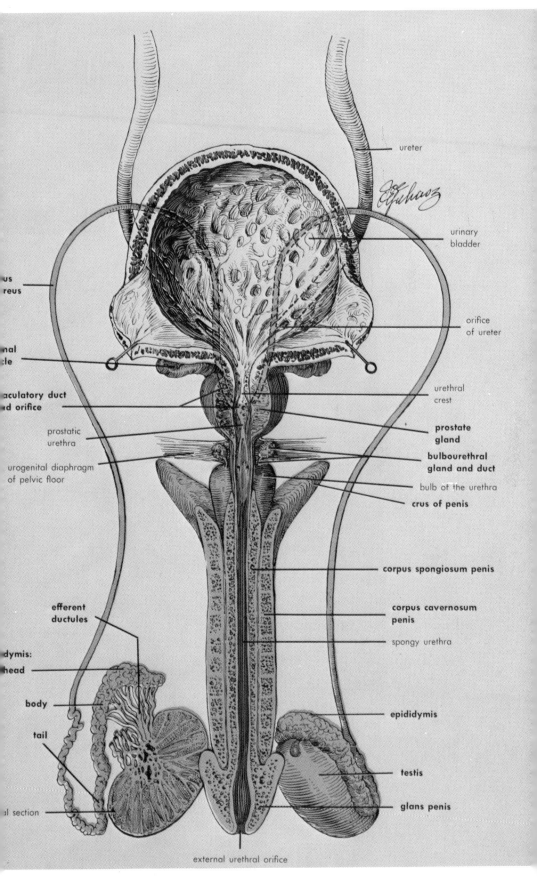

ureter

urinary
bladder

orifice
of ureter

...us
...reus

...nal
...:le

...aculatory duct
...d orifice

urethral
crest

prostate
gland

prostatic
urethra

bulbourethral
gland and duct

urogenital diaphragm
of pelvic floor

bulb of the urethra

crus of penis

corpus spongiosum penis

corpus cavernosum
penis

spongy urethra

efferent
ductules

...dymis:
...head

epididymis

body

tail

testis

...l section

glans penis

external urethral orifice

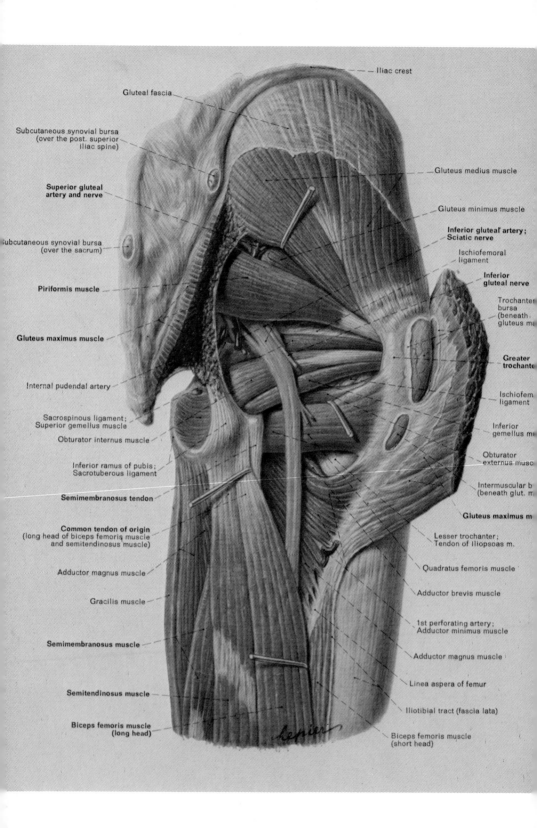

Iliac crest

Gluteal fascia

Subcutaneous synovial bursa
(over the post. superior
iliac spine)

**Superior gluteal
artery and nerve**

Subcutaneous synovial bursa
(over the sacrum)

Piriformis muscle

Gluteus maximus muscle

Internal pudendal artery

Sacrospinous ligament;
Superior gemellus muscle

Obturator internus muscle

Inferior ramus of pubis;
Sacrotuberous ligament

Semimembranosus tendon

Common tendon of origin
(long head of biceps femoris muscle
and semitendinosus muscle)

Adductor magnus muscle

Gracilis muscle

Semimembranosus muscle

Semitendinosus muscle

Biceps femoris muscle
(long head)

Gluteus medius muscle

Gluteus minimus muscle

**Inferior gluteal artery;
Sciatic nerve**

Ischiofemoral
ligament

**Inferior
gluteal nerve**

Trochanter
bursa
(beneath
gluteus ma

**Greater
trochante**

Ischiofem
ligament

Inferior
gemellus m

Obturator
externus musc

Intermuscular b
(beneath glut. m

Gluteus maximus m

Lesser trochanter;
Tendon of iliopsoas m.

Quadratus femoris muscle

Adductor brevis muscle

1st perforating artery;
Adductor minimus muscle

Adductor magnus muscle

Linea aspera of femur

Iliotibial tract (fascia lata)

Biceps femoris muscle
(short head)

Many athletes now inject themselves with anabolic steroids. Aside from greatly magnifying the risk of infection, hepatitis, and shock, an improperly placed needle may damage the nerves and blood vessels in the buttocks. These drawings depict the vulnerable structures in that area. Special attention should be paid to the large sciatic nerve, which if damaged could cause sharp pain and numbing sensations down the back of the leg. (From Clemente's *Atlas of the Human Body,* courtesy of Urban & Schwarzenberg, publisher.)

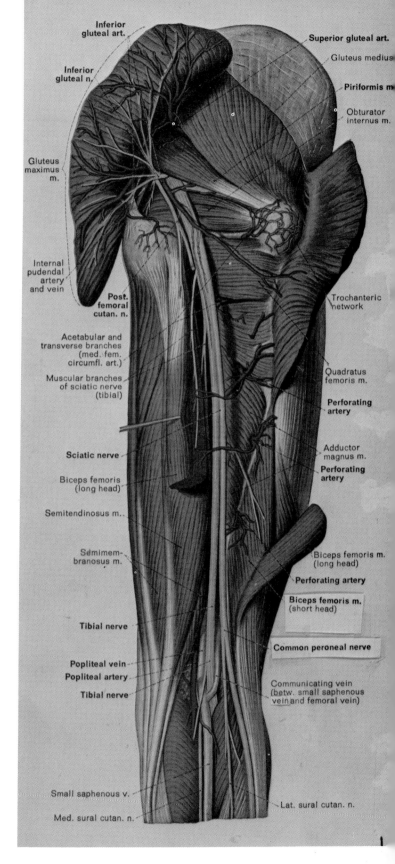

Inferior gluteal art.

Superior gluteal art.

Gluteus medius

Inferior gluteal n.

Piriformis m

Obturator internus m.

Gluteus maximus m.

Internal pudendal artery and vein

Post. femoral cutan. n.

Trochanteric network

Acetabular and transverse branches (med. fem. circumfl. art.)

Quadratus femoris m.

Muscular branches of sciatic nerve (tibial)

Perforating artery

Sciatic nerve

Adductor magnus m.

Perforating artery

Biceps femoris (long head)

Semitendinosus m.

Semimem- branosus m.

Biceps femoris m. (long head)

Perforating artery

Biceps femoris m. (short head)

Tibial nerve

Common peroneal nerve

Popliteal vein

Popliteal artery

Communicating vein (betw. small saphenous vein and femoral vein)

Tibial nerve

Small saphenous v.

Lat. sural cutan. n.

Med. sural cutan. n.

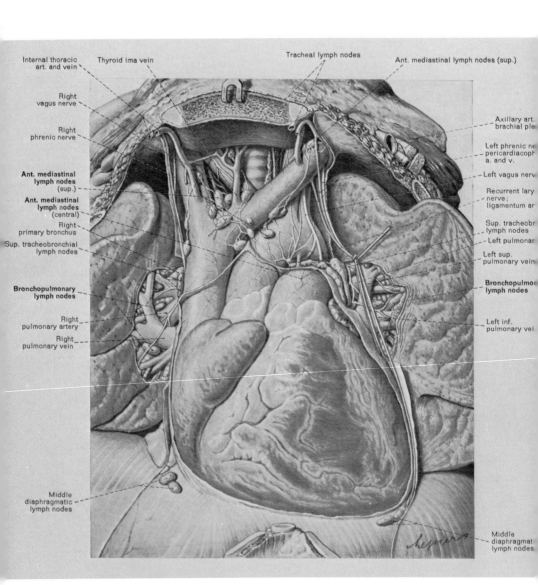

Internal thoracic art. and vein

Thyroid ima vein

Tracheal lymph nodes

Ant. mediastinal lymph nodes (sup.)

Right vagus nerve

Right phrenic nerve

Ant. mediastinal lymph nodes (sup.)

Ant. mediastinal lymph nodes (central)

Right primary bronchus

Sup. tracheobronchial lymph nodes

Bronchopulmonary lymph nodes

Right pulmonary artery

Right pulmonary vein

Axillary art. brachial ple

Left phrenic ne pericardiacoph a. and v.

Left vagus nerv

Recurrent lary nerve; ligamentum ar

Sup. tracheobr lymph nodes

Left pulmonar

Left sup. pulmonary vein

Bronchopulmo lymph nodes

Left inf. pulmonary vei

Middle diaphragmatic lymph nodes

Middle diaphragmat lymph nodes

The human heart, including surrounding structures. (From Clemente, *Atlas of the Human Body,* courtesy of Urban & Schwarzenberg, publisher.)

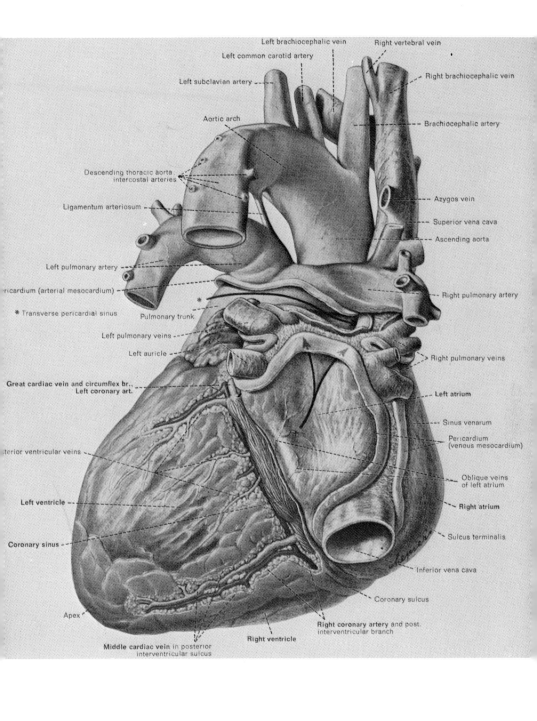

Left brachiocephalic vein

Right vertebral vein

Left common carotid artery

Right brachiocephalic vein

Left subclavian artery

Aortic arch

Brachiocephalic artery

Descending thoracic aorta
intercostal arteries

Azygos vein

Superior vena cava

Ligamentum arteriosum

Ascending aorta

Left pulmonary artery

...ricardium (arterial mesocardium)

Right pulmonary artery

* Transverse pericardial sinus

Pulmonary trunk

Left pulmonary veins

Left auricle

Right pulmonary veins

Great cardiac vein and circumflex br.,
Left coronary art.

Left atrium

Sinus venarum

Pericardium
(venous mesocardium)

...terior ventricular veins

Oblique veins
of left atrium

Left ventricle

Right atrium

Coronary sinus

Sulcus terminalis

Inferior vena cava

Coronary sulcus

Apex

Right coronary artery and post.
interventricular branch

Middle cardiac vein in posterior
interventricular sulcus

Right ventricle

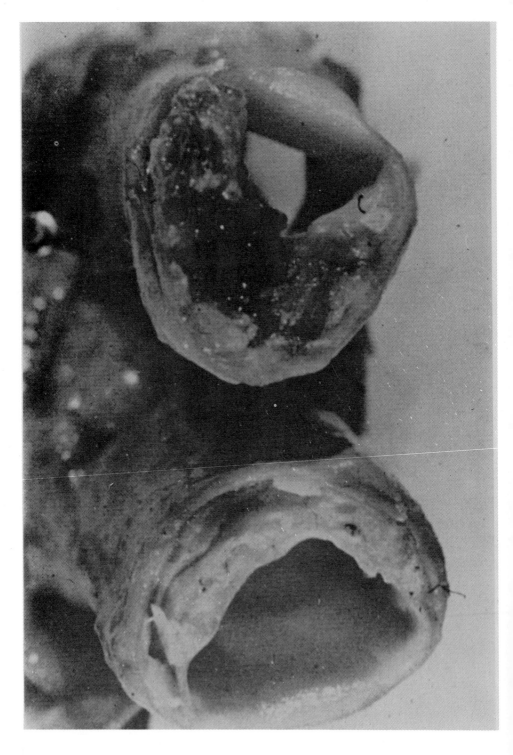

Above: Atherosclerotic plaque lesions in the major blood vessels. Right: Carotid artery of a dog with progressive atherosclerosis. (All photographs from *Atherosclerotic Vascular Disease/A Hahneman Symposium*, 1968, courtesy of Appleton—Century—Crofts.)

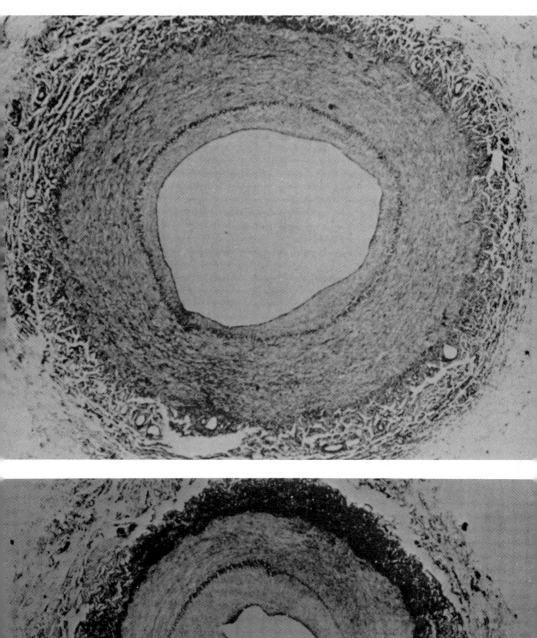

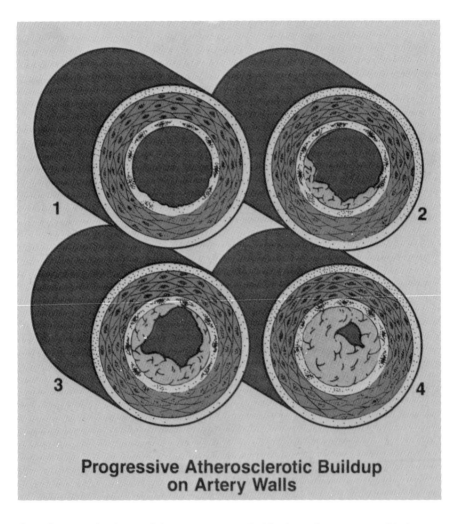

**Progressive Atherosclerotic Buildup
on Artery Walls**

Atherosclerosis, or hardening of the arteries, causes the blood vessels to narrow or block arteries. This serious disease is augmented with abuse of anabolic steroids. Reprinted with permission, ©American Heart Association.

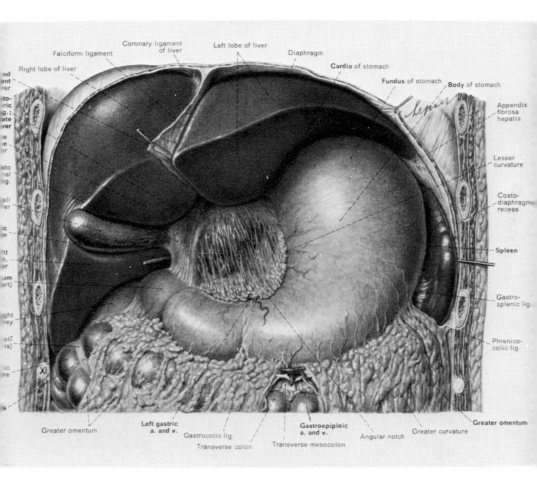

The liver and surrounding structures are beautifully shown in this drawing from Clemente's *Atlas of the Human Body*, Urban & Schwarzenberg, publishers.

Labels on the figure:

Coronary ligament of liver · Falciform ligament · Right lobe of liver · Left lobe of liver · Diaphragm · Cardia of stomach · Fundus of stomach · Body of stomach · Appendix fibrosa hepatis · Lesser curvature · Costo-diaphragmatic recess · Spleen · Gastro-splenic lig. · Phrenico-colic lig. · Greater omentum · Left gastric a. and v. · Gastrocolic lig. · Transverse colon · Transverse mesocolon · Gastroepiploic a. and v. · Angular notch · Greater curvature · Greater omentum

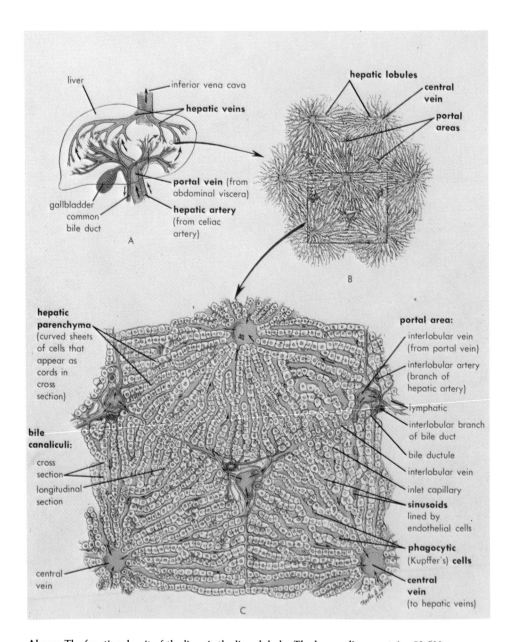

Above: The functional unit of the liver is the liver lobule. The human liver contains 50,000 to 100,000 individual lobule units. The liver lobule is constructed around a central vein that empties into the hepatic veins and then into the vena cava. Note the various structures in the diagrams. Thin plates of hepatic cells make up the liver lobules, and in between these cell plates are the sinusoids, which are channels that receive blood from the portal vein and hepatic artery. Kupffer cells line the sinusoids and function as protective cells. (From Crouch's *Essential Human Anatomy: A Text Atlas*, Lea & Febiger, publisher.) Right: Abdominal cavity, showing kidneys and surrounding structures. (From Clemente, *Atlas of the Human Body*, Urban & Schwarzenberg, publishers.)

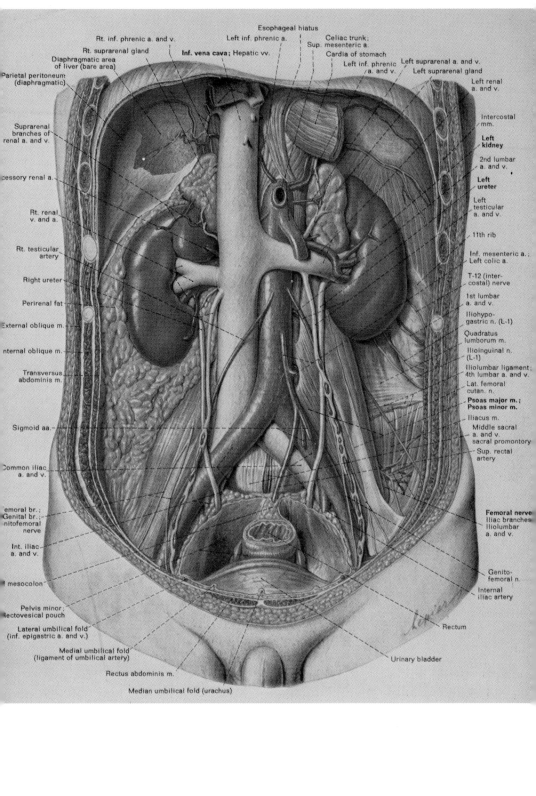

Esophageal hiatus

Rt. inf. phrenic a. and v.
Left inf. phrenic a.
Celiac trunk;
Sup. mesenteric a.
Rt. suprarenal gland
Cardia of stomach
Diaphragmatic area
of liver (bare area)
Inf. vena cava; Hepatic vv.
Left inf. phrenic
Left suprarenal a. and v.
a. and v.
Left suprarenal gland
Parietal peritoneum
(diaphragmatic)
Left renal
a. and v.

Intercostal
mm.
Suprarenal
branches of
renal a. and v.
Left
kidney
2nd lumbar
a. and v.
cessory renal a.
Left
ureter
Rt. renal
v. and a.
Left
testicular
a. and v.
Rt. testicular
artery
11th rib

Inf. mesenteric a.;
Left colic a.
Right ureter
T-12 (inter-
costal) nerve
Perirenal fat
1st lumbar
a. and v.
Iliohypo-
gastric n. (L-1)
External oblique m.
Quadratus
lumborum m.
nternal oblique m.
Ilioinguinal n.
(L-1)
Transversus
abdominis m.
Iliolumbar ligament;
4th lumbar a. and v.
Lat. femoral
cutan. n.
Psoas major m.;
Psoas minor m.
Iliacus m.
Sigmoid aa.
Middle sacral
a. and v.;
sacral promontory
Common iliac
a. and v.
Sup. rectal
artery
emoral br.;
Genital br.;
nitofemoral
nerve
Femoral nerve
Iliac branches
Iliolumbar
a. and v.
Int. iliac
a. and v.
Genito-
femoral n.
mesocolon
Internal
iliac artery
Pelvis minor;
Rectovesical pouch
Lateral umbilical fold
(inf. epigastric a. and v.)
Rectum
Medial umbilical fold
(ligament of umbilical artery)
Urinary bladder
Rectus abdominis m.

Median umbilical fold (urachus)

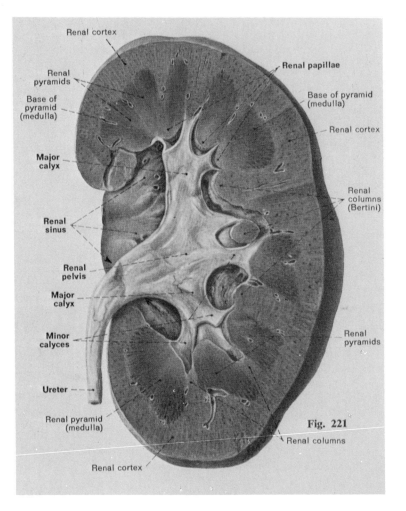

Renal cortex

Renal pyramids

Base of pyramid (medulla)

Major calyx

Renal sinus

Renal pelvis

Major calyx

Minor calyces

Ureter

Renal pyramid (medulla)

Renal cortex

Renal papillae

Base of pyramid (medulla)

Renal cortex

Renal columns (Bertini)

Renal pyramids

Renal columns

Fig. 221

Top Left: Left kidney, showing frontal section through the renal pelvis (Clemente, *Atlas of the Human Body,* Urban & Schwarzenberg). As the organs of the urinary system, the kidneys are involved in filtration and excretion of toxic body byproducts. High blood pressure, elecrolyte imbalances, and renal stone formation are some side effects of anabolic-steroid abuse that can seriously damage this organ. Wilm's tumor, a very serious cancer in adults, has been associated with steroid use. Flank pain and blood in the urine are early-warning signs that something is amiss. Bottom left photo shows Wilm's tumor (the actual kidney is shaded here, the rest being the cancerous tumor growth), a common kidney tumor in children but very rare in adults (less than 15 cases of such tumors in adults appear in the medical literature).

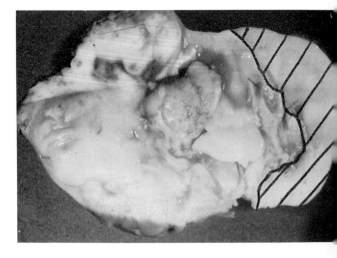

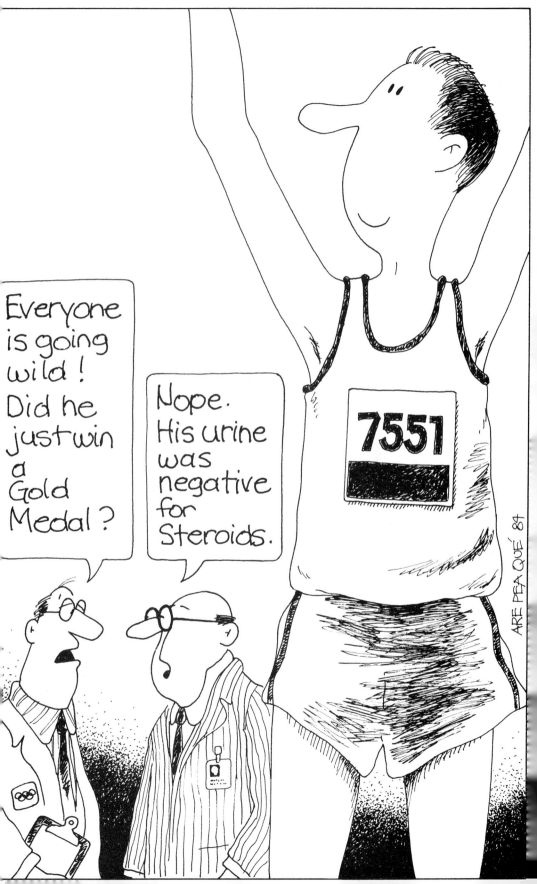

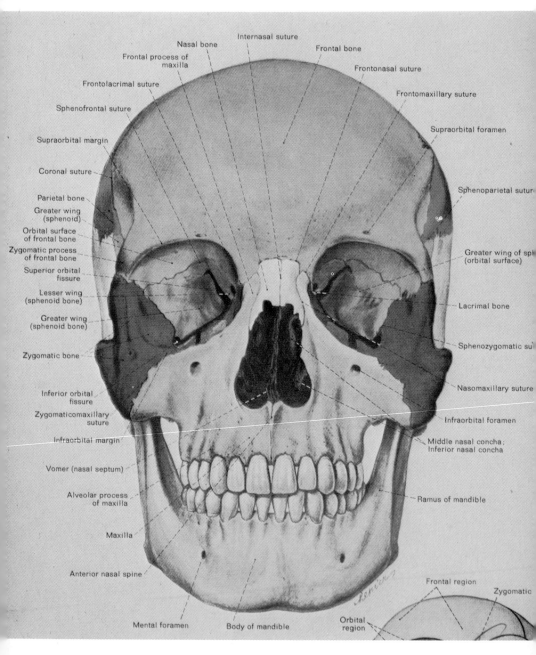

Internasal suture

Nasal bone

Frontal process of maxilla

Frontal bone

Frontonasal suture

Frontolacrimal suture

Frontomaxillary suture

Sphenofrontal suture

Supraorbital foramen

Supraorbital margin

Coronal suture

Sphenoparietal sutur

Parietal bone

Greater wing (sphenoid)

Orbital surface of frontal bone

Zygomatic process of frontal bone

Greater wing of spl (orbital surface)

Superior orbital fissure

Lesser wing (sphenoid bone)

Lacrimal bone

Greater wing (sphenoid bone)

Sphenozygomatic su

Zygomatic bone

Nasomaxillary suture

Inferior orbital fissure

Zygomaticomaxillary suture

Infraorbital foramen

Infraorbital margin

Middle nasal concha; Inferior nasal concha

Vomer (nasal septum)

Alveolar process of maxilla

Ramus of mandible

Maxilla

Anterior nasal spine

Frontal region

Zygomatic

Mental foramen

Body of mandible

Orbital region

This spread shows drawings of normal skulls (from Clemente, *Atlas of the Human Body* [Urban & Schwarzenberg, publishers] and Sobotta, *Atlas of Human Anatomy*, vol. 1, ed. H. Ferner and J. Staubesand [Urban Schwarzenberg, publishers]) compared with X-rays of male acromegalic patients (from *Atlas of Endocrine Diseases*, by Jerzy Kosowicz [Bowie, MD: Charles Press], courtesy of Dr. Kosowicz).

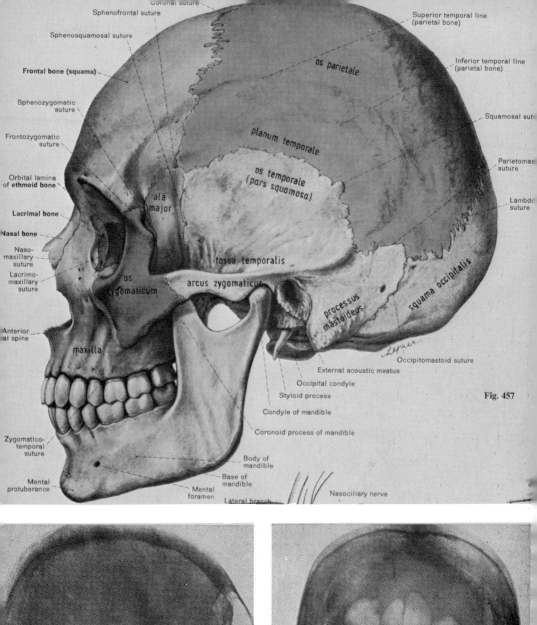

Coronal suture
Sphenofrontal suture
Sphenosquamosal suture
Frontal bone (squama)
Sphenozygomatic suture
Frontozygomatic suture
Orbital lamina of ethmoid bone
Lacrimal bone
Nasal bone
Naso-maxillary suture
Lacrimo-maxillary suture
Anterior nasal spine
maxilla
Zygomatico-temporal suture
Mental protuberance

Superior temporal line (parietal bone)
Inferior temporal line (parietal bone)
os parietale
Squamosal sut...
Parietomas... suture
planum temporale
os temporale (pars squamosa)
Lambda... suture
ala major
fossa temporalis
arcus zygomaticus
os zygomaticum
processus mastoideus
squama occipitalis
Occipitomastoid suture
External acoustic meatus
Occipital condyle
Styloid process
Condyle of mandible
Coronoid process of mandible
Body of mandible
Base of mandible
Mental foramen
Lateral branch
Nasociliary nerve

Fig. 457

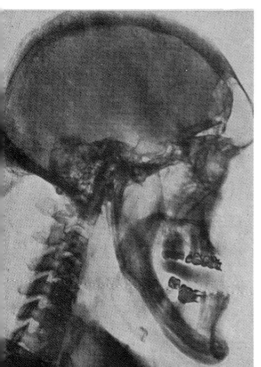

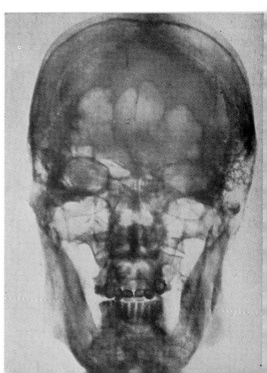

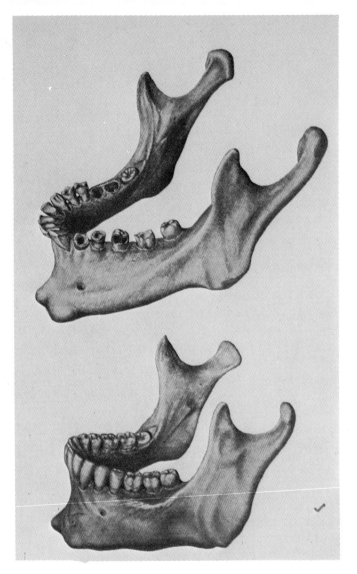

Left: Normal versus agromegalic jawbone, showing the incredible growth of the mandible (from Kosowicz' *Atlas of the Human Body,* Urban & Schwarzenberg, publishers). Below, left and right: X-ray and skull of acromegalic subject (from *Atlas of Clinical Endocrinology* [2nd ed.] by Lisser and Escamilla, courtesy of Elizabeth S. Escamilla).

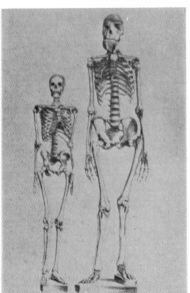

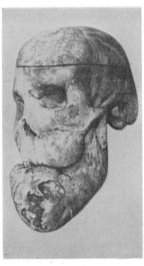

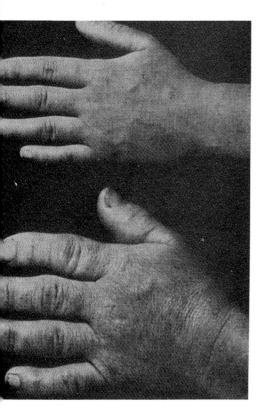
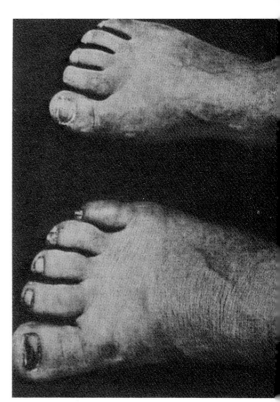
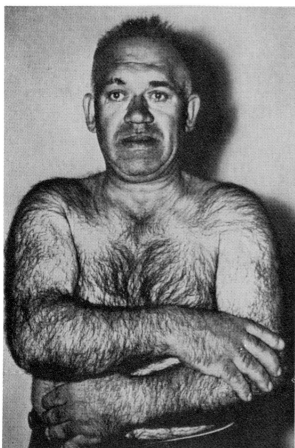

Above: Hands and feet of normal v. acromegalic subject. Left: Acromegalic man, showing coarse, enlarged features and extreme hair growth (from *Atlas of Endocrine Diseases*, by Jerzy Kosowicz [Bowie, MD: Charles Press], courtesy of Dr. Kosowicz).

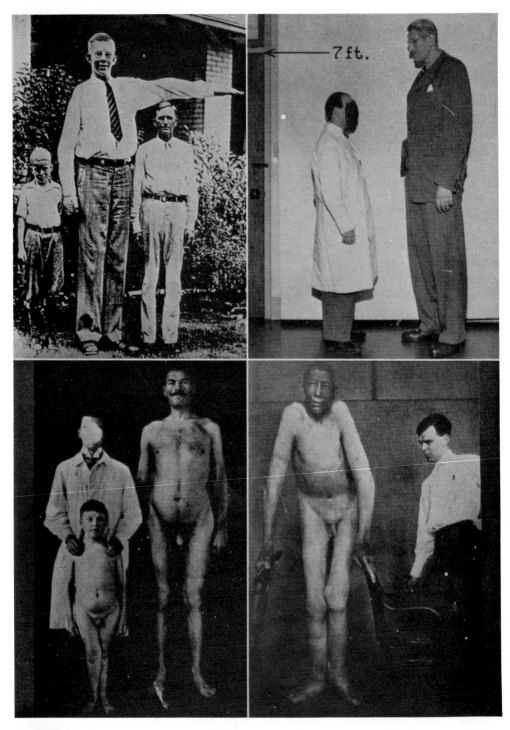

Left to right, top to bottom: The Alton giant, at age 14, when he was 7′ 6¹/₂″ in height and weighed 360 lbs. At age 18 he reached the height of 8′ 3¹/₄″, weighing 395 lbs. He is wearing a size 34 shoe here. The next subject is 43, 7′ 6¹/₂″, and weighs 359 lbs. The doctor beside him is 5′ 9³/₄″ tall. The Bulgarian giant of Falta at 24 (6′ 11¹/₂″, 429 lbs.) is posed with normal individual of over 6′ and a hypophyseal dwarf. Finally, the Cushing giant (8′ 3¹/₄″—although this has been disputed) has feeble, eunuchoid appearance (all from *Atlas of Clinical Endocrinology* [2nd ed.], by Lisser and Escamilla, courtesy of Elizabeth S. Escamilla). Most giants and acromegalics do not live long. With the abuse of HGH, a new fear arises. Once the body has reached full growth and HGH is taken, the visceral organs grow along with the soft tissues and bones of the hands, feet, and face, resulting in coarse, exaggerated features.

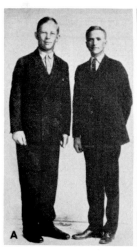
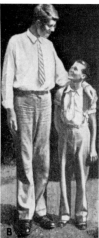
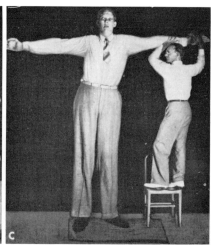

Above: A series of photos of the Alton giant, Robert Wadlow, who weighed only 9 lbs. at birth, but soon commenced in quick growth— he was 30 lbs. at six months, 62 lbs. at one year, and after his death at the age of 22, he was measured at 8′ 11″ and 475 lbs. (These photos are from Robert Williams' *Textbook on Endocrinology*, W. B. Saunders Co., 1981, which took them from F. Fadner, *Biography of Robert Wadlow*, Bruce Humphries, Publishers, 1944, and courtesy of C. M. Charles and C. M. MacBryde). Right: The face of a typical acromegalic male shows distortion of skull features and soft tissues of the face (from *Atlas of Endocrine Diseases*, by Jerzy Kosowicz [Bowie, MD: Charles Press], courtesy of Dr. Kosowicz).

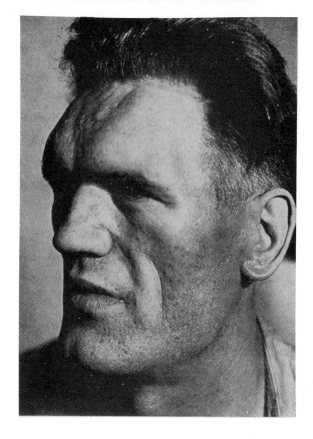

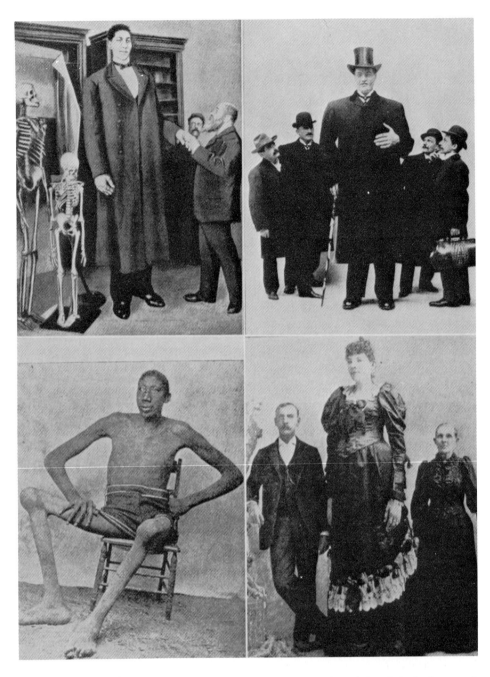

Left to right, top to bottom: The giant Machnow (7' 10") next to a short skeleton of a bushman and a tall one of a Patagonian. The giant Hugo (7' 6½") at age 25. The Tennessee giant (8' 6") at age 28. Note disproportionately long arms, legs, fingers, and feet. He had had severe arthritis. The Missouri giantess, Ella Ewing at age 25. Her alleged height was 8' 2". She stands between her father (6' 2") and mother (5' 1½"). From *Atlas of Clinical Endocrinology* (2nd ed.), by Lisser and Escamilla, courtesy of Elizabeth S. Escamilla).

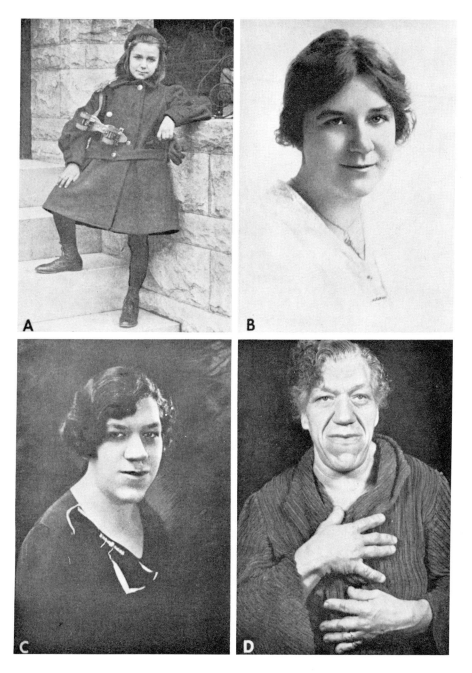

This series of photos from Williams' *Textbook on Endocrinology* (W. B. Saunders, 1981), show an acromegalic woman at ages, 9, 16, 33, and 52.

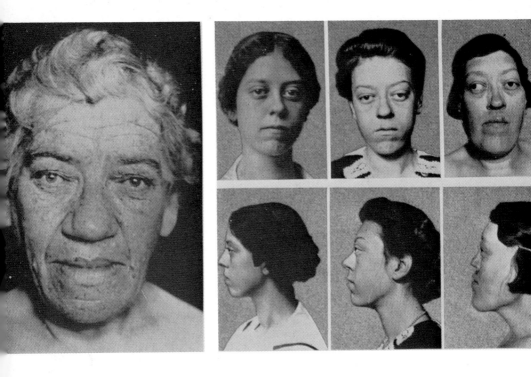

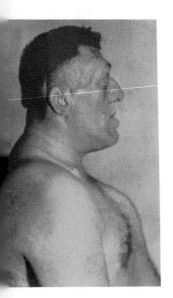

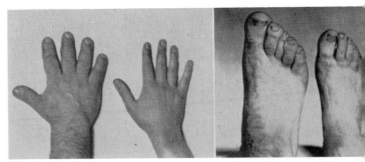

Top left: Acromegalic woman with typical facial features. Top, series of six photos: front and profile photos of young girl with acromegaly at ages 16, 25, and 44. Above left: Profile of same patient as on adjacent page. Center and right: Comparisons of hand and foot of normal and acromegalic male. (All photos from *Atlas of Clinical Endocrinology* [2nd ed.], by Lisser and Escamilla, courtesy of Elizabeth S. Escamilla).

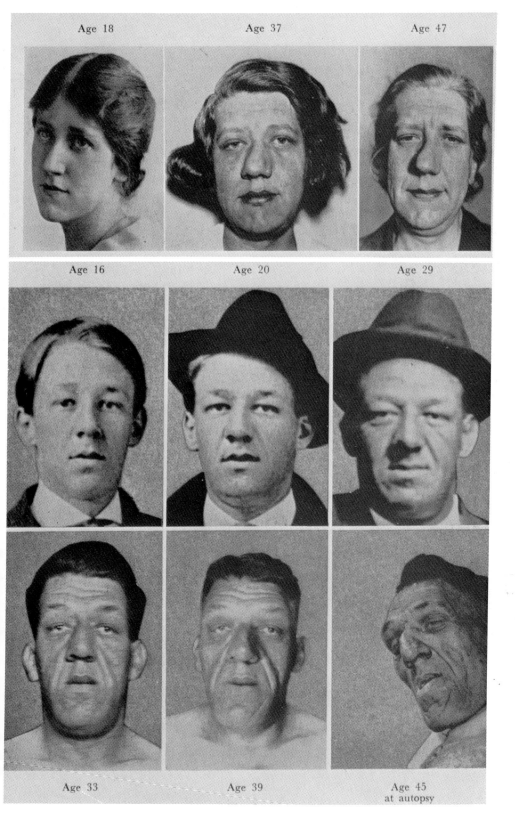

Age 18   Age 37   Age 47

Age 16   Age 20   Age 29

Age 33   Age 39   Age 45
at autopsy

Progressive coarsening of features of acromegalic female (at ages 18, 37, and 47) and male (at ages 16, 20, 29, 33, 39, and at autopsy at age 45). From *Atlas of Clinical Endocrinology* (2nd ed.), by Lisser and Escamilla, courtesy of Elizabeth S. Escamilla.

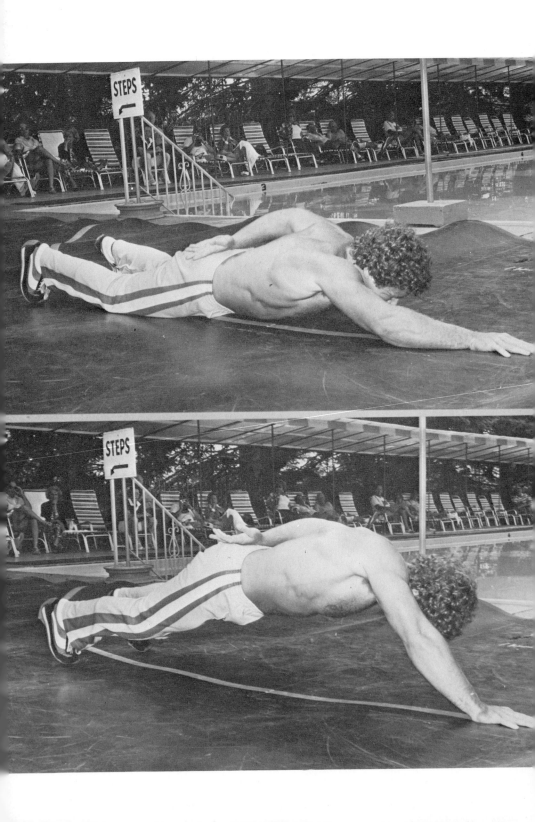

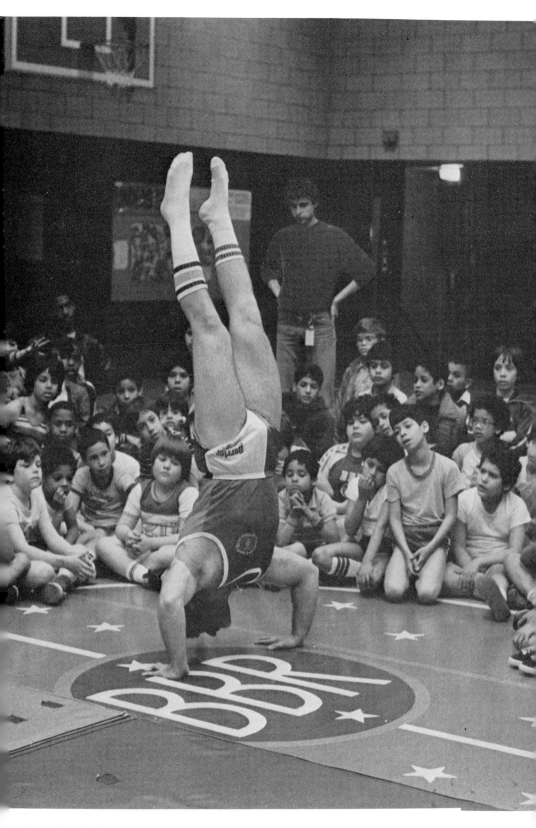

Author Bob Goldman en route to a record-setting 211 consecutive one-arm straight overhead extension push-ups (left) and demonstrating handstand push-ups, a strength feat in which he also holds world records, to underprivileged children (right). Overleaf: Goldman with some of his many strength-sport trophies.

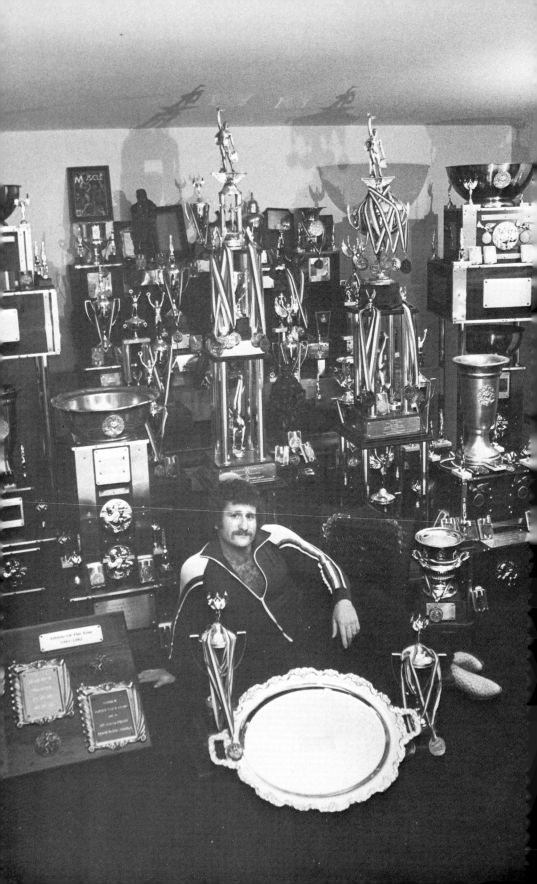

Med., 284 (1971):1135-1136.

6. R. Bowers and J. Reardon, "Effects of Methandro-stenolone (Dianabol) on Strength Development and Aerobic Capacity," Med. Sci. Sports, 4 (1972):54.

7. R.A. Burger and P.M. Marcuse, "Peliosis Hepatitis, Report of a Case," Am. J. Clin. Path., 22(1952):569-573.

8. H. Byerly, "Explaining and Exploiting Placebo Effects," Prosp. Biol. Med., 19 (1976):423-436.

9. S. Casner, R. Early and B.R. Carlson, "Anabolic Steroid Effects on Body Composition in Normal Young Men," J. Sports Med. and Phys. Fit., 11 (1971):98-103.

10. T.D. Fahey and C.H. Brown, "The Effects of an Anabolic Steroid on the Strength, Body Composition and Endurance of College Males When Accompanied by a Weight Training Program," Med. Sci. Sports, 5 (1973):272-276.

11. G.C. Farrell, D.E. Joshua, R.F. Uren, P.J. Baird, K.W. Perkins and H. Kraienberg, "Androgen-Induced Hepatoma," Lancet, 1 (1975):430-431.

12. W.M. Fowler, Jr., G.W. Gardner and G.H. Egstrom, "Effect of an Anabolic Steroid on Physical Performance of Young Men," J. Appl. Physiol., 20 (1965):1038-1040.

13. L.A. Golding, J.E. Freydinger, and S.S. Fishel, "Weight, Size and Strength—Unchanged by Steroids," Physician Sports Med., 2 (1974):39-45.

14. J.T. Guy and M.O. Auxlander, "Androgenic Steroids and Hepatocellular Carcinoma," Lancet, 1 (1973):148.

15. R.A. Harkness, B.H. Kilshaw and B.M. Hobson, "Effects of Large Doses of Anabolic Steroids," Brit. J. Sport Med., 9 (1975):70-73.

16. J.T. Henderson, J. Richmond and M.D. Sumerling, "Androgenic-Anabolic Steroid Therapy and Hepato-cellular Carcinoma," Lancet, 1 (1972):934.

17. F.L. Johnson, "The Association of Oral Androgenic-Anabolic Steroids and Life Threatening Disease," Med. Sci. Sports, 7 (1975):284-286.

18. F.L. Johnson, J.R. Feagler, K.G. Lerner, P.W. Majems, M. Siegel, J.R. Hartman and E.D. Thomas, "Association of Androgenic-Anabolic Steroid Therapy with Development of Hepato-cellular Carcinoma," Lancet, 2 (1972):1273-1276.

19. L.C. Johnson, G. Fisher, L.J. Sylvester and C.C. Hofheins, "Anabolic Steroid: Effects on Strength, Body Weight, O_2 Uptake and Spermatogenesis in Mature Males," Med. Sci. Sports, 4 (1972):43-45.

20. L.C. Johnson and J.P. O'Shea, "Anabolic Steroid: Effects on Strength Development," Science, 164 (1969):957-959.

21. L.C. Johnson, E.S. Roundy, P. Allsen, A.G. Fisher and L.J. Sylvester, "Effect of Anabolic Steroid Treatment on Endurance," Med. Sci. Sports, 7 (1975):287-289.

22. B.H. Kilshaw, R.A. Harkness, B.M. Hobson and A.W.M. Smith, "The Effects of Large Doses of the Anabolic Steroid, Methandro-stenolone on an Athlete," Clin. Endocr., 4 (1975):537-541.

23. W. Kintzen and J. Silny, "Peliosis Hepatitis after Administration of

Fluoxymesterone," *Canad. Med. Assoc. J.*, 83 (1960):860-862.

24. K.B. McCredie, "Oxymetholone in Refractory Anemia," *Brit. J. of Haemtology,* 17 (1969):265-273.

25. A.T. Meadows, J.L. Naiman and M.V. Valdes-Dapena, "Hepatoma Associated with Androgen Therapy for Aplastic Anemia," *J. Pediatr.*, 84 (1974):109-110.

26. J.P. O'Shea, "The Effects of an Anabolic Steroid on Dynamic Strength Levels of Weight Lifters," *Nutr. Report Internat.*, 4 (1971):363-370.

27. J.P. O'Shea and W. Winkler, "Biochemical and Physical Effects of an Anabolic Steroid in Competitive Swimmers and Weight Lifters," *Nutr. Report Internat.*, 2 (1970):351-362.

28. L. Recant and P. Lacy (eds.), "Fanconi's Anemia and Hepatic Cirrhosis," *Clinicopathologic Conference Am. J. Med.*, 39 (1965):464-475.

29. L. Sanchez-Medal, A. Gomez-Leal, L. Duarte and M. Guadalupe-Rico, "Anabolic-Androgenic Steroids in the Treatment of Acquired Aplastic Anemia," *Blood*, 34 (1969):283-300.

30. N.T. Shaidi, "Androgens and Erythropoiesis," *N. Engl. J. Med.*, 289 (1973):72-79.

31. S. Sherlock, "Disease of the Liver and Biliary System," 4th Edition, Philadelphia, *F.A. Davis*, (1968):371.

32. J. Silink and B.G. Firkin, "An Analysis of Hypoplastic Anaemia with Special Reference to the Use of Oxymetholone ('Adroyd') in Its Therapy," *Australian Ann. of Med.*, 17 (1968):224-234.

33. B.A. Stanford and R. Moffat, "Anabolic Steroid: Effectiveness as an Ergogenic aid to Experienced Weight Trainers," *J. Sports Med. and Phys. Fit.*, 14 (1974):191-197.

34. M. Steinbach, "Uber den Einfluss Anabolen Wirkstoffe und Korpergewicht Muskelkraft and Muskeltraining," *Sportarzt und Sport-medizin.*, 11 (1968):485-492.

35. L.T. Samuels, A.F. Henschel and A. Kays, "Influence of Methyltestosterone on Muscular Work and Creatine Metabolism in Normal Young Men.," *J. Clin. Endocrinol. Metab.*, 2 (1942):649-654.

36. S.B. Stromme, H.D. Meen and A.Aakvaag, "Effects of an Androgenic-Anabolic Steroid on Strength Development and Plasma Testosterone Levels in Normal Males," *Med. Sci. Sports*, 6 (1974):203-208.

37. P. Ward, "The Effect of an Anabolic Steroid on Strength and Lean Body Mass," *Med. Sci. Sports*, 5 (1973):277-282.

38. F.G. Zak, "Peliosis Hepatitis," *Am. J. Pathol.*, 26 (1950):1-15.

39. J. Ziegenfuss and R. Carabasi, "Androgens and Hepatocellular Carcinoma," *Lancet*, 1 (1973):262.

2
BRITISH ASSOCIATION OF SPORT AND MEDICINE POLICY STATEMENT ON DOPING, Published 1964

Bearing in mind the many implications of the use of chemical agents of one kind or another to modify artificially the performance of healthy human beings not only in sport but in all walks of life, the British Association of Sport and Medicine considers and recommends that:

1) The only effective and safe way of ensuring optimum performance in any activity is a proper programme of training and preparation.
2) No known chemical agent is capable of producing both safely and effectively an improvement in performance in a healthy human subject.
3) Every chemical agent taken by the healthy human subject with the intention of artificially improving his performance is in some degree harmful to the individual who takes it.
4) No purpose (other than medical—therapeutic or prophylactic) is properly to be served by the administration or use of chemical agents with the intention or effect of modifying human performance, except in cases of properly controlled experiment and research.
5) The use of chemical agents other than for medical purposes shall be regarded as doping.
6) Doping should be actively discouraged, and Governing Bodies of Sport and other interested parties should consider and implement what steps they can take appropriate to this end.
7) The public advertisement of chemical agents or preparations for purposes which fall within the definition of doping should cease and Parliamentary legislation to this end should be sought if necessary.
8) Appropriate methods should be evolved actively to curb the practice of doping, such methods to include an educational campaign, the prohibition of doping in the rules of Sports generally, the application of sanctions to offenders, and the introduction of suitable methods of test and control.
9) When a sportsman or woman is taking part in a competition while receiving drugs of any kind as a form of properly authorized medical treatment, the same should be made known in confidence to the duly authorized representatives of the body organizing the competition.
10) No drug included in the list shown in the second appendix to this draft shall ever be used for the properly authorized medical treatment

183

of any individual taking part in a sporting competition and where the use of any such prohibited drug is medically necessary the sportsman or woman concerned must be withdrawn from that competition. (Anabolic steroids fall into this category.)

The British Association of Sport and Medicine further considers that should its recommendations be put into effect the result can only be to the benefit of sport in particular, and the health of the community in general.

3
LIST OF DOPING SUBSTANCES TYPICALLY TESTED AT NATIONAL AND INTERNATIONAL SPORTING EVENTS

U. S. Olympic Committee on Sports Medicine List of Doping Substances

Psychomotor Stimulant Drugs, e.g.,
Amphetamine
Benzphetamine
Chlorphentermine
Cocaine
Diethylpropion
Dimethylamphetamine
Ethylamphetamine
Fencamfamin
Meclofenoxate
Methylamphetamine
Methylphenidate
Norpseudoephedrine
Pemoline
Phendimetrazine
Phenmetrazine
Phentermine
Pipradol
Prolintane
and related compounds

Sympathomimetic Amines, e.g.,
Chlorprenaline
Ephedrine
Etafedrine
Isoetharine
Isoprenaline
Methylephedrine
Methoxyphenamine
Pseudoephedrine

and related compounds

Miscellaneous Central Nervous System Stimulants, e.g.,
Amiphenazole
Bemegride
Doxapram
Ethamivan
Leptazol
Nikethamide
Picrotoxin
Strychnine
and related compounds

Narcotic Analgesics, e.g.,
Anileridine
Codeine
Dextromethorphan
Dextromoramide
Dihydrocodeine
Dipipanone
Ethylmorphine
Heroin
Hydrocodone
Hydromorphone
Levorphanol
Morphine
Methadone
Oxycodone
Oxymorphone
Pentazocine
Pethidine
Phenazocine
Piminodine
Thebacon
Trimeperidine
and related compounds

Anabolic Steroids, e.g.,
Methandienone
Stanozolol
Oxymetholone
Nandrolone decanoate
Nandrolone phenylpropionate
and related compounds

Other Lists of Doping Substances

Central Nervous System Stimulants and Psychomotor Stimulants
Imipramine *(antidepressant)*
  Imavate
  Janimine
  Presamine
  SK-Pramine
  Tofranil
Desipramine *(antidepressant)*
  Norpramin
  Pertofrane
Amitriptyline *(antidepressant)*
  Endep
  Elavil HCl
  Etrafon
  Triavil
Nortriptyline *(antidepressant)*
  Aventyl HCl
Doxeprin *(antidepressant)*
  Sinequan
  Adapin
Protriptyline *(antidepressant)*
  Vivactil
Amphetamine *(CNS stimulant, vasoconstrictor)*
  Benzedrine
  Levamphetamine
Dextroamphetamine *(central stimulant)*
  Daro, Preps
  Amphedex
  Dexampex
  Dexedrine
  Diphylets
  Ferndex
  Oxydess
  Robese-P
  Spancan #1, #4
  Tidex
  Amphadex
  Biphetamine $7^1/_2$, $12^1/_2$, 20
  Delcobese
  Dexamyl
  Dextroban
  Mingera

   Rotrim
   Trimex
   Trimex #2
   Obotan
   Obotan Forte
Methamphetamine (*central stimulant*)
   Desoxyn
   Methampex
   Methamphetamine HCl
   Obedrine-LA
   Stimdex
   Obe-Slim
   Span-RD
   Aridol
   Fetamin
   Oxydess
   Roxyn
   Meditussin-X
Phentermine (*anorexiant*)
   Adipex-P
   Fastin
   Ionamin
   Parmine
   Phentrol
   Rolaphent
   Tora
   Wilpo
   Wilpowr
Chlorphentermine (*appetite suppressant*)
   Lucofen
   Chlorophen
   Pre-Sate
Fenfluramine (*appetite suppressant*)
   Pondarex
   Pondimin
   Pendimin
Benzphetamine (*anorexiant*)
   Didrex
Phenmetrazine (*appetite suppressant*)
   Melfiat
   Preludin
Diethylpropion (*appetite suppressant*)
   Amfepramone
   Nudisproz

Ro-Diet
Ro-Diet Timed
Tenuate
Tepanil
Methylphenidate (*treatment for hyperactivity*)
Ritalin
Pemoline
Cylert
Tranylcypromine
Parnate
Phendimetrazine (*anorexic*)
Adphen
Anorx
Bacarate
B.O.F.
Bontril
Delcozine
Di-Ap-Trol
Dietabs
Dimetrix
Elphemet
Ex-Obese
Limit
Minus
Neo-Nilorex
Obacin
Obalan
Obepar
Obe-Tite
Obezine
Phenazine
Phendorex
Phen-70
Phentazine
Phenzine
Plegine
Reducto
Robese "P" Tabl. Vial
Ropledge
Slim Tabs
SPRX 1, 2, & 3
Statobex products
Stim-35
Stodex

Tanorex
Trimtabs
Weightrol
Iproniazid (*MAO inhibitors, treats depression, high blood pressure or angina*)
  Marslin Phosphate
Isocarboxazid (*MAO inhibitor*)
  Marplan
Phenalzine (*MAO inhibitor*)
  Nardil
Pargyline (*MAO inhibitor*)
  Eutonyl
Tranlcypromine (*MAO inhibitor*)
  Parnate
Picrotoxin (*respiratory stimulation*)
  Picrotoxin
Pentylenetetrazol
  Metrazol
Nikethamide (*CNS stimulant*)
  Coramine
Ethamivan (*respiratory stimulation*)
  Vandid
Doxapram (*respiratory stimulation*)
  Dopram
Flurothyl (*CNS stimulation*)
  Indoklon
Caffeine (*cardiac, respiratory, psychic stimulant*)
  Enerjits
  Femicin
  Nodoz
  Stim 250
  Tirend
  Vivarin
  Xantrinux (*stimulates spinal cord reflexes*)
  Caffeine-Citrated
  Caffeine Sodium Benzoate
  Caffeine Sodium Salicylate
  Theophylline
Aminophylline (*bronchodilator, smooth-muscle relaxant*)
  Aminodur
  Dura-Tab
  Lixaminol
  Rectalad-Aminophylline
  Somophyllin Oral Liquid

Somophyllin Rectal Solution
Amesec
Aminophylline and Amytal
Amphedrine Compound
Amsac
Amsacol
Asmadrin
Asminorel
Astmacon
B.M.E.
Bronchovent
Dainite
Lixaminol
Mini-lix
Mudrane
Orthoxine and Aminophylline
Quinamm
Romanhed
Strema
Theocomp
Theokaps
Verophylline
Amodrine
Kiaphyllin
Mudran GG
Aminophylline Injection
Aminophylline Suppositories
Aminophylline Tablets
Aminophylline-Phenobarbital
Aminophylline-Phenobarbital #1
Theobromine
　Thoeminal RS
　Harbolin
　Theocardone
　T.P.K. 1
　Theobromide Calcium Gluconate
　Theocalcin
　Athemol
　Doan's Pills
　Theolaphen

Sympathomimetic Amines

Levateranol (*CNS stimulant*)

Levophed Bitartrate
Dopamine (*as above and vasodilator*)
  Intropin
Epinephrine (*CNS stimulant*)
  Amolin
  Emergency AMA Kit
  Sus-Phrine
  Asthma Meter
Norepinephrine (*CNS stimulant*)
  Propadine
  Levophed bitartrate
Isoproterenol (*smooth muscle relaxant, brochodilator, asthma*)
  Iprenol
  Isuprel
  Norisodrine
  Aerotol
  Proterenol
  Vap-Iso
  Asminorel
  Aerolone compound
  Brondialate
  Isophed
  Iso-Asminyl
  Duohaler
  Duo-Medi-Haler
  Nebair
Phenylephrine (*vasoconstrictor, hypotensive agent, contained in nose-drops*)
  Alcon-Efrin
  Coricdin decongestant nasal mist
  Coryzine
  Ephrine
  Isophrin
  Neo-Synephrine HCl
  Pyracort-D
  Sinarest
  Superanahist Nasal Spray
  Synasal
  Acotus
  Allerest
  Anodynos
  Bellafedrol
  Bihisdin
  Bromo quinine cold tablets

Bar-Tuss expectorant
CDM expectorant
Cenahist
Cenaid
Chlor-Trimeton expectorant
Clistin-D
Conar
Conar-A
Congespirin
Contac nasal mist
Coricidin Demlets
Govanamine tablets
Dallergy
Demazin
Dri-Drip
Emagrin Forte
Extex K.I.
Expectico pediatric cough syrup
Eye-Gene
4-Way tablets, spray
Furacin nasal solution
Histabid
Histapp products
Histospan-D
Histospan-Plus
Kleer Products
Naal
Na-Co-Al
Nasahist
Noraphen-Plus Spamcap
Phenylzin drops (opthalmic solution)
PMP Preps
Presco nose drops
Phyraphed
Prysitan
Sinarest
Sinex
Singlet
Spectab
Spec-T sore throat decongestant lozenges
Sucrets cold decongestant lozenges
Tri-Ophtho solution
T-Spray
Turbilixir

Turpispan leisure caps
Valihist
Salbutamol (*CNS stimulator, brochodilator*)
Ventolin
Hyproxyamphetamine (*weak vasoconstrictor*)
Paredrine Hydrobromide
Mephentermine (*nasal decongestant*)
Synalgos
Wyamine
Metaraminol (*vasoconstrictor*)
Aramine
Pressonex
Methoxamine (*vasoconstrictor*)
Vasoxyl
Ephedrine (*brochodilator, for asthma*)
Ephedrine and procaine
Asthmaden
Airet-R
Airet-X
Amphed
Ephedrine
Anoiss Rectal
Asmadil-S Susp
Asma Lief
Asthmacon
Asthmadan
Bofedral
Bronsed
Brondialate
Calcidrine
Ceepa
Codel
Coryza brengle
Co-Xan
Dainite-DAY
Dainite-KL
Derma Medicone
Derma Medicone HC
Dilacap
Duovent
Ectasule
Emphysal
Epragen
Fedralen

For-Az-Ma
Golacal
Hemocaine
Histamead
Kie
Lardet expectorant
Lardet
Luftodil
Lufyllin-EP
Lyfylliln-EPG
Mudrane-GG
Mudrane
Myringacaine
Omnituss
Panaphyllin
Phedral
Phrralan
Quadrinal
Quelidrine
Quibron Plus
Tedfern
Tedral-25
T.E.P.
T.E.P. compound
Thalfed
Theofed
Theofenal susp.
Theokaps
Theospan
Verequad
Ephedrine HCl nasal jelly
Ephedrine and Numbutal-25 (*sedative, antispasmatic*)
Ephedrine and Phenobarbital
Ephedrine and Seconal Sodium (*nocturnal asthma*)
Ectasule Minus, Jr. & Sr.
Isofedrol
Slo-Fedrin
Slo-Fedrine
Aladrine
Asminorel
Aminul
B.M.E.
Bronkaid
Bronkolixir

Bronkotabs
CPC cough syrup
Ectasule caps
Ectasule Minus
Ephed Organidin
Eponel
Fednal
Flavihist
Hycoff-X
Isoasminyl
Luasmin
Marax DF
Marax
Masothylline
Nasus
Neogen
Neospect
Nyquil
Pazo
Pheno-Fed
Puribenzamine w/ephedrine
Pyribenzamine expectorant w/ephedrine
Rectacort
Thymodyne
Tri-Hist caps
Va-Trol-Nol
Wyanoids
Rynatuss
Pseudo Ephedrine (*antihistamine, antitussant*)
  Sudafed
  Besan
  Cenafed
  D-Feda
  Naldegesic
  Novafed
  Ro-Fedin
  Sudabid
  Actifed
  Asmidil Unicelles
  Actifed-C expectorant
  Asthmaspan
  Ayr
  Ayrcap
  Az-Cap

Brexin
Bronchobid
Chlorphen liquid and tablets
Control D
Co-Tylenol
Co-Tylenol liquid cold formula
Deconamine
Dilorbron
Dimacol
Emprazil
Fedahist
Historal
Intensin
Isoclor
Novafed-A
Phenergan comp.
Phenergan-D
Rhinosyn
Rondec (drops, tablets, syrup, filmtab)
Rondec DM
Sinacet
Sudahist
Suda-Proll
Theo-Sed
Trifed
Trifed tablets
Tussfed Expectorant
Phenylpropanolamine (*sympathomimetic*)
Propadrine HCl
Alclear Antiallergy Tablets
Alcon Decongestant
Algecol
Algetuss
Allerest products
Allergesic
Allerstat
Amaril "D" Span Capsules
ARM Tablets
Bayer Products
Blu-Hist
Bowman decongestant comp. inj.
Breacol cough medication
Bur-Tuss Expectorant
Chexit

Contac
Contac Jr.
Cophene #2
Rynatussadine
Sanhist
Santussin
Sinacol
Sinahist
Sinaphen
Sine-Aid
Sine-Off
Soltice Products
Sinubid
Sinudan
Sinulin
Sinutab
Spec-T sore throat decongestant lozenges
Sto-Caps
Sucrets cold decongestant lozenges
Super Anahist tablets
Symptomax
Symptrol
Teragen
Triaminic
Triaminicin tablets, chewable, spray
Triaminicol
Tricongestic
Trihistin Expectorant
Trinade
Turbilixir
Turbispan Leisure Caps
Tusquelin
Tussagesic susp., tablets
Tussaminic
Tusscaps
Tusstrol
U.R.I. caps, liquid
Vernate

List of Doping Substances in the U.S. Olympic Committee on Sports Medicine But Not Pharmacology Texts

CNS Stimulants and Psychomotor Stimulants

Cocaine (*surface anaesthetic, used in opthalmic and otolaryngologic surgery*)
    Cocaine and Homatropine oily eyedrops
    Cocaine and mercuric chloride oily eyedrops
    Cocaine oily eyedrops
    Atropine and cocaine eye ointment
    Cocaine, adrenaline and zinc eyedrops
    Cocaine eyedrops
    Cocaine and adrenaline eyedrops
    Strong (or weak) cocaine eyedrops
    Cocaine paste
    Pasta cocainae composita
    Bonain's anaesthetic mixture
    Bonain's anaesthetic mixture w/adunaline
    Cocaine solution
    Nebula cocainae et ephedrinae
Dimethylamphetamine (*unlisted*)
Ethylamphetamine (*unlisted*)
Fencanfamin (*CNS stimulant, appetite suppressant*)
    Euvitaol
    Reactivin
Meclofenoxate (*cerebral stimulant*)
    Lucidril
    Helfergin
    Lutiaron
    Ropoxyl
Norpseudophedrine (*CNS stimulant*)
    Mirapront N (cathine)
Pipradrol (*CNS stimulant*)
    Meratran
Prolintane ("tonic")
    Villescon
    Promotil
Amiphenazole (*respiratory stimulant*)
    Daptazole
    Daptazile
Bemegride (*medullary respiratory stimulant*)
    Megimide
    Eukraton
Leptazol (*medullary respiratory stimulant*)
    Pentylenetetrazol
    Cardiazol

Metalex-P
Metrazol
Strychnine (*no therapeutic justification, rodenticide*)

Sympathomimetic Amines

Chlorprenaline HCl (*bronchodilator*)
Etafedrine HCl (*relief of asthma bronchitis*)
  Nethaprin Dospan
  Nethaprin expectorant
Methylepedrin HCl (*bronchodilator*)
  Metheph
Methoxyphen Amine (*bronchodilator*)
  Orthoxine HCl
  Orthoxine and aminophylline
  Pyrrotate
  Orthoxicol
  Statuss
  Medrol
  Metasma

4
THERAPEUTIC USES OF ANABOLIC STEROIDS

When used correctly and with caution, anabolic steroids have some very fine therapeutic uses, such as: treatment of osteoporosis, for patients recovering from an illness, or after surgery; for fracture healing; severe burns; protein tissue building and myotrophism; to stimulate the appetite; and for muscular dystrophy. They are mostly used as adjunctive therapy and are also effective in treating pituitary dwarfism when the growth hormone is not available, control of metastatic breast cancer, and as adjunctive therapy in special cases of refractory anemia and aplastic anemia.

1. *Surgery.* Steroids aid and promote healing; improve appetite; increase protein synthesis; serve as a protective aid for blood producing bone marrow after malignant tumors have been treated with radiation therapy.
2. *Skeletal Disorders.* Anabolic steroids aid and stimulate the formation of the protein matrix of the bone; they help to retard the effects of osteoporosis which occurs in the elderly as a bone loss.
3. *Starvation and Malnutrition.* For individuals who have an insufficient intake of dietary protein. This occurs most in the elderly. Improved appetite results allowing the stimulation of cellular growth. Negative nitrogen balance can be corrected. The patient has an uplifted psychological disposition and may experience a feeling of well-being.
4. *Balance Therapy.* For patients who might have a low hormonal production rate.
5. Therapeutic use for *muscular dystrophy* and *diabetes.*

Many athletes feel that the use of anabolic steroids will increase their strength. It is a possibility that the studies involving men over 50 that showed increased strength levels for the subjects might have been due to the fact that these men might have had below normal testosterone levels as a result of their age. Hettinger reported a direct relationship between the urinary excretion of 17-ketosteroids (which are lower in older individuals) and the amount of strength possible during training.

The use of steroids helps prevent nitrogen loss, an important factor in subjects trying to gain weight. There has been a trend towards manufacturing anabolic steroids that are highly anabolic with little of the androgenic properties. This would add to the muscle-building qualities while cutting down on the chance of harmful side effects. Steroids aid the utilization of protein and can prove useful in patients with nutritional problems.

6. For patients suffering from *rheumatoid arthritis.*
7. For patients suffering from irretractable *Reynaud's Syndrome* noted in collagen vascular diseases.
8. For patients with *chronic anemias.*
9. For *kidney dialysis* patients.
10. For patients with *osteoporosis,* androgens can improve the calcium balance and increase bone resorption (see 2.)
11. In *aging men with reduced libido* and sexual activity.
12. For treatment of *endometriosis,* a disorder where endometrial tissue is found outside the uterus. This tissue may cause dysmenorrhea or even sterility.
13. For men who are subject to male-pattern baldness.
14. To accelerate growth in in childhood, e.g., girls with Turners Syndrome or children of short stature. However, the younger the child, the greater the risk or compromising the final mature height. This is a much-debated area of use.

5
ANABOLIC ANDROGENIC RESEARCH STUDIES

ABSTRACTS OF RESEARCH PAPERS

There are a number of critical weaknesses in much of the research that has been done in this area.

1. The dosages used are well below what is common practice among athletes. In addition, many athletes "stack" or use several different drugs at the same time for what they feel will provide synergistic or exponential gains.
2. There is not proper control in some studies.
3. Many studies lack cross-over designs.
4. The subjects might be untrained, and if they do train with resistance exercise, their workouts might be limited in duration and modality.
5. The protein and caloric intake might be below what the body needs to grow.
6. Many studies are not double-blind ones.
7. Oftentimes, these studies use a small population pool or one that does not correspond to the individuals actually using the drugs.
8. Sometimes, manipulation of the statistics, measurement methods, or other parameters give erroneous results.

WHEN ORAL DRUGS HAVE BEEN USED

1. Some oral agents may withstand proper degradation by the liver on the first pass, not allowing proper resorption of the metabolites into the bloodstream.
2. The acid secretions of the stomach may destroy much of the drug used, if not properly prepared.
3. The drug must have metabolites that can be properly absorbed in the gastrointestinal tract and small bowel.
4. Following absorption, the metabolites of the drug must retain their characteristics and binding capacities.
5. Oral drug half-life (time in body) is generally shorter than depot injections. In order to maintain therapeutic levels, orals might have to be taken every few hours as the drugs are metabolized.

The following are abstracts of some of the principal research studies performed in this area on human beings.

Dr. Gideon Ariel, while at the University of Massachusetts in the 1970s, explored the residual effect of anabolic steroids upon isotonic muscular force. He tested male weight lifters from the university with a double-blind technique. He gave a placebo for four weeks to one group, followed by 15 mg. of methandrostenolone (an anabolic steroid) for the next four weeks of the study. He noted significant increases in strength in athletes during the time they were taking the steroids.

In another study, Dr. Ariel tested six male athletes for another double-blind study. The drug used was 10 mg. of 17-beta-hydroxy-17-alpha-methyl-androsta-1,4-diene-3-one (Dianabol), which again produced statistically significant gains in strength.

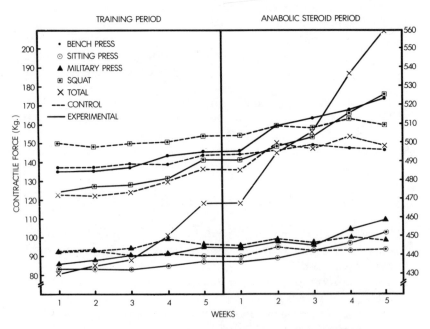

Journal of Sports Medicine & Physical Fitness, 13 (1973):187–90.

In another study, Ariel tested the effect Dianabol had on reflex components. He noted statistically faster reflex times and significantly lower latencies. From this, he extrapolated that anabolic steroids affect the central nervous system and biochemical processes involved in reflexes.

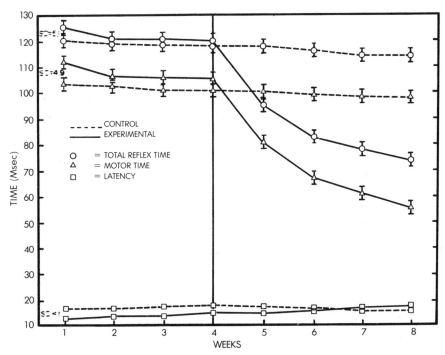

Medicine and Science in Sports, 4 (1972):120–23.

Drs. Simonson, Kearns, and Enzer studied the effects of methyl testosterone on the muscular performance and central nervous system in older men (aged 48–67). They used 30–40 mgs. of methyl testosterone and found an increase in back-muscle strength over the placebo group. They noted no increase in strength of the arm extensor and only a slight increase in handgrip strength in two of the six subjects.

David Freed et al. utilized the double-blind cross-over technique to test the effects of anabolic steroids on weight lifters. They picked thirteen male lifters on high protein diets and administered 10 to 25 mg./day of methadienone and a placebo. The drug caused numerous side effects, which prompted three of the subjects to withdraw from the study. They noted significant gains for the steroid over the placebo group.

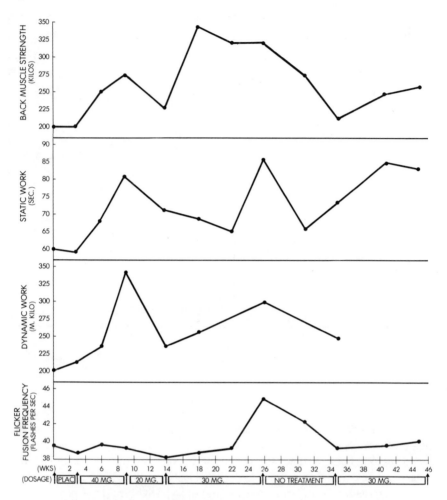

Effect of methyl testosterone dosage upon (a) back-muscle strength, (b) endurance in static-work performance, (c) dynamic-work performance, and (d) fusion frequency of flicker. The beginning and variation of treatment are indicated by arrows beneath the abscissa (weeks). Placebo administration does not show significant effects. In all muscle-performance tests (a, b,c), there is a peak at the end of the 40 mg. period (ninth week); a drop during the following 20 mg. period; a renewed increase during the 30 mg. period, with the peak of back-muscle strength in the eighteenth week and of static and dynamic performance in the twenty-sixth week; a drop after cessation of treatment; and increase again after renewal of treatment with 30 mg. (back-muscle strength and static performance only). The fusion frequency (d) shows no significant reaction before twenty-two weeks; a peak is reached at the end of 30-mg. period (twenty-sixth week), from which it drops after cessation of treatment and slowly increases again after renewal of 30-mg. administration.

Journal of Clinical Endocrinology and Metabolism, 4 (1944):528–34.

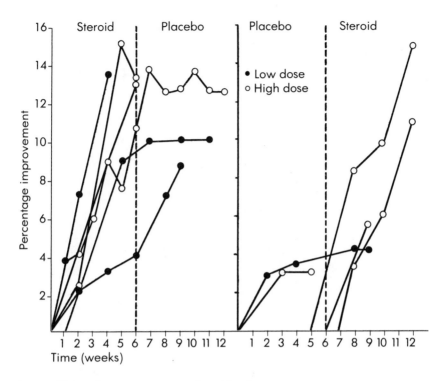

Average athletic performance as percentage of pretrial performance.

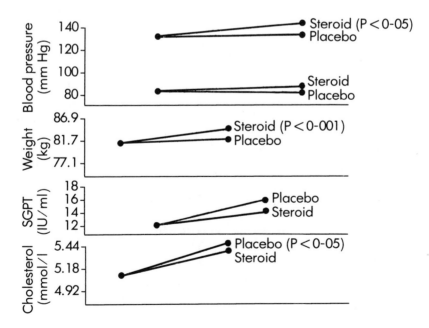

Mean changes in weight, blood pressure, and biochemical values during trial.
Conversion: SI to Traditional Units—Cholesterol: 1mmo/1 = 38.7 mg/100 ml.

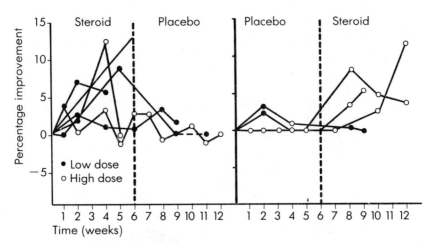

Average athletic performance as percentage of performance reported on previous visit. Any point greater than zero means that improvement has continued since then.

British Medical Journal, May 31, 1975.

One of the first contemporary studies was done in 1965 by Dr. William Fowler, Jr., and associates. This study involved forty-seven healthy men as subjects, ranging from eighteen to twenty-five years old. Ten of the subjects competed in rugby during the study, while the rest were untrained college students. The untrained men were placed in four randomly selected treatment groups. Nine men received androstenolone, eight were given a placebo, ten more were given exercise with the placebo, and the final ten were given exercise and androstenolone. The rugby players were divided into two groups of five—one receiving the drug and the other a placebo. This was a double-blind study and even the staff aiding the experiment was not aware who was getting the drug or placebo.

This study was for sixteen weeks. The exercise consisted of thirty minutes of physical conditioning five days a week. The drug dosage was 20 mg./day.

A cable tensiometer was used to test the isometric muscle strength of thirteen muscle groups. Along with the testing for physical working capacity, skinfold thickness, weight, height, limb circumference, and various tests for motor performance (reflexes) were also measured. These measurements were done three times, and the best of the three was taken. Blood samples were also taken to note any less overt physiological alterations.

SIMPLE PATELLER REFLEX

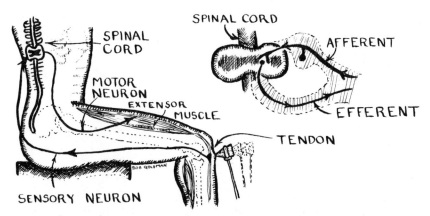

Methandrostenolone (Dianabol) was used to study the effects of steroids on the nervous system by measuring the knee jerk reflex. The use of anabolics seemed to affect the central nervous system. There seemed to be three separate components:

Reflex Arc — started by striking the patellar ligament.

1) *Reflex Latency* — "time from mechanical stimulation of patellar ligament to appearance of an action potential at the motor point of the rectus femoris muscle."

2) *Motor Time* — "period from the appearance of an action potential at the motor point to the mechanical movement of the leg by the muscle."

3) *Total Reflex Time* — "time from the mechanical stimulation of the tendon to the mechanical movement of the leg."

A majority of the factors measured remained unchanged during the course of study. While improvement of performance was noted in those groups given exercise, no significant differences were noted between the placebo and steroid groups.

Casner, Early, and Carlson (1971) tested twenty-seven males randomly divided into four groups as follows: steroid therapy and normal daily activity; steroid therapy and progressive-resistance weight training; placebo and normal daily activity; placebo and progressive weight training. In this double-blind study, the experimental groups were given 2 mg. of Stanozolol three times per day on days 1–21 and 28–49 of the fifty-six-day experiment. The control placebo group had the same schedule. They found that the groups on anabolic steroids gained significantly more weight than the two placebo groups, but much of the weight gain noted was not muscle but, rather, water weight. Over the entire period, the placebo group lost .9 liters of body water while the steroids groups gained 1.2 liters of body water. There were no significant changes in isometric strength between the groups.

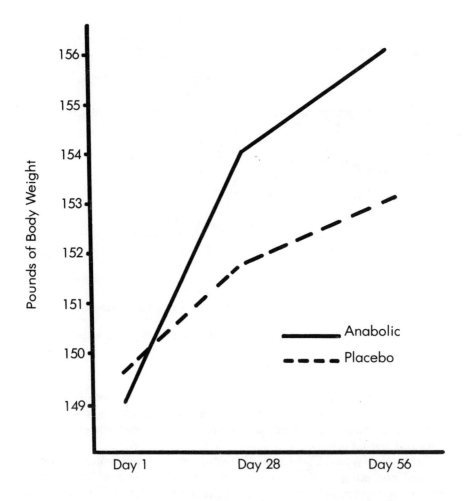

Fahey and Brown (1972) conducted a double-blind test at the University of California at Berkeley, utilizing two matched groups of fourteen males on the criteria of strength and body weight. All subjects were placed on a progressive weight-training program. An injection of 1 mg./kg. body weight of Deca-Durabolin was administered to half the subjects during weeks 2, 5, and 7 of the nine-week study. The Universal Weight gym and standard Olympic barbells were used in the weight training. Both groups improved in the ability to perform the bench press, latissimus pull, and curl, but there were no significant differences between the groups when tested on the Cybex Isokinetic Dynamometer. The Cybex is an isokinetic computer hooked up to a resistance-testing machine and measures force exerted by an extremity by recording the torque of force capabilities of the subject tested. The steroid group increased its bench press and dead lift by thirty and thirty-two pounds respectively, while the control group increased its lifts by twenty-two and thirteen pounds respectively. Statistically, there were no significant differences noted.

Golding, Freydinger, and Fisher (1974) tested forty amateur weight lifters with Dianabol (methandrostenolone). All subjects were in good physical shape and trained eighty minutes four times per week. They recorded the subjects' food and fluid intake to better note any change with a steroid-protein supplement program. Workout schedules for the subjects ranged from sixty to a maximum of three hours per day and from three to seven times per week. The steroid group was given 10 mg. of Dianabol per day for twelve weeks (three weeks on followed by one week off). Protein supplements were given in relation to the athlete's body weight.

No significant change in fat as measured by skinfolds and underwater weighing were noted. There were also no statistically significant differences between steroid and control groups, with all groups showing improvement in the pre- and post-study period.

Munson (1970) conducted a double-blind study at the University of Southern California, testing the effects of 20 mg./day of Anavar for four weeks on skinfold thickness, strength, body weight, and oxygen consumption on sixteen college students training thirty-five to forty minutes twice weekly. The exercises performed were the leg press, bench press, and arm curl. No significant differences were noted between the steroid and control groups in oxygen consumption and muscle strength.

One of the most important studies performed was done in 1974 by scientists at the Norwegian College of Physical Education and Sport. They evaluated the effects of Mestoranum administered over an eight-week period, giving 75 mg./day for weeks 1–4 and 150 mg./day during weeks 5–8. The double-blind study utilized eleven control subjects and ten experimental ones, testing static strength and aerobic work capacity. The subjects exercised ninety minutes three times per week on basic weight-training exercises and were given vitamin-mineral and protein supplements. Even at this high dosage, no significant differences were noted between the control and steroid groups in body weight and aerobic work capacity. Both groups benefited from the study with increased strength and limb circumferences.

To further support this, another study was published by S. Solberg at the University of Tromsø in Norway in 1982. The mean body weight and mean weight-lifting results for the ten best Norwegian weight lifters were studied. Solberg studied the body weight and weight-lifting results of Norwegian champions from 1962 to 1982. He was also able to obtain data on the sale of anabolic steroids from 1963 to 1981 and the sale of testosterone from 1974 to 1981 from the records of Norsk Medisinaldepot (the state wholesale drug monopoly).

A series of correlations was made to determine whether doping tests at competitions were cutting down on the use of anabolic steroids and, further, what effect this had on testosterone consumption.

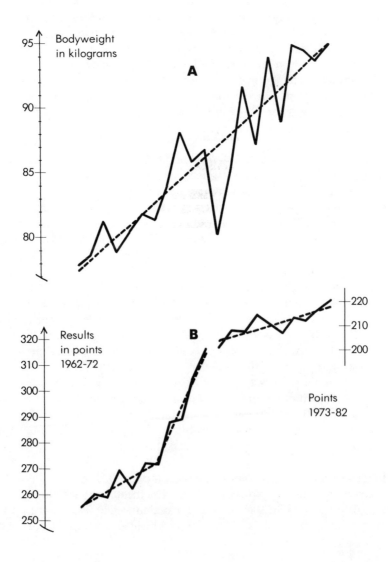

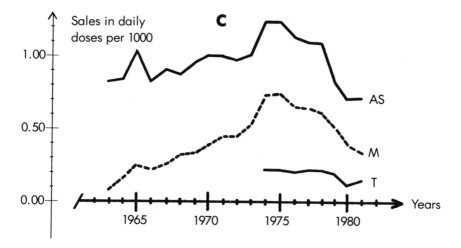

Part A: Mean bodyweight for the ten best weight-lifters at the annual Norwegian championships 1962-82. The dotted line is the regression line.

Part B: Mean points (kilograms lifted x coefficient) for the ten best weightlifters at the annual Norwegian championships 1962-82. The dotted lines are the regression lines for 1962-68, 1968-72 and 1973-82. Note the discontinuity and shift of scale 1972-73, caused by elimination of press from 1973 onwards.

Part C: Annual sale of androgens in Norway. AS: Entire group of anabolic steroids 1963-81. M: Metenolone (to selling preparation in the AS group), T: Testosterone preparations 1974-81.

British Journal of Sports Medicine, 16, no.3 (September 1982):170.

Interestingly, the introduction of testing was followed by a drop in anabolic-steroids sales of 42 percent in a six-year period (1975-82). The author goes on to state:

> The exact use of hormones in sports is difficult to determine, but some data exist: In Sweden, Ljungqvist (1975) found in a questionnaire sent to 144 top male athletes that 99 (69%) answered, and among these, 31% confirmed the use of anabolic steroids. Most of the users were throwers, and a few runners or jumpers were included. At the Nordic championship in 1974, 25 (68%) of the 37 participating weightlifters answered a questionnaire, and 6 (24%) of these said that they used anabolic steroids (Solberg, 1974). Haug et al, (1974) asked the 40 best Norwegian weightlifters about their use of anabolic steroids. Fifteen (38%) answered, and 13 (87%) confirmed use. Each of these 15 estimated the percentage of hormone-users at the World Championships to be about 75%. Nine of the 13 had decided themselves to start to use anabolic steroids, and 4 started after advice or pressure from others. The 13 had started their use from 1968 to 1973. I have calculated the reported use of these 13 to be 0.003 daily doses per 1,000 inhabitants. A rough estimate that these 13 represent between 1% and 10% of the total use in Norwegian sports implies that the sale for doping purposes in 1975 was between 2.4% and 24% of the total sale that year.
>
> A tentative conclusion is that the doping tests may have had their intended effect, namely, a reduction in the use of anabolic steroids by athletes and a slower rate of result improvements. Testosterone sale has decreased slightly in recent years. This development gives no support to the theory that introduction of doping tests for anabolic steroids would switch the problem to abuse of testosterone.

Johnson and O'Shea (1969) studied twelve matched pairs of subjects, fed a high-protein diet and trained with weights for six weeks. During the final three weeks, twelve of the subjects received 5 mg. of Dianabol twice daily. The subjects trained three times a week for one hour, utilizing a weight-resistance program that worked the major muscle groups. The strength of steroid-treated subjects was found to increase over the control group significantly, as did oxygen intake and nitrogen retention by the blood.

Crist, Stackpole, and Peake (1983) examined the effects of anabolic steroids on neuromuscular power and body composition in nine volunteers experienced with progressive-resistance weight training. The double-blind technique was used with the placebo group receiving 1 ml. of sesame oil intramuscularly once weekly for three weeks. The experimental groups received 100 mg. of testosterone cypionate USP (100 mg./ml.) or 100 mg. of nandrolone deconate NF (100 mg./ml.) intramuscularly once weekly for three weeks. All injections were given in the gluteal muscles. Protein and caloric intake was sufficient for muscular growth, yet no significant differences were noted between the control and steroid-treated groups. Of the nine healthy adults aged 19-31, the one female volunteer's results were comparable with some of those obtained from the male subjects.

Win-May and Mya-Tu (1975) from the Department of Medical Research in Rangoon, Burma, conducted a study to assess the effects of anabolic steroids on the various areas included under physical fitness. Thirty-one university male students aged 18-23 volunteered for this double-blind study, in which one group was given a placebo while the test group was administered 5 mg. of Dianabol daily for three months. The steroid group experienced significant increases in both dynamic and static strength, but there were no significant differences between the placebo and control groups in balance, coordination, flexibility, or cardiorespiratory endurance.

Bowers and Reardon (1972) studied eighteen subjects in equally matched weight lifters to study strength, age, and size. The subjects went through a six-week training program consisting of squats, forearm curls, bench presses, and tricep extensions. They were given 30 gm. of 90 percent protein supplements daily. The steroid group was administered 10 mg. of Dianabol for the last twenty-one days of the training, while the control group received a placebo. There were significant gains for the steroid group in the bench press and squat. The growth of forearm and bicep girths were not significant, but body weight increases in the steroid group were significant. No improvement in aerobic capacity was found.

Ward (1970) attempted to determine the effects of anabolic steroids on strength and lean body mass. He took sixteen healthy male college students, 16-26, and tested them before and after a five-week training period for strength and body-composition gains. Dianabol was used in this double-blind test.

The author found strength and body mass to increase significantly during the course of the study for the steroid group.

Stamford and Moffatt (1974) used twenty-four male weight lifters, who had trained for two years prior to submitting to this study. Twelve of the subjects were prisoners (criminals) and had taken steroids before, while the remaining twelve subjects were from the same area in the state. The four divided groups were assigned according to their ability on the bench press and their body weight. Diet was not monitored or controlled. Exercises consisted of bench press, deadlift, squat, curls and maximum poundage on these barbell lifts for two hour sessions. Group 1 was given 20 mg. of Dianabol five days a week, along with 30 gm. of a 90 percent protein supplement; Group 2 was given a placebo and a protein supplement; Group 3 received only the protein supplement; Group 4 received nothing.

Strength-testing maximums were done by measuring peaks in the bench press; maximum repetitions for the bench press with 80 percent of the previous top lift. Dynamometers were used to measure static strength in back, legs, and grip strength, as well as measurements of flexed arm and thigh. These measurements were taken after the first and second four-week periods of the study. Blood pressure and blood test samples were also taken.

The only area where the steroid group excelled over the control groups was in body weight. There was increased appetite and strength found in members of all the groups due to the exercise there were no significant strength gains by the steroid group.

Steinbach (1968) performed a random study for three and one-half months using 125 men, aged 17-19. Some were given anabolic steroids, some were not given steroids, some of them trained, some were given a placebo, and some were given nothing at all. There were five groups. Group 1—steroid, but no training; Group 2—received nothing and no training; Group 3—received steroid and training; group 4—placebo and training; Group 5—placebo and no training. Body weight was taken at the beginning and end of the study. Single isometric contraction strength was taken with one leg and one arm being measured. The steroid groups received 3 mg. of Dianabol twice a day. The groups then underwent physical training and performed an isometric contraction at 40 percent of their maximal isometric strength. This exercise program was done twice a day for three seconds, five times a week. Of the two groups training, one of them was trained in arm exercise only, the other group in leg exercise only. This researcher found a significant increase in leg and arm strength, as well as body weight, for the groups given Dianabol as compared to the other groups in the study.

O'Shea (1971) used twenty university students, 19-26, who had at least a minimum of one year of continuous weight training experience. The subjects were paired according to their strength levels, which were determined as a dynamic strength level discovered during a pretest period prior to the test training period.

Random selection was the method for determining placebo and steroid groups in this double-blind study. Even the investigator did not know who was really receiving the drug so as to assure a strict double-blind procedure.

The study was for a four-week period, and the anabolic steroids used was methandrostenolone in a dose of 10 mg./day. The control group received a placebo of 10 mg./day of calcium lactate. In addition, a high protein supplement was given to all which contained 92 percent protein in the amount of 0.5 gm./kilogram of body weight/day.

A progressive weight-training program was given to all through a triweekly cycle. By progressive overload weight training, we mean that the resistance is gradually increased so that the muscles can be worked to their maximum. The bench press and full squat were two of the main exercises used. The workouts were difficult since they lasted for one and one-half hours, three times a week. There was constant supervision of all workouts to ensure that the strict procedures were followed.

Strength was tested every week of the study utilizing maximum lifting (one repetition maximum in the bench press and squat). These lifts were performed according to the AAU rules for lifting. The steroid group was found to have significant increase in body weight, but no difference between placebo and control groups in the dynamic strength lifts of squat and bench press. Again no strength increase.

Berg and Keul (1974) studied fifteen weight lifters, 20-38, and ten male students, 18-23. The experiment lasted for about six weeks, and the steroid used was nandrolone decanoate given intramuscularly (by injection) in doses of 50 mg. at intervals of 10-14 days. During this time the participants were engaged in a physical-training program to increase dynamic strength. The exercises used were back lifts (dead lifts), bench press, and squats. Blood tests were taken, and changes noted. There were no significant changes in improved performance between control and steroid groups.

Harvey and Hutchinson used Dianabol (methandienone) on eleven athletic men during the course of their weight-training activities. This experiment was double blind. Dianabol was given in the dose of 100 mg./day for six weeks. Body composition and weight, muscular strength and performance, and assorted endocrine functions were measured. The athletes improved but not significantly between placebo and steroid groups. An accumulation of potassium was noted as a result of steroid use, and any increase in muscular size seemed to be attributed to water retention and retention of intracellular fluid.

Loughton and Ruhling studied twelve male college students, half of whom were unathletic, the other six athletic students from the Utah University wrestling team. These subjects were divided into three-man groups with the following qualifications: trained placebo; untrained placebo; trained Dianabol; untrained Dianabol. The study was for a period of seven weeks. The volunteers were randomly placed in the groups and trained six days a week in running and weight training. Weight training was three days a week and the weight-training sessions included push-ups, sit-ups, and various other calisthenics.

The weight-training sessions consisted of squat, bench press, military press, knee flexion and extension, overhead pulls, calf raises, arm curls, leg press, three sets of each exercise for four repetitions. Maximum weight was always used for each set. In order to assure a maximum effort, the largest amount of weight that could be handled was used. The type of weights used were the Universal Gym and Olympic Barbells. Throughout the study all subjects were given 20 gms. of 92 percent protein as a dietary supplement. The average caloric intake of the subjects was 3,200-3,500 per day.

The anabolic steroid used was Dianabol (methanadrostenolone). The placebo was lactose. During the first three weeks, the steroid group received 10 mg./day; and 5 mg./day the last three weeks. There were no significant results obtained among the four groups.

Johnson and Roundy (1975) studied twenty-one volunteer college students, 19-33. These subjects were divided into three randomly picked groups of seven. Their diets were supplemented with 90 percent protein powder in this double-blind study. They performed an interval running program, six days a week that lasted for the three-week duration of the experiment. The steroid group received 6 mg. of stanozolol/day. Tested and measured were the following: maximum oxygen uptake; time in mile run; static strength increases in knee extension and elbow flexion; skinfold thickness; and body weight. The results showed no improvement with steroid use.

SUPPLEMENTAL CONCLUSIONS

Some other factors to consider when evaluating the results of anabolic steroid studies are that you *cannot* always use animal studies and apply them to man because there are species differences in responses to target organs. In correlating animal studies with rats to human potential gains with the use of steroids, it was discovered by a Michigan State research team that animal studies served as very poor "models."

One of the first studies in 1942, by Professor L.T. Samuels, found no muscular performance increase with the administration of methyl testosterone to non-training subjects.

Simson, in 1941, found no increase in dynamic work performance with the administration of 30-40 mgs./day of methyl testosterone. The subjects ranged from 48 to 67 years old.

When noting effects of steroid administration on weight in men, Dr. Ryan, in 1974, found no significant betterment with the use of steroids. He also found that many of the athletes in this study had been using steroids for about three years.

One theory among steroid proponents is that they feel that trained muscles have more receptor proteins for steroids. Along with this fact, those individuals who train especially hard may be in negative nitrogen balance. Usually, the average individual would require 20-30 gms. of protein a day if they are active. Athletes in training usually ingest 50-150 gms./day so that there is no loss of any lean muscle mass. This high protein requirement can only be satisfied by nutritional supplements and that is why most serious athletes take them.

Again, there are many non-drug factors which effect the results of these tests, such as the assumption that athletes who work at very high tension levels might be more apt to benefit from the use of anabolics than those who are low-stress individuals.

There is cause to believe that androgens have fat mobilizing properties. Women characteristically have more fat and lower androgen levels than men. It is possible that the use of androgens in treating subjects may lead to a long term effect of fat mobilization in those subjects.

This means that even years later, after you have stopped taking steroid drugs, you may have a problem losing weight (fat).

6

ANDROGENIC-TO-ANABOLIC RATIO: THE THERAPEUTIC INDEX

There is a ratio between the androgenic (male characteristics) and anabolic (growth producing) qualities of anabolic-steroid preparations. The ratio of these two properties is known as the *therapeutic index* of the drug.

The *androgenic factor* has been defined as the steroid's ability to stimulate growth of the rat prostate gland and seminal vesicles, while the *anabolic character* is the growth noted in the rat's levator ani muscle.

Medical researchers have come to various interpretations of the factors involved in calculating the therapeutic index (TI). Testosterone is generally give the TI value of 1. Therefore, theoretically, the greater the therapeutic index of a drug compound, the higher the anabolic qualities. Various terms have been related to this concept, such as:

1. the androgenic response v. the levator ani muscle hypertrophy (growth);
2. the androgenic properties v. the body nitrogen balance;
3. androgenic v. renotrophic (growth of the kidney) responses;
4. androgenic v. the mytrophic (muscle growth).

Certain anabolic steroids have had their chemical structure altered in order to enhance the anabolic (versus androgenic) effect. This has created the 19-Nor drugs, where the constituent group on the 19th carbon has been altered.

So, in calculating a therapeutic index, one may note, for example, that the levator ani muscle has grown four times that of the standard, while the seminal vesicle has grown two times the standard; this would give us $4 \div 2 = 2$ for our TI. The end results of these types of calculations and their true effects on the body are dubious, to say the least.

To complicate matters, there are different and unscientifically proven methods of taking the drugs.

1. *shotgunning:* a hit or miss method;
2. *stacking:* using more than one drug at the same time—injectables combined with orals; the synergistic or increased effects athletes feel they achieve surely augments the toxic effects as well;
3. *tapering:* gradually decreasing the intake;
4. *plateauing:* when the drug no longer is working in the desired manner at a particular dosage.

You also have *blending* (mixing of drugs), *cycling, rebounding,* and a host of other methods, none of which have been successfully documented in literature as yet.

7
ANABOLIC-STEROID RESEARCH PERTAINING TO THE LIVER

NITROGEN BALANCE AND RETENTION

One of the most important aspects of androgenic anabolic steroid usage has to do with nitrogen retention. the use of steroids causes a marked increase in nitrogen retention along with extra water retained in the body, which is sometimes mistaken for a positive weight gain. One method for determining this nitrogen content is the system of the Kjeldahl analysis (82). One of the often used formulas for measurement: (206, 207, 208) of nitrogen balance is:

STEROID PROTEIN ACTIVITY INDEX (SPAI)

$$SPAI = \frac{NBSP}{NISP} - \frac{NBCP}{NICP} \times 100$$

where:
NBSP equals nitrogen balance in steroid period
NISP equals nitrogen intake in steroid period
NBCP equals nitrogen balance in control period
NICP equals nitrogen intake in control period

Thus, the ratios

$$\frac{NBSP}{NISP} \quad \text{and} \quad \frac{NBCP}{NICP}$$

"indicate the fraction of dietary protein retained by the body during the steroid and control periods, respectively."

The SPAI levels are effected by the amount of protein and calorie content of the foods ingested. In some cases the SPAI level decreases with the prolonged use of anabolic steroids, and in some cases can be used to determine the various nutritional effects of some catabolic and anabolic steroids.

SPAI results are important in that they help determine the best dosage of anabolic steroid that could offset the protein catabolic effects of exercise and training while aiding the need for increased biosynthesis of protein in building muscle tissue.

Nitrogen retention cannot only be achieved with anabolic steroids such as testosterone propionate (Bartlett & Garber, 1952, 1953), but also with growth hormone. This again is characterized by a lowered rate of amino acid catabolism along with a higher rate of protein synthesis.

In some cases an increased appetite and increased food intake may increase the nitrogen content, as well as the administration of anabolic steroids. But it was found that even doubling the dosage of anabolic steroids did not further increase the nitrogen retention (209, 212) significantly. Sometimes after steroid administration has been stopped a rebound effect occurs where there is an increase in nitrogen excretion, which may continue for several days (209, 213, 214).

To eliminate the point of diminishing returns it has been noted that 25 to 50mg. of Norethandrolone will provide maximum nitrogen retention (213, 215, 126, 217, 218).

In a comparison of three derivatives of the anabolic steroids comparing norethandrolone propionate, testosterone propionate and norethandrolone it was found that the nitrogen retention levels were independent of age, sex, nitrogen uptake, physical activity, and steroid induced variables (219).

NITROGEN BALANCE

The amino acids that are taken into the body are either excreted or incorporated into protein due to the fact that they are stored only temporarily. This is the theory of nitrogen balance. One can therefore study protein metabolism by comparing the excreted nitrogen end products with that of the nitrogen content of ingested protein. If one's body mass remains at a constant level the amount of nitrogen excreted equals the amount of nitrogen ingested. In the normal health individual this is known as nitrogen balance. If one increases one's body mass protoplasm more nitrogen is ingested than excreted due to the retained nitrogen in the form of new protein. This is positive nitrogen balance which usually occurs during periods of recuperation from special ailments, growth, pregnancy or just a general increase in body protein.

Negative nitrogen balance occurs when the nitrogen excretion is more than the nitrogen ingested. One would lose body protoplasm during this phase which might occur during fever, starvation or in the case of extensive burns to the body. It might occur for a period after surgery, or when the biosynthesis of proteins is impaired or when there is excessive loss of proteins.

Anabolic steroids tend to produce a positive nitrogen balance which is why they are recommended therapy for weight gain in some cases. Anabolic steroids also cause a retention of a number of basic minerals (electrolytes) such as calcium ad sodium which causes the retention of fluid so commonly seen as a form of edema.

HYPERBILIRUBINEMIA ASSOCIATED WITH THE USE OF ANABOLIC STEROIDS IN HUMANS

Anabolic-Androgenic Steroid	Reference
Fluoxymesterone	Werzne (1960)
Methandienone	Wernze (1960)
Metribolone	Kruskemper and Noell (1966)
Methyltestosterone	Arias (1962)
	Carbone et al (1959)
	Koszalka (1957)
	Lloyd-Thomas and Sherlock (1952)
	Peters et al (1958)
	Seelen (1958)
	Werner et al (1950)
	Wood (1952)
Norethandrolone	Arias (1962)
	Datta and Sherlock (1963)
	Dunning (1958)
	Schaffner et al (1959)
	Scherb et al (1963)

BSP RETENTION ASSOCIATED WITH THE USE OF ANABOLIC STEROIDS IN HUMANS

Anabolic-androgenic Steroid	Reference
Fluoxymesterone	Marquardt et al (1961)
	Wernze (1960)
Methandienone	Aly (1961)
	Liddle and Burke (1960)
	Marquardt et al (1961)
	Wernze (1960)
	Wernze et al (1961)
	Wynn et al (1961)
Methenolone Acetate	Kruskemper (1966a)
	von Oldershausen and Schweiger (1964)
Methyltestosterone	Carbone et al (1959)
	Foss and Simpson (1959)
	Heaney and Whedon (1958)
	Kruskemper (1968)
	von Oldershausen and Schweiger (1964)
	Werner et al (1950)
Metribolone	Kruskemper and Noell (1966)
Norethandrolone	Dowben (1958)
	Heaney and Whedon (1958)
	Kory et al (1957)
	Kory et al (1959)
	Marquardt et al (1961)
Testosterone Propionate	Heaney and Whedon (1958)

STUDIES OF THE EFFECT OF ANABOLIC STEROIDS ON BSP RETENTION AND SGOT LEVELS

Reference	Number of subjects	Type of subject	Liver function before steroid administration	Steroid administered	Dose of drug (mg per day)	Length of administration	% showing 45-min retention of BSP above 6%	% showing elevation of SGOT
Carbone et al (1959)	17	Patients	Normal	Methyltestosterone	67	3 weeks	90	40
Heaney & Whedon (1958)	5	Patients	Normal	Methyltestosterone	100	Not given	100	40
	11	7 patients & 4 healthy controls		Norethandrolone	20-100	Not given	100	40
Dowben (1958)	6	Healthy laboratory workers	Normal	Norethandrolone	30	6 weeks	100	100
Kory et al (1959)	47	Patients	Normal	Norethandrolone	25 or 50	6 months	72	100
	10	Patients	Normal	Norethandrolone	25	5 weeks	90	70
Schaffner et al (1959)	27	Chronically ill elderly patients	Normal	Norethandrolone	50	3 weeks	90	70
Wynn et al (1961)	19	Patients	Normal in 23, Abnormal in 7	Methandienone	10-100	70 days	62	20
	14	Patients		Methandienone	10-100	70 days	80	45

EFFECTS OF ANDROGENS AND RELATED STEROIDS
ON SOME LIVER ENZYMES

Activity	Anabolic Steroids	Reference
Alkaline phosphatase		
Increase	Methyltestosterone	Koszalka (1957)
(mild)	Norethandrolone	Dunning (1958)
		Schaffner et al (1959)
No effect	fluoxmesterone	Wernze (1960)
	Methandienone	Liddle and Burke (1960)
		Schwarting and Neth (1960)
		Werner et al (1961)
		Wernze (1960)
		Wynn et al (1961)
	Metenolone	Kruskemper (1966a)
	Metenolone acetate	Kruskemper (1966a)
	Methyltestosterone	Wood (1952)
	Metribolone	Kruskempler and Noell (1966)
	Nandrolone	Wernze (1960)
SGOT		
Increase	Acetythiomethyl-testosterone	Kruskemper (1966b)
	1,17 α-Dimethyltestosterone	Kruskemper (1966b)
	Fluoxymesterone	Wernze (1960)
	Methandienone	Werner et al (1961)
		Wernze (1960)
		Wernze and Schmidt (1961)
		Wynn et al (1961)
	Methenolone	Pohle (1966)
	Methyltestosterone	Petera and Lahn (1960)
		Petera et al (1962)
	Metribolone	Kruskemper and Noell (1966)
	Norethandrolone	Kory et al (1959)
		Shaffner et al (1959)
No effect	Mesterolone	Schnack and Wewalka (1966)
	Methenolone	Kruskemper (1966a)
	Methenolone acetate	Kruskemper (1966a)
		Gramsch (1963)
	Methenolone enanthate	Gramsch (1963)
	Norethandrolone	Dowben (1958)
SGPT		
Increase	Acetylthiomethyl-testosterone	Kruskemper (1966b)
	1,17 α-Dimethyltestosterone	Kruskemper (1966b)
	Methandienone	Werner et al (1961)
	Mehtyltestosterone	Petra and Lahn (1960)
		Petera et al (1962)
	metribolone	Kruskemper and Noell (1966)
No effect	Mehtenolone	Kruskemper (1966a)
	Methenolone acetate	Kruskemper (1966a)
		Gamsch (1963)
	Methenolone enanthate	Gramsch (1963)
Lactic Dehydrogenase (LDH)		
Increase	Methyltestosterone	Petera et al (1962)
	Norenthandrostenolone	Dowben (1958)

		Marquardt *et al* (1961)
No effect	Methyltestosterone	Marquardt *et al* (1961)
	Methandienone	Marquardt *et al* (1961)
	Methenolone acetate	Marquardt *et al* (1961)
	Methenolone enanthate	Marquardt *et al* (1961)
	Nandrolone phenylpropionate	Marquardt *et al* (1961)

Aldolase

Increase	Norethandrolone	Dowben (1958)
No effect	Methenolone	Kruskemper (1966a)
	Methenolone acetate	Kruskemper (1966a)
		Marquardt *et al* (1964)
	Methenolone enanthate	Marquardt *et al* (1964)
	Nandrolone phenylpropionate	Marquardt *et al* (1964)

All the above charts are from James E. Wright, *Anabolic Steroids in Sports*, vol. 2.

REPORTED CASES OF ANDROGEN ASSOCIATED PELIOSIS (AAP)

Case reports	Age & sex	Disease treated	Androgen used	Total dose*	Length of treatment (months)
Burger & Marcuse (1952)	39F	carcinomatosis	'oral testosterone'	6g	12
Gordon *et al* (1960)	43M	pemphigus	norethandrolone	5.8g	6.5
	57F	anaemia	norethandrolone	6.6g	11
Kintzen & Silny (1960)	60F	carcinomatosis	fluoxymesterone	10.2g	17
Yanoff & Rawson (1964)	73F	osteoporosis	norethandrolone	0.7g	5
Weir *et al* (1969)	39F	anaemia	norethandrolone	—	—
McGiven (1970)	75M	aplastic anaemia	oxymetholone	—	12
			methandienone	—	
Port *et al* (1971)†	21M	Fanconi's anaemia	oxymetholone	—	9
Berstein *et al* (1971)†	20M	Fanconi's anaemia	IM testosterone	—	—
			oxymetholone	30g	12
Necheles & Robins (1971)	6M	aplastic anaemia	S testosterone proprionate	13g	8
			oxymetholone	22g	9
	9M	Fanconi's anaemia	oxymetholone	35g	17
Naeim *et al* (1973)	26M	Fanconi's anaemia	fluoxymesterone	5.2g	3.5
Groos *et al* (1974)	33F	aplastic anaemia	oxymetholone	118g	19
Meadows *et al* (1974)†	6F	aplastic anaemia	oxymetholone	72g	48
			nandrolone decanoate	10.6g	
Bagheri & boyer (1974)	64M	Pancytopenia	IM testosterone enanthate	0.6g	13
			fluoxymesterone	15g	
	68M	pancytopenia	oxymetholone	40g	15
	49F	carcinomatosis	fluoxymesterone	2.2g	5
			methyltestosterone	1.5g	1
	37F	pancytopenia	IM testosterone enanthate	4.8g	2
	69M	Hodgkin's disease	oxymetholone	92g	27
	43M	malignant thymoma	norethandrolone	3.6g	4.
			IM testosterone propionate	1.2g	1.5

Kühböck et al (1975)	19M	aplastic anaemia	oxymetholone	—	15
Usatin & Wigger (1976)	11M	cystic fibrosis	methandrostenelone	—	—
Kessler et al (1976)†	17M	aplastic anaemia	oxymetholone	171g	36
Kew et al (1976)	13F	Fanconi's anaemia	oxymetholone	144g	48
	12M	Fanconi's anaemia	oxymetholone	90g	50
			methyltestosterone	22g	36

*Approximate total dose received assuming uninterrupted treatment with the doses and for the periods of time stated in the text. When several different doses are mentioned the mean dose has been used for the calculation.
†In these cases peliosis and tumours were present. IM: intramuscular, S:sublingual.

From Paradinas et al., *Histopathology*, 1 (1977): 240.

Finally, an important recent letter published in the *Annals of Internal Medicine:*

TO THE EDITOR: An association between primary hepatic tumors and androgen therapy was first noted in 1965 (1). In a recent review of the literature, 33 cases of patients with androgen-associated hepatic tumors were reported (2); 14 of these patients had received androgens as therapy for Fanconi's anemia, and 19 patients, for various other, potentially androgen-responsive illnesses. We have recently cared for a young man who developed a primary hepatic malignancy after taking androgens to increase his skeletal muscle mass. This patient represents the first reported case of such a malignancy in an otherwise healthy athlete taking androgens for this purpose.

On 6 July 1983, a 26-year-old white man was hospitalized for evaluation of weight loss and generalized malaise. He had no history of liver disease. For years he had competed in body-building contests, and had taken anabolic steriods to increase his muscle mass. During the 4 years before his admission, he had consumed methandrostenolone, oxandrolone, stanozolol, nandrolone decanoate, and methenolone.

On physical examination, the patient was wasted, had dullness and decreased breath sounds over the right posterior chest wall, and had marked hepatomegaly. Laboratory findings included eosinophilia of 18%; sedimentation rate, 80 mm/h; hyperglobulinemia, 4.8 g%; alpha-fetoglobulin, 375 ng/mL; and carcinoembryonic antigen, 36 ng/mL. Bloody fluid was obtained from the right hemithorax. Pleural biopsy showed undifferentiated carcinoma, and liver biopsy showed hepatic carcinoma with both cholangio and helpatocellular elements. The patient refused chemotherapy and died 27 September 1983. Autopsy revealed near-total replacement of the liver by tumor and pulmonary and intraabdominal metastases.

This occurrence of androgen consumption and subsequent primary hepatic malignancy is notable because of the absence of any preceding disease (1-5). The prolonged period of androgen consumption is in agreement with current reports of primary hepatic tumors in patients with illnesses other than Fanconi's anemia (3). Our finding of distant metastases differs from those of several recent reports (2); our patient is also unusual because the alpha-fetoprotein level was elevated (4). This case further supports a direct relation between the consumption of C-17 alkylated androgens and hepatic carcinoma (2). The potential relation between steroids and hepatic carcinoma is important to recognize because of the interest expressed by some athletes in taking these drugs.

Wylie L. Overly, M.D.
Joseph A. Dankoff, B.S.
Barbara K. Wang, M.D.
Usha D. Singh, M.D.

Latrobe Area Hospital; Latrobe, PA 15650

REFERENCES
1. RECANT L, LACY P. Fanconi's anaemia and hepatic cirrhosis. *Am I Med.* 1965; 39: 466-75.
2. WESTABY D, WILLIAMS R. Androgen and anabolic steroid related liver tumours. In: DAVIS M, TEDGER JM, WILLIAMS R, EDS. *Drug Reactions and the Liver.* London: Pitman Medical; 1981:284-9.
3. SWEENEY EC, EVANS DJ. Hepatic lesions in patients treated with synthetic anabolic steroids. *J Clin Pathol,* 1976; 29:626-33.
4. FARRELL GC, UREN RF, PERKINS KW, JOSHUA DE, BARID PJ, KRONENBERG H. Androgen-induced hepatoma. *Lancet.* 1975; 1:430-1.
5. MOKRHISKY ST, AMBRUSCO DR, HATHAWAY WE. Fulminant hepatic neoplasia after androgen therapy. *N Engl J Med* J Med. 1977; 296;1411-2.

From
Annals of Internal
Medicine (January 1984)

The above case history is critically important. A number of years ago, I stated that this disorder would begin to surface in previously healthy athletes with no history of liver disease. My critics claimed this was ridiculous and the only cases in the literature were of patients treated with androgens for serious diseases. It is now obvious that my critics were incorrect, but the reason this is very frightening is because there are no doubt hundreds and maybe thousands of other young athletes almost on the verge of this fatal disorder. Hepatomas (liver cancers) warning signs many times don't surface until it's too late—two months later, you're a death statistic. I hope physicians will be aware of this, and attempt to catch it early as well as report cases which may soon begin to surface in clusters.

8
ANABOLIC-STEROID RESEARCH PERTAINING TO THE HEART

CHOLESTEROL AND LIPOPROTEIN
RISK FACTOR PROFILES MULTIPLIERS*

Total Cholesterol

300 mg/dl	Almost three times standard risk: very probably a type of hyperlipoproteinemia
260 mg/dl	Twice the standard risk: possibly a type of hyperlipoproteinemia
234 mg/dl	1.4 × standard risk: average cholesterol of CHD cases in the Framingham study
225 mg/dl	Standard risk: average cholesterol
220 mg/dl	0.95 × standard risk: average cholesterol of non-CHD cases in the Framingham study
200 mg/dl	0.9 × standard risk
185 mg/dl	0.8 × standard risk
150 mg/dl	Probable cholesterol threshold for CHD (below this value no cases appear except in unusual lipoprotein disorders, i.e., Tangiers Disease)

HDL Cholesterol

Plasma Level (mg/dl)	Risk Factor Multiplier	
	Males	Females
25	2.00	—
30	1.82	—
35	1.49	—
40	1.22	1.94
45	1.00 (Avg Risk)	1.55
50	0.82	1.25
55	0.67	1.00 (Avg risk)
60	0.55	0.80
65	0.45	0.64
70	—	0.52
75	Longevity Syndrome	

HDL + Total Cholesterol

If both HDL and total cholesterol values are known, the risk of CHD can be more accurately assessed by computing the ratio of these two values.

Total cholesterol/
HDL cholesterol   Risk

3.43		$^1/_2$ Average
4.97	MEN	Average
9.55		2× Average
23.99		3× Average
3.27		$^1/_2$ Average
4.44	WOMEN	Average
7.05		2× Average
11.04		3× Average

HDL + LDL Cholesterol

The most definitive assessment of coronary heart disease risk available from a lipid profile is determined using a ratio of LDL to HDL cholesterol.**

**LDL cholesterol/
HDL cholesterol   Risk**

1.00		$^1/_2$ Average
3.55	MEN	Average
6.25		2× Average
7.99		3× Average
1.47		$^1/_2$ Average
3.22	WOMEN	Average
5.03		2× Average
6.14		3× Average

**If LDL cholesterol is not measured it can be calculated from triglyceride values using the equation:

$$\text{LDL Cholesterol} = \text{Total Cholesterol} - \text{HDL Cholesterol} = \text{Triglycerides}/5$$

*Keep in mind that, given our current CHD incidence, the "standard" or "average" risk is by no means the optimal risk for an active, health conscious person.

From James E. Wright, *Anabolic Steroids in Sports*, Vol. 2.

So you can see the importance of using polyunsaturated oils, like Crisco Oil or Wesson Oil, to decrease the risk of cholesterol plaque formation.

ATHEROSCLEROSIS

All quotes and graphs that follow are from *The Framingham Study* by Thomas R. Dawber (Cambridge: Harvard University Press, 1980).

The long-standing hypothesis that blood lipids contribute to the development of atherosclerosis has been strongly supported by numerous studies, both clinical and epidemiologic. The determination by pathologists that the major constituent of the atheromatous lesion is cholesterol strengthened the concept that cholesterol in the circulating blood, through some unknown mechanism, is deposited in the arterial wall. Other changes—fibrosis and calcification—are considered inflammatory reactions to the presence of this substance. Seventy-five years ago (Marchand, 1904) simple filtration of the lipid from the blood through the intimal wall was proposed as the means by which the atheromatous lesion was produced. Later suggestions have been that the lipid in the arterial wall develops in situ, or that it is derived from the incorporation of arterial wall thrombi into the intima (Duguid, 1949). Hemorrhages from capillaries in the wall have also been suggested, as have combinations of the above mechanisms.

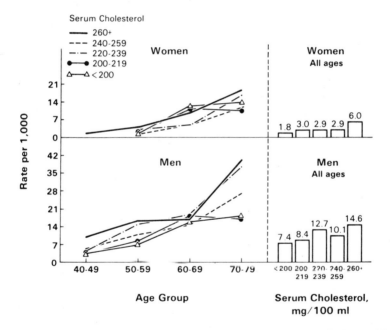

Average annual incidence of coronary heart disease, by serum cholesterol level.

One must remember that it is not only the blood cholesterol level that is important. The way the body handles the cholesterol is also very important. Anabolic steroids have proven to increase both blood lipid and cholesterol levels, as well as low-density lipoproteins, while they decrease the protective high-density lipoproteins.

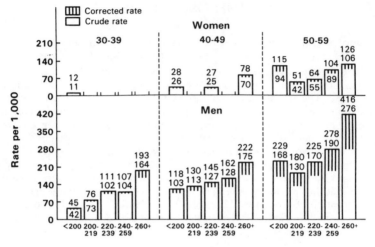

24-year incidence of myocardial infarction, by serum cholesterol level.

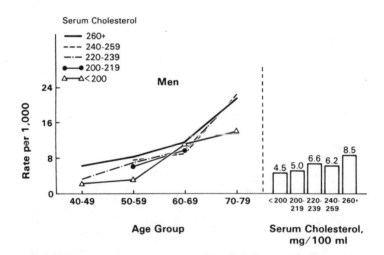

Average annual incidence of myocardial infarction in men, by serum cholesterol level.

The most recent interest has been in the possible value of determining the cholesterol in certain lipoprotein fractions and using this as a measurement of risk. Preliminary studies suggest that the level of cholesterol in the low-density lipoprotein fraction (LDL) is positively related to coronary heart disease development, while the cholesterol in the high-density lipoproteins (HDL) is negatively related (Castelli *et al.*, 1977; Gordon *et al.*, 1977).

HYPERTENSION (HIGH BLOOD PRESSURE)

The Framingham Study explored blood-pressure elevations.

It was logical to assume that the greater the pressure against the arterial walls, the more likely that they would rupture or that mechanical damage which might lead to atherosclerotic changes would occur. It was also reasonable to believe that the heart that had to pump blood against an increased pressure would fail much earlier than if the pressure were lower....

Several theories to account for the role of blood pressure in atherosclerosis have been considered. A direct pressure effect might damage the intimal cells, leading to earlier deposition of atheromatous material. The pressure in the arterial lumen might affect the rate of filtration of cholesterol into the intimal arterial cells (if that is the process that actually takes place). Repeated stretching of the arterial walls via a wide pulse pressure might damage the intima. And it has been suggested that the loss of elastic tissue in the arterial wall might be one of the earlier changes in the atherosclerotic process (Dawber, Thomas, and McNamara, 1973).

There is little medical doubt as to the hazards of elevated blood pressure's link with cardiovascular disease.

101

HYPERTENSION AS A RISK FACTOR

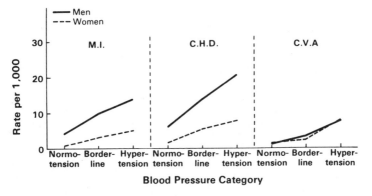

Average annual incidence of cardiovascular disease, by blood-pressure category. M.I. = myocardial infarction; C.H.D. = coronary heart disease; C.V.A. = cardiovascular accident.

These elevations are particularly important in athletes that weight train at high levels. A medical research group from McMaster University reported in the September 1983 issue of *Medical Tribune* the dramatic blood-pressure elevations of athletes undergoing heavy weight training.

HYPERTENSION AS A RISK FACTOR

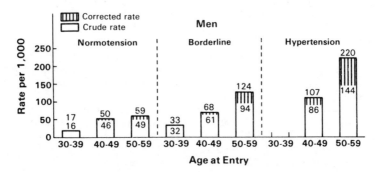

24-year incidence of sudden death in men, by blood-pressure category.

Headaches, dizziness, and problems with vision, coordination, and speech in these athletes are warning signs demanding immediate medical attention. Dr. John R. Sutton described two suspected cases of subarchnoid hemorrhage.

One 33-year-old weight lifter who ignored his intermittent symptoms for three years was admitted to the hospital after experiencing a sudden, severe occipital headache, neck stiffness, and photophobia following three attempts to set a world record lifting 1,600 lbs. with his calves. For the previous decade, he had emphasized calf training and had managed to increase the girth of each lower leg to 52 cm.

Systolic blood pressures as high as 450 mmHg and diastolic values exceeding 300 were recorded through a brachial artery catheter during the active exercise phase involving 90 minutes of simulated weight training in five of the iron pumpers," said exercise physiologist Duncan MacDougall, Ph.D., professor of physical education and medicine, McMaster University, Hamilton, Ontario.

The training exercises involved a single arm curl, overhead press, and single and double leg presses, all performed while seated. Each exercise was repeated until failure at 80%, 90%, 95%, and 100% of a previously determined maximum capacity for each subject. The five lifters were 20-25 years of age and averaged five years' experience with the sport.

The greatest peak pressures were observed with the double leg press exercise, where the mean was 355/281 mmHg. One subject reached 450/310. The lowest increases were seen with single arm curls. The mean: 293/230 mmHg.

Now, when one is to combine the fluid retention and elevated blood pressures from androgens, the decrease in HDL's, and the increase in LDL's, and combine this with the increase blood lipids, cholesterol, and atherosclerosis (topped off with amphetamines that some athletes take to train harder and faster), you have a situation with tragic potential.

9
PSYCHOLOGICAL EFFECTS OF STEROIDS

Psychological stress has been proven to lower plasma testosterone levels.

There is also indirect evidence in humans that psychological stress results in suppression of androgen activity. Rose et al. studied soldiers in basic training and special forces personnel anticipating imminent combat in Vietnam. These men showed lowered urine excretion of testosterone, epitestosterone, androsterone, and etiocholanolone.

Taken together, these studies suggest that male animals and men respond to stress with suppression of androgens.

From *Archives of Gender Psychiatry*, 26 (May 1972).

[In addition], it has been observed that sex hormones, by means of a variety of direct and indirect influences, act on the central nervous system and other organ systems involved in the execution of sexual and aggressive behavior. It is also well known that sexual and aggressive behavior in humans is accompanied by changes in affect; that is, alterations of a subjective nature that are reported as feelings or emotions, such as excitement or anger.

The notion that aggressive behavior might be associated in some way with a chemical substance circulating in the blood has intrigued observers of human and animal behavior for many centuries. Hippocrates suggested that an excess of yellow bile was responsible for the aggressiveness and irritability of the choleric individual....Furthermore, among the many variables involved in aggressive behavior, the influence of androgens on the central nervous system and other organ systems may be a significant factor in providing both the capacity and the impulse to act in certain ways, given certain stimuli.

There is an obvious way in which male sex hormones influence behavior, and that is in their influence on physical stature, musculature, and strength that in most species gives males a clear-cut advantage over females in fighting....

[Further it has been noted] that early exposure to testosterone sensitizes the central nervous system in such a way that subsequent exposure to androgen in adulthood results in fighting behavior *when the animal is confronted with an appropriate external stimulus to fight.* Perhaps there is a lowering of a threshold of a response tendency that is present, but latent, in untreated, castrated adults. Although androgen may affect the "internal urge" to fight, it seems clear that appropriate external stimuli are necessary, if not sufficient, prerequisites for actual fighting to occur. Hinde (1967) has criticized Lorenz' suggesting that aggressive behavior may arise spontaneously from irresistible internal urges. Tinbergen (1968), however, reconciles the "internal vs. external causation" arguments in his discussion of the interplay between the two classes of variables. It seems obvious, and yet one needs to be reminded, that "fighting is started by a number of variables, of which some are internal and some external... fighting behavior is not like the simple slot machine that produces one platform ticket every time one three-penny bit is inserted" (Tinbergen, 1968).

[Finally, we must realize that] the effects of androgens on the CNS and behavior, is good reason to believe that, as with other steroid hormones, the CNS-androgen relationship is a two-way street; i.e., the CNS can influence androgen secretions as well as be influenced by exposure to circulating androgens.

From the work of D. Lunde and D. Hamburg
of Stanford University

A fascinating experiment demonstrating the testosterone response to stress involved taking a dominant male monkey from his own colony and introducing him to a strange colony where he lost status. The move was associated with a striking drop in plasma testosterone concentration. If the same monkey was returned to his own colony and harem of female monkeys, however, his testosterone secretion quickly returned to normal levels. Perhaps a somewhat comparable situation for humans is the experience of basic training. Recruits in basic training judged to be having the greatest difficulty in adapting had significantly lower urinary testosterone excretion than those who were coping well.

From *Hospital Practice* (July 1975)

10
PHYSIOLOGY AND REGULATION
OF TESTICULAR FUNCTION

The testis consists of two components—a system of spermatogenic tubules for the production and transport of sperm and clusters of interstitial or Leydig cells that lie between the tubules and produce androgenic steroids.

THE LEYDIG CELL Testosterone synthesis The biochemical pathway by which the 27-carbon sterol cholesterol is converted to androgens and estrogens is depicted in Fig. 1. Cholesterol can either be synthesized de novo in the Leydig cell or derived from plasma lipoproteins. Five enzymes or enzyme complexes are required for the conversion of cholesterol to testosterone. In this process the side chain of cholesterol is cleaved in two steps to reduce the size from 27 to 19 carbons, and the A ring of the steroid is con-

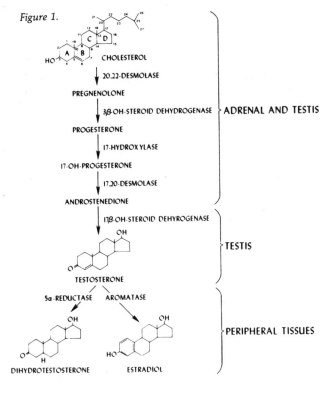

Figure 1.

Pathways of androgen formation in the testis and the conversion of androgens to other active hormones in peripheral tissues.

HORMONE RELEASE & PRODUCTION
FEED-BACK LOOP

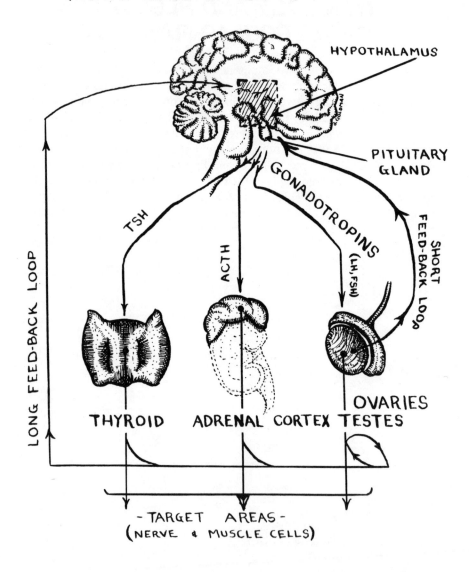

verted to the Δ^4-3-keto configuration. The five enzymes are the 20,22-desmolase, the 3β-hydroxysteroid dehydrogenase-$\Delta^{4,5}$-isomerase complex, 17α-hydroxylase, 17,20-desmolase, and 17β-hydroxysteroid dehydrogenase. The first four enzymes are also present in the adrenal.

The rate-limiting reaction in testosterone synthesis is the conversion of cholesterol to pregnenolone by the 20,22-desmolase; luteinizing hormone (LH) from the pituitary acts at this step to regulate the rate of testosterone formation. Several other steroids including estradiol are synthesized within the Leydig cell, but the significance of these in the normal man is thought to be minor.

Testosterone secretion and transport Only about 0.02 mg of testosterone is stored in the normal testes so that the total hormone content turns over about 200 times each day to provide the average of 5 to 6 mg that is secreted into plasma in normal young men (Fig. 2). As is true for other steroid hormones, testosterone is transported in plasma bound to protein, largely to albumin and to a specific steroid hormone transport protein, testosterone-binding globulin (TeBG). The bound and unbound fractions in plasma are in dynamic equilibrium, only about 1 to 3 percent being present in the free fraction.

Peripheral metabolism of androgens A special feature of testosterone metabolism is that it serves as a circulating precursor (or prohormone) for the formation of two other types of active metabolites which mediate many of the physiological processes involved in androgen action (Fig. 1). On the one hand, testosterone can be converted by 5α-reduction to dihydrotestosterone, which is believed to perform many of the differentiative, growth-promoting, and functional actions involved in male sexual differentiation and virilization. On the other hand, circulating androgens in both sexes can be converted to estrogens in the peripheral tissues. In men estrogens act in some instance in concert with androgens but can also have effects independent of or opposite to those of androgens. Thus, the physiological effects of testosterone are the result of the combined effects of testosterone itself plus those of the active androgen and estrogen metabolites of the parent molecule. (In normal men small amounts of estradiol and dihydrotestosterone are also derived by direct secretion from the testis and indirectly from the weak adrenal androgen and androstenedione.)

The quantitative relation between circulating androgens and the formation of estrogen in normal young men is illustrated diagrammatically in Fig. 2. The production rates of testosterone and androstenedione average about 6 and 3 mg., respectively, per day. All of estrone production (averaging about 60 μg per day) can be accounted for by formation from circulating precursors. The mean estradiol production rate is about 45 μg per day; about 35 percent of this amount is derived from circulating testosterone, 50 percent is derived from the weak estrogen estrone, and 15 percent is secreted directly into the circulation by the testes. When gonadotropin levels are elevated the amount of estradiol secretion by the testis is increased.

The 5α-reduced and estrogenic metabolites can exert local actions in the tissues in which they are formed or enter the circulation and act as hormones at other sites. Circulating dihydrotestosterone is formed principally in the androgen target tissues, whereas estrogen formation takes place in

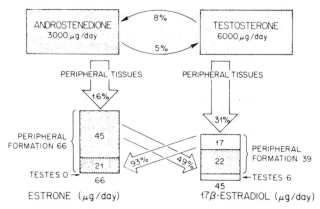

Figure 2.   *Androgen and estrogen production in normal young men.*

many peripheral tissues, the most significant site being adipose tissue. The overall rate of peripheral estrogen formation increases with increasing amounts of adipose tissue and with age.

Plasma testosterone and its active metabolites are converted into inactive metabolites in the liver and excreted predominantly in the urine; approximately half of the daily turnover is excreted in the form of urinary 17-ketosteroids (primarily androsterone and etiocholanolone), and the remainder is excreted as a series of polar compounds (diols, triols, and conjugates).

Gonadotropin regulation and testosterone secretion Testosterone secretion is regulated by pituitary LH (Fig. 3). Follicle-stimulating hormone (FSH) may also augment testosterone secretion, possibly by regulating the number of LH receptors on the plasma membrane of the Leydig cell. Testosterone feeds back on the pituitary to alter the sensitivity of the gland to the hypothalamic-releasing factor luteinizing hormone-releasing hormone (LHRH). Although the pituitary can convert testosterone to dihydrotestosterone and to estrogens, testosterone itself is the primary regulator of gonadotropin secretion. Whether testosterone also acts in the central nervous system to regulate the rate of LHRH formation or secretion is not known. Under ordinary circumstances, LH secretion is exquisitely sensitive to the feedback effects of testosterone, with complete suppression following the administration of amounts of exogenous androgen that approximate the normal daily secretory rate of testosterone (about 6 mg). However, prolonged elevation of plasma LH (as in testicular deficiency) renders the pituitary less sensitive to negative feedback control by exogenously administered androgens.

Neither the plasma concentration of testosterone nor that of LH is constant, each showing fluctuations of a pulsatile nature that reflect changes in secretory rates (Fig. 4). In the pubertal male major sleep-related surges in the pulsatile secretion of both LH and testosterone signal the initiation of puberty. In the adult the diurnal variation in the magnitude of this episodic secretion of LH and testosterone is minor with peak levels in the morning only about 10 to 15 percent higher than during the rest of the day.

Androgen action The major functions of androgen are the regulation of gonadotropin secretion, the initiation and maintenance of spermatogenesis, the formation of the male phenotype during sexual differentiation, and the induction of sexual maturation and function following puberty. The cellular mechanisms by which androgens perform these functions are summarized

Figure 3.

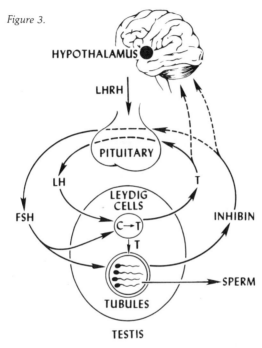

Regulation of testosterone and sperm production by LH and FSH. (C, cholesterol; T, testosterone.)

schematically in Fig. 5. Testosterone (T) enters the cell by passive diffusion. Inside the cell T can be converted to dihydrotestosterone (D) by the 5α-reductase enzyme. T or D is then bound to the androgen receptor protein in the cytosol (R). The hormone-receptor complex (TR or DR) is translocated to the nucleus where it attaches to specific chromosomal sites; as a result, new messenger RNA is transcribed, and ultimately new protein appears within the cytoplasm of the cell.

Although testosterone and dihydrotestosterone bind to the same receptor their physiological roles differ. The testosterone-receptor complex regulates gonadotropin secretion and is responsible for spermatogenesis and for the Wolffian stimulation phase of sexual differentiation whereas the dihydrotestosterone-receptor complex is responsible for external virilization during embryogenesis and the major portion of androgen action during sexual

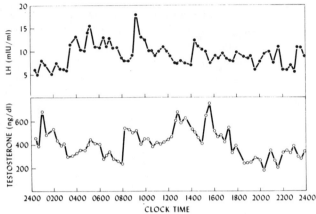

Figure 4.

Twenty-four-hour pattern of plasma LH and testosterone in a normal man sampled every 20 min. (Reprinted from Griffin and Wilson, 1980.)

maturation and adult sexual life. The mechanism by which testosterone and dihydrotestosterone mediate these different functions is not known. The mechanisms by which estrogens act to augment or block androgen effects are also not known. It is presumed that estradiol acts by a mechanism similar to that of androgens but involving its own receptor protein.

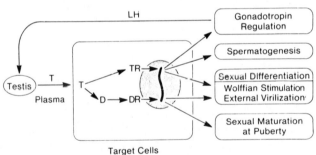

Figure 5.

Current concepts of androgen action. (T, testosterone; D, dihydrotestosterone; R, receptor protein.)

THE SEMINIFEROUS TUBULE AND SPERMATOGENESIS Normal function of the seminiferous tubule is dependent both on the pituitary and on normal function of the adjacent Leydig cells, both FSH and testosterone being essential for spermatogenesis (Fig. 3). The major site of FSH action is the Sertoli cell component of the seminiferous tubules. The seminiferous tubule is also a target for testosterone and contains specific androgen receptors. Testosterone appears to be essential for the initial phase of spermatogenesis, whereas FSH is required for the terminal phases of spermatid development. In the normal adult male this machinery produces more than 100 million sperm per day.

The Sertoli cell cannot synthesize steroid hormones de novo and is dependent on testosterone that diffuses in from adjacent Leydig cells. Isolated Sertoli cells (as well as Leydig cells) can convert testosterone to estradiol and to dihydrotestosterone. The role of these various metabolites in spermatogenesis is unclear.

The seminiferous tubules also produce the hormone inhibin that regulates the secretion of FSH by the hypothalamic-pituitary axis (Fig. 3). This hormone is a peptide that is formed during the late phase of spermatogenesis. Whether the hormone acts primarily at the level of the pituitary or hypothalamus to regulate FSH secretion is unknown.

The interlocking system in which two pituitary hormones regulate testicular function provides a precise dual-control mechanism by which plasma testosterone and sperm production feed back upon the hypothalamic-pituitary system to regulate their own rates of production (Fig. 3).

ASSESSMENT OF TESTICULAR FUNCTION

LEYDIG CELL FUNCTION The presence of male secondary sex characteristics clearly indicates that testosterone levels have been normal at least in the past, and normal libido and normal ejaculate indicate that testosterone levels are currently normal. However, the degree of virilization—for example, beard growth—among men with similar plasma testosterone levels is extremely variable. In addition, sexual function is influenced by many nonendocrine factors. Consequently, the laboratory assessment of Leydig cell function is frequently useful in separating endocrine from nonendocrine causes of male sexual dysfunction and in following the response to replacement therapy in patients with endocrine disorders.

Plasma testosterone and dihydrotestosterone levels Plasma testosterone is measured by a specific radioimmunoassay. Testosterone is secreted into plasma in a pulsatile fashion every 20 to 30 min (Fig. 4); a single random sample provides a result within ± 20 percent of the true mean value only two-thirds of the time while three equally spaced samples 6 to 18 min apart provide a more accurate assessment. The samples do not need to be assayed separately, and aliquots of the three samples can be pooled for a single determination. The range of plasma testosterone in normal adult men is 300 to 1000 ng/dl. In adult men the plasma values vary slightly throughout the day and at different times of the year, but these variations are not as great as those for plasma cortisol and are not significant in routine clinical assessment. Plasma levels of testosterone correlate in general with testosterone secretory rates as measured by isotope infusion.

The plasma testosterone value in normal prepubertal children is statistically higher in boys than girls, the range in both being 5 to 20 ng/dl. The major change of plasma testosterone at the beginning of puberty occurs as a result of sleep-related nocturnal gonadotropin surges so that during the initial phases of plasma testosterone and LH are higher at night than during the day. The random daytime levels of plasma testosterone increase gradually as puberty progresses and reach adult levels at about age 17.

Dihydrotestosterone can also be measured by radioimmunoassay. In normal young men the plasma dihydrotestosterone level is about a tenth that of the testosterone value and averages around 50 ng/dl. In older men with benign prostatic hyperplasia, plasma dihydrotestosterone levels are higher and average about 90 ng/dl.

Urinary 17-ketosteroids The measurement of urinary 17-ketosteroids is not a valid way to assess testicular function. Urinary 17-ketosteroids are mainly weak adrenal androgens or their metabolites, and testosterone contributes only about 40 percent of daily 17-ketosteroid production in men.

Plasma LH Plasma LH is measured by specific radioimmunoassay. LH is also secreted in a pulsatile fashion and fluctuates more widely than does plasma testosterone so that in adult men an isolated random plasma LH is likely to be within ± 20 percent of true mean value only a third of the time. Again, assay of a pool of plasma comprised of equal portions of three samples drawn 6 to 18 min apart as described above provides a value approaching the true mean. In early puberty plasma LH secretion increases only during sleep, but the pulsatile secretion in the adult is of similar magnitude during sleep and waking periods. The normal plasma LH values should be established for a given laboratory. The usual normal range in adult men is 26 ± 18 ng/ml SD (5 to 20 mIU/ml). A low plasma testosterone concentration can be interpreted correctly only if plasma LH is also measured simultaneously, and likewise the "appropriateness" of a given plasma LH must be interpreted in relation to the plasma testosterone. For example, a low plasma testosterone coupled with a low LH implies pituitary disease, whereas the finding of a low plasma testosterone and a high LH suggests primary testicular insufficiency.

Response to gonadotropin stimulation Leydig cell function is difficult to assess prior to puberty when both LH and testosterone levels are low, and it is common to measure response of plasma testosterone to gonadotropin stimulation as an index of Leydig cell capacity. A standard test is to administer human chorionic gonadotropin (HCG) 2000 IU intramuscularly daily for 4 days and to measure plasma testosterone before the first dose and 24 h after the fourth dose. Normal prepubertal boys respond by an increase in plasma testosterone to about 300 ng/dl.

Response to luteinizing hormone-releasing hormone The response of plasma LH (and/or FSH) to the administration of luteinizing hormone-releasing hormone (LHRH) is utilized in some centers to assess the functional integrity of the pituitary-testicular axis. In normal men LHRH, when given intravenously in a 100-μg bolus, leads to a four- to eightfold increase in plasma LH and a one- to twofold increase in the plasma FSH. Three baseline samples should be obtained in the half hour preceding the injection and again at 30 and 45 min after the injection to allow determination of the peak values of both the LH and FSH. Plasma testosterone does not change significantly after a single bolus of LHRH. However, continuous infusions of 10 μg of LHRH over a 1- to 2-h period result in an increase of plasma testosterone of approximately 20 percent above base line. LHRH is not available for routine use, and in most clinical situations assessment of response to LHRH is not necessary since basal gonadotropin levels correlate adequately with the stimulated response.

SEMINIFEROUS TUBULE FUNCTION Examination of the testes Evaluation of the testes is an essential portion of the physical examination. The seminiferous tubules account for about 95 percent of testicular volume. The prepubertal testis measures about 2 cm in length and 2 ml in volume and increases in size during puberty to reach the adult proportions by age 16. When damage to the seminiferous tubules occurs prior to puberty the testes are small and firm, whereas the testes are usually small and soft following postpubertal damage (the capsule, once enlarged, does not contract to its previous size). Testes average 4.6 cm in length (range, 3.5 to 5.5 cm), corresponding to a volume of 12 to 25 ml in normal adults. Advanced age alone does not influence testicular size, so that the significance of small testes is the same at all ages in the adult.

Semen analysis Seminal fluid analysis is performed after 24- to 36-h abstinence on samples obtained by masturbation into a glass container. Analysis should be performed within an hour. The normal ejaculate volume is greater than 2 ml. Immediately after ejaculation, coagulation of the seminal fluid occurs, followed within 15 to 30 min by liquefaction. Estimation of motility should be made on undiluted seminal fluid; more than 60 percent of the sperm should be motile and of normal morphology. The normal range for sperm density is generally considered to be 20 to 100 million per milliliter with a total count per ejaculate of more than 60 million, but a major difficulty in the interpretation of a semen analysis is the definition of the minimally adequate ejaculate. Some men documented to have low sperm counts are nevertheless fertile. This uncertainty as to the lower level of sperm density, percent motility, and percent normal forms in fertile semen stems from two issues. First, many factors produce temporary aberrations in sperm count, and in men who present with semen of equivocal quality it may be necessary to examine three or more ejaculates to determine whether abnormal findings are permanent or temporary. Second, at present fertilizing capacity can only be assessed by indirect means. A valid in vitro test of the capacity of human spermatozoa to fertilize ova is needed. Until such a test is available, the best functional assessment of spermatozoa is obtained from the cervical mucus penetration test, which is sometimes helpful in the evaluation of infertile couples when the routine semen analysis is normal.

Plasma FSH Plasma FSH as measured by specific radioimmunoassay usually correlates inversely with spermatogenesis. In normal adult men, the range of plasma FSH is 102 ±55 ng/ml SD (5 to 20 mIU/ml). Men with intact hypothalamic-pituitary axes have elevations of FSH when damage to the germinal epithelium is severe.

Testicular biopsy Testicular biopsy is useful in some patients with oligospermia and azoospermia both as an aid in diagnosis and as an indication of feasibility of treatment. For example, a normal testicular biopsy and a normal FSH in an azoospermic man suggest the diagnosis of obstruction of the vas deferens, which may be surgically correctible. Tissue culture of the biopsy material with subsequent karyotypic analysis is necessary to identify those instances of Klinefelter syndrome secondary to chromosomal mosaicism in which the abnormality is limited to the testes. Testicular biopsy is often followed by a transient decrease in sperm counts, but no permanent adverse effects are usually encountered.

ESTRADIOL Plasma estradiol is measured by radioimmunoassay and in normal men ranges from 20 to 42 pg/ml. As discussed above most estradiol produced in normal men is formed by extraglandular formation from circulating androgens. Elevated estradiol production and elevated plasma levels can be due to elevations in plasma precursors (liver disease), to increases in peripheral aromatization (obesity), or to increased production by the testes (androgen resistance syndromes). The level of plasma estradiol is not always a good index of estradiol production rate in men. One reason is technical difficulty in accurately measuring the low levels normally present in men. Another cause for the poor correlation may be episodic secretion in some men with enhanced estradiol production.

From *Harrison's Principles of Internal Medicine*, 10th edition, McGraw-Hill, 1982.
Reprinted with permission.

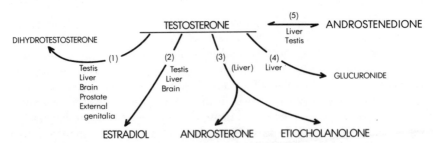

The diverse fates of testosterone illustrate the critical role of hormone metabolism in determining hormone effects. Although a potent androgen in itself, testosterone also serves as a prohormone for the stronger androgen dihydrotestosterone (1) and for the estrogen estradiol (2). Certain tissues can make both transformations. In addition, testosterone is converted to a weak androgen (3) or excreted as the glucuronide (4). Finally, testosterone can be interconverted to androstenedione (5), which is also aromatized (to esterone).

From Williams, *Textbook of Endocrinology*

11
RISK OF BIRTH DEFECTS

Anabolic steroids have been noted in the literature to effect not only the number of sperm produced but also the genetic integrity. In a fine paper by D.T. Lunde and D.A. Hamburg they noted:

In Primates. A significant series of experiments based on the discoveries in rodents of the effects of early exposure to androgens has been done by Goy, Phoenix, and their colleagues at the Oregon Regional Primate Research Center. Pregnant female rhesus monkeys have been given daily injections of testosterone proportionate during the presumptive period of sexual differentiation (from about day 39 to day 90 of the 108-day gestational period). Pseudohermaphrodite female monkeys have resulted from these pregnancies, and their behavior has been closely studied over a period of years through the various stages of development. Observations of eight such animals through infancy and adolescence have shown that they exhibit behavior in the aggressive sphere (initiating play, threats, rough-and-tumble play, and chasing) which resembles that of the male of the species rather than the female (Goy, 1968). Other forms of behavior that are not sexually dimorphic (e.g., huddling, grooming, withdrawing, and fear-grimacing) are not affected by testosterone treatment.

Sexual behavior is masculinized in these pseudohermaphrodite monkeys with an increase in mounting behavior the most striking difference between normal females. On the other hand, hormonal puberty is female in these animals, and they have menstrual cycles. This is in contrast to the findings in rats and guinea pigs, where early androgen treatment has produced anovulatory, acyclic females. It would appear that the effects of testosterone on the developing central nervous system are not limited to the hypothalamic-pituitary centers as originally suggested but also include other centers or circuits of the brain, which are involved in such activities as play and aggression.

In Humans. The preceding experiments in small mammals and subhuman primates raise the question of possible androgen effects in the early development of human females. Studies of two groups of females who were exposed to androgenic compounds *in utero* suggest that sexually dimorphic behavior in humans may be subject to early hormonal influence in a way analogous to the observations in animals. One such group consists of ten young girls ("progestin-induced hermaphrodites") whose mothers received either 17-ethynyltestosterone or 19-nor-17-ethynyltestosterone during pregnancy as a treatment for threatened abortion (Ehrhardt and Money, 1967).

Additional reference data:

Binding of Steroids to Human Spermatozoa and Its Possible Role in Contraception. Hyne R.V.: Boettcher B.—*Fertil. Steril.* 30(3):322-8, Sept. 78.

"A correlation between progestogens that bind to steroid-binding sites on human spermatozoa and progestogens that inhibit sperm migra-

SPERMATOZOON

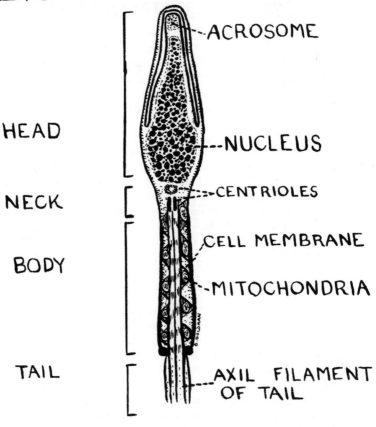

HEAD

NECK

BODY

TAIL

ACROSOME

NUCLEUS

CENTRIOLES

CELL MEMBRANE

MITOCHONDRIA

AXIL FILAMENT
OF TAIL

tion was established. The results indicated that there is a direct and specific effect on human spermatozoa..." Further..."The significance of these findings was discussed in relation to the contraceptive action of steroids applied directly to the lumen of the female genital tract."

"The major drawback to the development of chemical contraceptives for men is the fear of **genetic damage** and impotence." *Canadian Medical Assoc. Journal* 119(7):757-9 Oct. 78.

The metabolism and motility of human spermatozoa in the presence of steroid hormones and synthetic progestations, Hyne R.V.; Murdoch R.N.; Boettcher B. *Journal of Reproductive Fertility* 53 (2), July 78. "Progesterone and norethynodrel appeared to act on the plasma membrane of human spermatozoa to increase its permeability and hence to facilitate the loss of essential cofactors required for the glycolytic and oxidative processes." On the development of different morphologic abnormalities human spermatozoa:

"Morphologic comparison of the live and dead sperm population gives information concerning non-lethal and lethal abnormalities...

this indicates that no significant abnormalities develop after sperm maturation within the epididymis. Cyproterone acetate was shown to affect midpieces and tails of the living spermatozoa within two weeks of treatment. *Andrologia* 10(1): 43-8, Jan-Feb 78

12
RESEARCH STUDIES ON REPORTED CANCER TUMORS ASSOCIATED WITH ANABOLIC STEROIDS

Man lives in justifiable fear of anything potentially endangering his health or even life. No wonder that the worst fear is that of war, in the light of the dreadful experience from both of the last two World Wars. An individual, on the other hand, is most acutely afraid of potential malignancy.

Athletes, although healthy and full of zest of life, are no exception in this respect. Each case of death of a prominent athlete in consequence of a malignant tumor arouses profound sympathy in the others, as illustrated recently when several stars of the world athletic firmament died of cancer.

L. Schmid, *Journal of Sports Medicine*, 15 (1975)

There are many unknown aspects of the feared word *cancer*. One day we may find that which we considered healthy habits to be exactly the opposite. Perhaps chocolate cake is not as bad as we think or perhaps one day orange juice will be taboo.

Dr. L. Schmid of the Institute of Sports Medicine in Prague, Czechoslovakia, explored the fascinating links between vigorous athletic activity and the incidence of malignancy and tumor growth. He has published numerous papers in this area, and his study published in 1975 is probably the most extensive examination of this concept. As of 1973, his files contained 780 postmortem protocols of athletes who had died a natural death in Czechoslovakia, not including those who had died from accidents, violent acts, or in war. Then he chose those athletes who had a minimum of ten years of some physical athletic discipline. Dr. Schmid felt that this was ample time to have initiated significant morphological and physiological changes in those individuals.

He found that of the 780 subjects, 218, or 27.9 percent, had been treated for malignant tumors, which diagnosis was also confirmed by necropsy (autopsy). Of these, 86.4 percent were carcinomas and 13.6 percent were tumors of others types.

This brought to light the possibility of a link between chronic intense physical exertion and the development of tumor growth.

Discipline	Total number of athletes who died	Number of athletes who died of malignant tumors	In %
Track and Field	47	30	63.9
Gymnastics	105	14	13.3
Cycling	49	10	20.4
Rowing	19	7	36.8
Wrestling, Weight-Lifting	33	10	30.3
Soccer	200	89	44.5
Other games	48	31	64.5
Varia	61	27	44.2

He questioned whether the interferences athletic training and competition impose on the human metabolism and function might initiate or perpetuate tumor growth through homeostatic disturbances, fluid and electrolyte imbalances, dehydration, and metabolic disturbances. Mind you, this is not a frequent study design, since it is difficult to accumulate autopsy data or even research that many deceased athletes. This is not a pleasant thought for those of us straining and sweating through our daily torturous workouts. If anything, we tend to study the detrimental effect of a sedentary life and obesity.

The 28 percent noted in his study was well above the norm death rate due to cancer in the Czechoslovakian population and greater than the 20-22 percent incidence in the free world.

Malignant tumors as causes of death of former athletes.

F. W. Bickert[2]	(1929)	232 gymnasts	8.8%
		32 rowers	9.4%
C. J. Mervennee[16]	(1941)	100 soccer players	9.0%
A. Rook[22]	(1954)	99 cricket players	10.1%
		110 track and field	13.6%
		130 rowers	18.4%
		100 rugby players	12.0%
H. J. Montoye[19]	(1956)	66 athletes	14.0%
L. Schmid[25]	(1959)	514 athletes	16.9%
L. Schmid	(1973)	780 athletes	27.9%

If anything, most literature points to the fact that intense physical activity and muscular effort delays the inception and impedes tumor growth due to a rich oxygen supply to the tissues and supposedly retards malignant tumors. Other researches feel that histamine, which is produced in the tissues during exercise, inhibits tumor growth in laboratory animals.

Selye was the first to demonstrate that a disturbance of homeostasis leads to a mobilization of defensive forces of the organism, mainly by hypophyseal activation of the adrenals. In Selye's opinion, the potential of the adaptation energy is determined

SUMMARY OF REPORTED TUMORS ASSOCIATED WITH ANABOLIC STEROIDS

Author(s)	Reference	Diagnosis	Drug(s)
Bernstein et al.	1	Fanconi's anemia	Oxymetholone
Port et al.	2	Fanconi's anemia	Oxymetholone
Johnson et al.	3	Aplastic anemia	Oxymetholone
Johnson et al.	3	Aplastic anemia	Oxymetholone
Recant et al.	4	Fanconi's anemia	Methyltestosterone
Johnson et al.	5	Fanconi's anemia	Methandrostenolone
Zeigenfuss et al.	6	potency problem	Methyltestosterone
Henderson et al.	7	Hypoplastic anemia	Methyltestosterone Norethandrolone Oxymetholone Stanozolol
Meadows et al.	8	Aplastic anemia	Oxymetholone Deca-Durabolin
Farrell et al.	9	Paroxysmal nocturnal hemoglobinuria	Oxymetholone
Farrell et al.	9	Hypopituitarism	Methyltestosterone
Farrell et al.	9	Cryptorchidism	Methyltestosterone
Mulvihill et al.	10	Fanconi's anemia	Oxymetholone
Holder et al.	11	Acquired hypoplastic anemia	Methandrostenolone Oxymetholone Fluoxymesterone Deca-Durabolin
Bruguera et al.	12	Paroxysmal nocturnal hemoglobinuria	Oxymetholone
Sarna et al.	13	Fanconi's anemia	Norethandrolone Oxandrolone Oxymetholone
Lesna et al.	14	Aplastic anemia	Testosterone Oxymetholone
Sweeney et al.	15	Fanconi's anemia	Methyltestosterone Oxymetholone Deca-Durabolin
Sweeney et al.	15	Aplastic anemia	Oxymetholone
Kew et al.	16	Fanconi's anemia	Methyltestosterone Depo-testosterone Methyltestosterone Oxymetholone
Mokrohisky et al.	17	Fanconi's anemia	Oxymetholone
Sale et al.	18	Aplastic anemia	Testosterone Oxymetholone Methyltestosterone Fluoxymesterone
AFIP Case 1	19	Aplastic anemia	Methyltestosterone Oxymetholone

Dosage mg/day	Duration (months)	Transfusions	Abnormal liver function tests
100	100	no	yes
?	9	no	?
30–100	46	yes	no
150–250	28	yes	yes
20	40	yes	yes
10–50	89	no	yes
?	360	no	yes
40–80	21	yes	yes
10	3		
100	35		
15	18		
60	41	yes	no
50/wk	6		
100–150	6	yes	yes
25–50	20	no	yes
50	96	no	no
20–60	37	no	yes
?	2	yes	yes
?	13		
?	?		
50/wk	?		
?	36	?	?
56.7g(total)	88	yes	yes
2.1 (total)	88		
1.2 (total)	88		
?	?	yes	?
68	?		
20	36	yes	yes
?	?		
25/wk	12		
100–300	3	no	yes
100	12	yes	yes
100	9		
20	24		
150	48		
?	2	no	?
?	35	yes	yes
100–150	?		
75	?		
?	?		
70	60	yes	yes
70–210	24		

genetically. If this potential is spent by strenuous training, sometimes leading to complete exhaustion, the defensive forces decrease or even completely disappear in consequence thereof. In such a situation, in subjects possibly thus predisposed, at certain sites of the organism a malignant cellular degeneration takes place.

Journal of Sports Medicine, 15 (1975)

To further support the oxygen-deficiency theory in cells, some authors feel the prime cause of cancer is disturbed cell respiration. They were able to prove this by producing cancer cells in the lab by intermittent withdrawal of oxygen.

This can cause one to speculate that exhaustive exercise procedures without proper rest, oxygenation of tissue, and nutrition could lead to degradation of nucleic acids in cell nuclei that may initiate the activation of cellular oncogenous genes.

The body has a delicate nuclear balance. Anabolic steroids, although used in therapy to rejuvenate the body and blood constituents, might lead to some imbalance and predispose one to tumor growth. So train hard, get the oxygen those cells need, and leave the hormones to your adrenals and testes.

Some athletes say that the birth-control pill is more dangerous than taking anabolic steroids. They are probably correct. However a woman does not consume a month's supply of pills per day!

1. M.S. Berstein, R.L. Hunter, S. Yachnin, "Hepatoma and peliosis hepatis developing with Fanconi's anemia," *New Engl. J. Med.*, 284 (1971):1135-36.
2. R.B. Port, J.P. Patasnick, K. Ranniger, "Angiographic demonstration of hepatoma in association with Fanconi's anemia," *Am. J. Med.*, 39 (1965):464-75.
3. F.L. John, "Androgenic-anabolic steroids and hepatocellular carcinoma," in *Hepatocellular Carcinoma*, K. Okuda, R.L. Peters, eds. New York: Wiley (1976):95-103.
4. L. Racant, and P. Lacey, "Fanconi's anemia and hepatic cirrhosis," *Clinicopathologic conference. Am. J. Med.*, 39 (1965):464-75.
5. F.L. Johnson, J.R. Feagler, K.G. Lerner, P.W. Majerus, M. Siegel, J.R. Hartman, and E.D. Thomas, "Association of androgenic-anabolic steroid therapy with development of hepatocellular carcinoma," *Lancet*, 2 (1972):1273-76.
6. J. Ziegenfuss, and R.Carabasi, "Androgens and hepatocellular carcinoma," *Lancet*, 1 (1973):262.
7. J.T. Henderson, J. Richmond, and M.D. Sumerling, "Androgenic-anabolic steroid therapy and hepatocellular carcinoma," *Lancet*, 1(1973):934.
8. A.T. Meadows, J.L. Naiman, and M. Valdes-Dapena, "Hepatoma associated with androgen therapy for aplastic anemia," *J. Pediatr.*, 84 (1974):108-10.
9. G.C. Farrel, D.E. Joshua, R.F. Uren, J.J. Baird, K.W. Perkins, and H. Kronenberg, "Androgen-induced hepatoms," *Lancet*, 1 (1975):430-32.
10. J.J. Mulvihill, R.L. Ridolfi, F.R. Schlutz, M.S. Borzy, and P.B.T. Haughton, "Hepatic adenoma in Fanconi anemia treated with oxymetholone," *J. Pediatr.*, 87 (1975):122-24.

11. L.E. Holder, D.J. Gnarra, B.C. Lampkin, H. Nishiyama, and P. Perkins, "Hepatoma associated with anabolic steroid therapy," *Am. J. Roentgenol*, 124 (1975):638-643.

12. M. Bruguera, "Hepatoma associated with androgenic steroids," *Lancet*, 1 (1975):1295.

13. G. Sarna, P. Tomasulo, M.J. Lotz, J.G. Bubinak, and H.R. Shulman, "Multiple neoplasms in two siblings with a variant form of Fanconi's anemia," *Cancer*, 36 (1975):1029-33.

14. M. Lesna, I. Spencer, and W. Wolker, "Liver nodules and androgens," *Lancet*, 1 (1976):1124.

15. E.C. Sweeney, and D.J. Evans, "Hepatic lesions in patients treated with synthetic anabolic steroids," *J. Clin. Pathol.*, 29 (1976):626-33.

16. M.C. Kew, B. Van Coller, C.M. Prowse, B. Skikne, J.I. Wolfsdorf, J. Isdale, S. Krawitz, H. Altman, S.E. Levin, and T.H. Bothwell. "Occurrence of primary hepatocellular cancer and peliosis hepatis after treatment with androgenic steroids," *S. Afr. Med. J.*, 50 (1976):1233-37.

17. S.T. Mokrohisky, D.R. Ambruso, and W.E. Hathaway, "Fulminant hepatic neoplasia after androgen therapy," *New Engl. J. Med.*, 296 (1977):1411-12.

18. G.E. Sale, and K.G. Lerner, "Multiple tumors after androgen therapy," *Arch. Pathol. Lab. Med.*, 101 (1977):600-603.

19. K.G. Ishak, "Hepatic neoplasms associated with contraceptive and anabolic steroids,"

From William N. Taylor, M.D., *Anabolic Steroids and the Athlete*, which was adapted from K.G. Ishak, "Hepatic Neoplasm Associated with Contraceptive and Anabolic Steroids," *Recent Results in Cancer Research*, 66 (1979):73–128.

13
DIET AND STEROIDS

In order for anabolic steroids to be of use in increasing muscular strength and size an adequate amount of foodstuffs, especially protein, must be taken in. The normal individual usually requires about one gram protein/kg. body weight per day. When taking protein supplements during training they must be of high biological value, the quality of which depends on the proportions of certain amino acids and their digestibility. The degree of intensity of training will better define the needs.

Chloride is very important since it plays a major role in acid-base relationships in the body and the maintenance of body water. It comprises 65% of the total extracellular anions, and is ingested as a potassium, calcium, sodium or magnesium salt in food. Serum chloride levels are determined in cases where there is serious dehydration, edema or electrolyte problems which are sometimes the case in retention of water with the use of anabolic steroids. Some of the negative results in anabolic steroid studies may have been due to not supplying an adequate diet.

Nitrogen retention was found to be better on a diet of natural food rather than simulated artificial foods. An example is using whole egg rather than a mixture of amino acids mimicking egg protein (224), and other foods such as whole egg (225, 226), milk (227) and peanut butter, and oats (228) instead of their equal amounts of amino acids simulating these foods. There might be other additives in the natural foods that better facilitate their metabolic use.

In an animal study using adult male castrated rats it was found that increasing the protein content of the diet by replacing some of the carbohydrate in diet with an equal amount of protein (casein) did not change the nitrogen retention or growth for the animals on anabolic steroids.

Vitamin B and folic acid, along with vitamin B_1, B_2, and B_{12}, have been noted to decrease with the administration of oral contraceptives. It is strongly suggested that an athlete undergoing intensive training take a high-potency B-complex vitamin with 500-1,000 mg. of vitamin C daily to maintain protective and growth levels of these vitamins for nervous-system tissue and muscle growth. Some good trustworthy brands are Centrum and Theragram M. Maximum lifespan vitamins are just now becoming available and can be looked into.

Finally, good snacks are Kraft hard cheeses, Del Monte raisins and prunes, or Dannon yogurt.

14
HUMAN GROWTH HORMONE (HGH)

Human growth hormone is a polypeptide hormone with a molecular weight of 21,000 and is produced by the pituitary gland.The metabolic processes controlled by growth hormone are multiple and complex. Back in the early 1920s, H. M. Evans and J. A. Long found that following an injection of alkaline extracts of ox pituitary glands, normal rats reached abnormally huge body proportions. Along with the growth of skeletal muscle and bone, there was organomegaly (growth of the visceral organs and tissues).

The hormone is extracted from the pituitary glands of cadavers and is also known as somatotrophic hormone (STH) or somatotrophin. It comes from the anterior portion of the pituitary gland and makes up about 8 milligrams, or 10 percent of the dry weight of the gland. Fortunately, the human pituitary and the somatotrophic granules resist autolytic dissolution after death.

As with most laboratory experimentation, the rat model is most commonly used, since this species responds well to growth hormone because the epiphyses (ends) of the long bones remain open and viable throughout the life of the animal. This is not the case with humans. Growth hormone seems to effect virtually every cell in the body except the eyeballs and the brain. It has been noted that the abdominal and thoracic viscera, such as the GI tract, lungs, heart, and liver, may grow in an even greater proportion than the musculo-skeletal system.

Growth hormone has been used for the past twenty-five years to treat children with growth-hormone deficiency. The supply in the past has always been short and not all needy children could receive the needed medicine to lead a normal life.

Fortunately for these children, a synthetic laboratory source of GH is now available. The October 1983 issue of *Hospital Practice* examines the clinical uses of synthetic growth hormone. It has been found that more than 1 percent of the protein synthesized by genetically manipulated E. Coli is growth hormone. Thus, 10 liters of bacterial suspension produce 10 grams of the hormone.

This is very exciting for me as a scientist but frightening in my role of athlete. This means that the high cost of the drug—$500–1,000 for a six-to-ten-week treatment—now costs $2,500 in the natural state, but it might plummet the way of pocket calculator prices, and this will lead to abuse. We could soon be looking at the land of the giants, or *Acromegalic City.*

Before going into the dangers, let us explore further how growth hormone works. HGH stimulates the liver to produce somatomedins, which are messenger molecules sometimes referred to as "growth factors." Somatotrophin is both an anticatabolic as well as a protein anabolic hormone. This in-

Natural V. Synthetic Human Growth Hormone

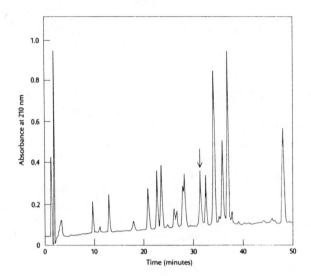

High-pressure liquid chromatography of rDNA-derived growth hormone (above) and human pituitary-derived growth hormone (below), each broken into 17 fragments by trypsin digestion, showed that elution patterns corresponded exactly, except for 12th peak (arrows). Fragment contains first nine amino acids, including additional methionine in rDNA-derived hormone molecule. (From Kohr WJ, Keck R, Harkins RN: Characterization of intact ad trypsin-digested biosynthetic human growth hormone by high-pressure liquid chromatography. Anal Biochem 122:348, 1982)

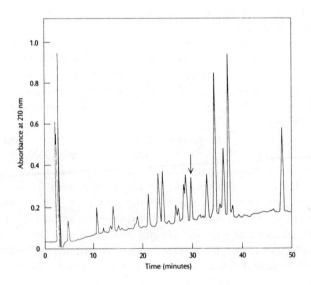

creases the incorporation of amino-acid uptake in the body, leading to protein anabolism in body cells, creating a positive nitrogen balance.

FACTORS INFLUENCING NORMAL GH SECRETION

	GH Secretion	
	Augmented	Inhibited
Neurogenic	1. Stages III and IV sleep	1. REM sleep
	2. Stress (traumatic, surgical, infectious, psychogenic)	2. Emotional deprivation
	3. α Adrenergic agonists	3. β Adrenergic agonists
	4. βAdrenergic antagonists	4. αAdrenergic antagonists
	5. L-Dopa	
Metabolic	1. Hypoglycemia (fasting)	1. Hyperglycemia
	2. Falling fatty acid level	2. Rising fatty acid level
	3. Amino acids*	3. Obesity
	4. Uncontrolled diabetes	
	5. Uremia	
	6. Hepatic cirrhosis	
Hormonal	1. Low somatomedin(?)	1. Somatostatin
	2. Estrogens	2. Hypothyroidism
	3. Glucagon	3. Large doses of corticosteroids
	4. Vasopressin	4. Medroxyprogesterone

From Williams' *Textbook on Endocrinology*

Arginine and Ornithine

The Dangers of Growth Hormone

Now with the advent of synthetic HGH, the obsessed abusers can pick up the ball and run with it. Witness Dr. Kerr's recent statement in *Muscle Digest*: "The bulking gains I've described have been quite excellent. The main feature is that with twenty to fifty pounds of weight gain, there is to be found little fat or fluid weight gain!" He goes on:

> Some athletes find that while bulking with STH and using a highly androgenic oral anabolic drug such as Anadrol, Dianabol or Maxbolin [sic], some cutting features are to be found. Little or no change in the waist size can be seen while the athlete is undergoing a weight gain of 40 lbs. . . . As far as its bulking effect it would appear now that STH is just about mandatory for competing in the Universe and Olympia and probably beginning this year for the America.

What aspiring and obsessed young athlete wouldn't give his left testicle and part of his liver for forty pounds of solid muscle? But now, back to reality.[1] Here is what the young athletes read and take as fact. The following is from *The Underground Steroid Handbook for Men and Women*, which bears no author's name but can be purchased through a post office box from magazine ads.

There comes a time for many in competitive athletics where winning is more important than those initial goals of health, recreation, and relaxation. If you don't like the use of drugs in competitive athletics, you shouldn't have bought this book and you shouldn't be reading it now; we're trying to help you, not antagonize you. There are always people who are genetically near perfect for a particular sport and would probably win without steroids. Steroids mostly help those (ourselves included) with poor to just good genetic predispositions. The real truth is, that if used correctly (and most people don't use steroids correctly), steroids can give you permanent weight gains.

Let's tell you some straight facts on steroid usage. ONE: The more that you take, the more you'll grow (if you eat enough and train right). TWO: Some brands work better than others. THREE: Orals do more damage to your liver than injectables. FOUR: The less toxic an oral is to your liver, the less effective it is for growth. FIVE: There is no such thing as taking too much steroid. It varies from person to person. 'Too much' for one may not be enough for another. SIX: 'Too much' is only related to your health. No doctor, no researcher, no one has determined the optimum dosage for athletic performance. SEVEN: Most of the people who have taken massive amounts of steroids and shot their blood test results past the normal reference ranges didn't get ill, didn't die and had the test results drop into the normal range after the cessation of the drugs. EIGHT: Never assume that you are like 'most people' until you prove it.

GROWTH HORMONE (aka GH and STH) Injectable, 10 unit vials, 4 to box. Wow, is this great stuff! It is the best drug for permanent muscle gains. It is the basic pituitary hormone that makes your whole body grow. People who use it can expect to gain 30 to 40 lbs. of muscle in ten weeks if they can eat about 10,000 calories per day. It is about $600-$800 per 4 vials, and we think this to be another best buy. It has been very hard to get in the past as it was made from the pituitary glands of rhesus monkeys and is illegal for general sale in the USA. It is now being made from 'smart' E Coli bacteria at Baylor Medical School in Texas. Usual dosage has been 2 units every three days. This is the only drug that can remedy bad genetics as it will make anybody grow. A few side effects can occur, however. It may enlongate your chin, feet and hands, but this is arrested with cessation of the drug. Diabetes in teenagers is possible with it. It can also thicken your ribcage and wrists. Massive increases in weight over such a short time can, of course, give you heart problems. We have heard of a powerlifter getting a heart attack while on GH. GH use is the biggest gamble that an athlete can take, as the side effects are irreversable [sic]. Even with all that, we LOVE the stuff.

This —not medical journals—is what the kids take as fact.

Some problems one may encounter are antibody formation against HGH, a sort of allergic reaction to a foreign substance in the body. Hepatitis is a possibility, since the hormone is extracted from human tissue. Hypoglycemia and diabetes with the chance of diabetic coma in susceptible individuals is also a possibility. Finally, the one area I fear the most is acromegaly, which I call the *Frankenstein Syndrome.*

Acromegaly

Acromegaly is a disorder that occurs when excess growth hormone is secreted by a pituitary tumor. Its symptoms can be induced with abuse of this substance. The bones of the feet, hands, fingers, nose, and jaw grow, along with the soft tissue of the face—the nose, lips, naso-labial folds, forehead, and tongue—increase in size to give one a Frankenstein look.

At first you might notice a progressive increase in ring, shoe, or hat size. There is a coarsening of facial features with increased size of the nose, lips, tongue, and soft facial tissues. An underbite is noted with enlargement of the mandible and jaw. The forehead grows with prominent orbital ridges and enlarged frontal sinuses. The voice develops a deep, husky, cavernous quality. The fingers and toes widen into a spade-like appearance. An increase in sweating and sebaceous-gland activity, along with small patches of increased skin pigmentation, known as fibromata mollusca. There may also be an increased growth of coarse body hair.

Joint pain comes next with a widening of the joint spaces because of the growth of cartilage and soft tissues. When an adult of full height takes HGH, his or her bone ends are already fused, so they get a widening and distortion of the boney structures, which leads to all sorts of problems and disfigurement. Later on, osteoarthritis and limitation of joint range or motion occur. The increased growth hormone causes the heart to enlarge so that congestive heart failure may occur.

I hope athletes of the future will not resemble the individuals pictured in this book, but with the advent of synthetically produced, inexpensive growth hormone and the abuse of it, there will be a price to pay.

Levodopa

As though this were not bad enough, it has become common practice for athletes on growth hormone to also take L-Dopa (Levodopa), a drug used for the treatment of Parkinson's Disease, to enhance the effects of HGH. L-Dopa is a dangerous medication in a healthy body and has been known to cause:

* gastrointestinal bleeding
* phlebitis (inflammation of the veins)

* activation of melanoma (skin cancer)
* cardiac arythmias and irregularities
* hemolytic anemia
* agranulocytosis
* orthostatic hypotension (a dangerous drop in blood pressure)
* mental changes such as depression, paranoia, and dementive episodes
* anorexia (loss of weight)
* nausea and vomiting
* symptoms of abdominal distress
* vertigo (dizziness)
* narrow-angle glaucoma could worsen
* headaches, insomnia, blurred vision

In addition, some respiratory and endocrine disturbances could well occur. This drug was created to help people who cannot manufacture sufficient dopamine and not for GH-crazy jocks.

15
HUMAN CHORIONIC GONADOTROPIN (HCG)

Human Chorionic Gonadotropin (HCG) is secreted from the trophoblastic cells of the placenta into the mother's plasma and excreted in the urine. This natural protein hormone is produced by the placenta of pregnant women, where its function is to maintain the corpus luteum (the hormone-secreting ovary). HCG is composed of two subunits: The alpha subunit is akin in structure to LH (luetinizing hormone) and FSH (follicle-stimulating hormone).

In males, LH stimulates the interstitial cells of the testes, which cause them to produce androgen (gonadal steroids, such as testosterone). In women, both LH and FSH work together to aid development of the egg (ovarian follicle), which usually occur at the middle of a woman's cycle. When a woman becomes pregnant, the HCG is secreted by the placenta so that the corpus luteum is maintained after the decrease in LH secretion. This allows the body to continue putting out progesterone and estrogen to help maintain the uterus and child—thereby preventing menstruation.

Serum levels of HCG are highest during the first three weeks of pregnancy. Some of the other functions of HCG are: (1) used by men whose testes require stimulation to increase spermatogenesis (increased sperm production); (2) as a stimulant to women with ovarian dysfunction; (3) to detect pregnancy in women; (4) to detect tumor growth to help evaluate the pathological progression of such diseases as Oat cell lung carcinoma, hydatiform moles, and choriocarcinoma; (5) to stimulate testes function after endogenous production of male hormones have decreased from taking anabolic steroids. When you take exogenous steroids, you decrease your body's own natural production of androgens. This is also the case when clomid (clomiphene citrate) is used to rejuvenate atrophied testicular function.

When anabolics are taken, you get a negative feedback, shutting off the LH and FSH secretion by the pituitary gland. HCG is not a male hormone but a substance derived from the urine of pregnant women. One interesting aspect is that with abuse of this drug men might finally realize what it feels like to be pregnant, for with enough use, they may experience the nausea, vomiting, and "morning sickness" syndrome women enjoy, and with long-term abuse, men may begin to develop changes in adipose (fat) distribution and induce gynecomastia (female breast tissue). These abuses are still in their infantile stage and have yet to manifest enough to hit the literature. But time will tell.

16
CLOMID (CHLOMIPHENE CITRATE)

Clomid is a woman's fertility drug that has been used to help women get pregnant; it has also been used to increase men's sperm counts. The drug initiates increased release of luteinizing hormone, which triggers ovulation. In the 1970s, David Paulson, M.D., of Duke University found that low doses of clomid increase male sperm counts (1). He found that clomid "disrupts normal feedback inhibition of the anterior hypothalamus and hypophysis [the pituitary gland] so as to enhance release of follicle-stimulating hormone [FSH] and luteinizing hormone [LH] by binding or occupying steroid-binding receptors at these sites and thereby inducing the release of hypophyseal [pituitary] gonadotropin-releasing hormones." (1)

Thomas Jones, M.D., staff endocrinologist at the University of Chicago, has found that individuals on anabolic steroids, especially the androgenic variety, have exhibited a significant decrease in sperm production and very significant testicular atrophy. Of even greater concern is the change in quality and size of the prostate. There is a clear correlation between the increase in size (benign prostatic hypertrophy) and the risk of prostatic cancer. "I would guess," said Dr. Jones, "that those individuals who abuse anabolics as young athletes might present with prostatic cancer at a much younger age. Instead of being in their seventies, they might present in their forties or fifties."

Dr. Jones performed his own study utilizing clomid (1980) and noted increases in sperm count and testosterone. His study noted an increase of body testosterone from 599 ng/dl (nanograms/deciliter) to 1,104 ng./dl. after one cycle of 25 milligrams of clomid daily for three weeks, followed by one week with no drug. The group average sperm count went from 11 to 39 million per cc. (2)

However, in an earlier study with this drug, it was found that increasing dosages caused decreased sperm counts by damaging the spermatids. (3)

Clomid has no effect on a woman's testosterone level because she doesn't have androgen-producing organs as a man does—unless, of course, she has a testosterone-secreting tumor, at which point she would, no doubt, pass for someone's brother. It should be noted, however, that testosterone itself retains much of the unwanted androgenic-male characteristics that safer anabolic agents attempt to subdue.

Some athletes who have damaged their testes and lowered sperm production with anabolic abuse might be able to salvage possible fatherhood with proper and supervised administration of clomid.

Notes
1. D. F. Paulson and J. Wacksman, "Clomiphene Citrate in the Management of

Male Infertility," *Journal of Urology*, 115 (January 1976): 73-76.
2. T. M. Jones, V. S. Fang, R. L. Rosenfield, et al., "Parameters of Response to Clomiphene Citrate in Oligospermic Men," *Journal of Urology*, 124 (July 1980): 53-55.
3. C. H. Heller, J. R. Mavis, and G. V. Heller, "Clomiphene Citrate: A Correlation of Its Effect on Sperm Concentration and Morphology, Total Gonadotropins, ICSH, Estrogen and Testosterone Excretion, and Testicular Cytology in Normal Men," *Journal of Clin. Endocrin. Metab.*, 29 (1969): 638.

17
PRINCIPLES OF CARBOHYDRATE LOADING
by Dr. Ben Londeree

1. During prolonged heavy exercise, the carbohydrate stores are gradually depleted. Energy for exercise is derived almost entirely from fats and carbohydrates. Whereas the supply of fats is virtually inexhaustible, carbohydrates, due to volume requirements, are stored in limited quantities.

2. Depletion of carbohydrates leaves only fats available for energy, with the result that the intensity of activity must be reduced considerably (1–3 minutes per mile). Optimal performance requires that the runner avoid depletion during competition.

3. The rate of glycogen depletion is a function of the relative intensity (percent of maximal oxygen consumption). Below an intensity representing 50 percent of maximal oxygen consumption, about 50 percent of the energy is derived from fat. At higher intensities, an increasing proportion of the energy is obtained from carbohydrates. This means that glycogen depletion can be delayed by reducing the speed.

4. The time to exhaustion and glycogen depletion is directly related to the initial concentration of glycogen in the muscles. In other words, with higher beginning muscle glycogen levels, an individual can work at a particular intensity of exercise for a longer period of time.

5. In order to bring about glycogen super-compensation, the body first must be stimulated to synthesize extra glycogen-storing enzyme through depletion of the present supply of glycogen. A high-carbohydrate diet without prior glycogen depletion will not produce super-compensation.

6. Whereas live glycogen is readily depleted by starvation, a low-carbohydrate diet, and/or prolonged exercise, the only way to deplete muscle glycogen is through exercise. Carbohydrate cannot escape once inside of a muscle fiber.

7. Depletion of muscle glycogen stores occurs only in the active muscle fibers. Consequently, a significant amount of the depletion activity must be identical with the activity for which the individual is preparing.

8. The greater the glycogen depletion, the greater the stimulation for the synthesis of glycogen-storing enzyme will be. This, in turn, will increase the potential for super-compensation.

9. The longer the depletion is maintained, the greater the stimulation

for the synthesis of glycogen-storing enzyme will be. As above, this increases the potential for super-compensation.

10. Depletion can be maintained with a low-carbohydrate diet and continued training. In fact, such an approach will make it less necessary for complete initial depletion via exhaustive exercise and thereby reduce the risk of incurring fatigue injuries.

11. A small amount of carbohydrates (about 60 grams per day) is essential during the depletion phase for adequate functioning of several important systems in the body, e.g., the nervous system, red blood cells, and kidneys.

12. Before commencing the high-carbohydrate diet, redeplete through appropriate physical activity. This is to make sure that you are depleting as much as possible and probably will require only 5–10 miles, depending upon the carbohydrate content of your diet since the previous depletion run. If you have not used the low-carbohydrate diet, then this depletion run must be much longer (15–20 miles). This latter approach, of course, exposes the individual to an injury very close to the time of competition.

13. Glycogen super-compensation (following depletion) will occur only to the extent that carbohydrates are made available in the diet. The greater the percent of carbohydrates in the diet, the greater the super-compensation will be. Adequate proteins (2–3 ounces per day), minerals, vitamins, and lots of water should be included in the diet also.

14. *Do not overeat* when on the high-carbohydrate diet. Although you will need a positive caloric balance in order to store energy in the form of glycogen, the reduced activity will more than take care of this if you eat your normal amount of food. The important point is to increase the dietary carbohydrate percent.

15. Drink a large excess of fluids while on the high-carbohydrate diet. About 3–4 grams of water are stored with every gram of glycogen. If an inadequate supply of water is drunk the extra water is withdrawn from other body sources and a relative dehydration will occur. It is not uncommon for infections to result from such dehydration. A good indicator of proper water intake is clear urine. An amber urine means that you need more water.

16. Activity will tend to reduce super-consumption and should be avoided while on the high-carbohydrate diet. Stay off of your feet as much as possible.

17. Once super-consumption occurs, the excess glycogen-storing enzyme is inactivated and the muscles will tend to burn off the excess glycogen during normal activities. Therefore, timing of the peak super-consumption is rather critical and varies among individuals— typically 2–4 days on the high-carbohydrate diet. The time will depend on individual genetic differences and will tend to be shorter for

those persons who regularly deplete and super-compensate during their normal training and diet regime. Some symptoms that the peak super-compensation has passed include: bloated feeling, loose bowels, and excessive urination.

18. Reduce the quantity of carbohydrates as well as other foods in the diet during the several hours before the event. There is evidence that a large amount of carbohydrates at this time may impair performance.

19. It is not necessary to fully super-compensate for all competitions. For short activities, it probably would be beneficial to increase the percent of carbohydrates in the diet for one or two days only for the purpose of ensuring that glycogen stores are not low. For events lasting 30–60 minutes, moderate super-compensation would suffice (e.g., ten-mile run forty-eight hours before competition followed by a high-carbohydrate diet and rest). For longer periods of competition, moderate super-compensation would be beneficial, but utilization of the full protocol would produce better results.

20. If, after weighing all the pros and cons, you decide to super-compensate, try it in stages during your training. For example, start with a long run followed by a high-carbohydrate diet (start with principle 12). Keep a detailed log of what you do and what happens. If satisfied, then try the entire series (depletion, low-carbohydrate diet, re-depletion, high-carbohydrate diet) but stay on the low-carbohydrate diet only for one day. If there are no adverse effects, then extend the low-carbohydrate diet gradually to a maximum of three to four days. Do not take short-cuts. Remember, you are playing with biochemical dynamite.

Reprinted with permission from "Food for Fitness" published by *Runner's World Magazine, Mountainview, CA.*

Good sources of ruffage carbohydrates include natural grain breads, like Pepperidge Farms whole wheat breads, and whole-grain cereals, such as Nabisco Shredded Wheat, Allbran, Bran Chex from Ralston Purina, and Post Grape Nuts.

18
THE SKELETAL SYSTEM AND STEROIDS

Bone cells carry on metabolic activities and must meet homeostatic requirements just as any system of cells or tissue in the body. Unlike other connective tissues, bones possess a mineral intercellular matrix (material base).

Minerals account for two-thirds of the weight of bone and give it hardness and rigidity. The remaining portion (ground substance, fibers and cells) are basically protein and give bone a degree of flexibility and toughness.

If one is to examine bone that has been burned (incinerated), only the inorganic material, an ash-like remaining portion, will still retain the original shape of the bone. The organic portion has been oxidized. The inorganic portion is very brittle, as can be seen by the way the ash will disintegrate upon impact. However, if bone is immersed in acid, the inorganic mineral portion will be removed leaving only organic material. Basically, all organic means is carbon compound. With the mineral (inorganic portion) gone, the decalcified bone can be bent and twisted like a pretzel into a knot.

The bone has now lost its rigidity but still looks like ordinary bone.

Bones make up the skeletal framework and supportive system for the body and most of the internal viscera is attached to the skeleton directly or indirectly. Bones *articulate* (fit together) and with the muscles attached to them form levers for body movement. The bones also serve as a protective function for fragile and soft tissues (such as the brain encased in the cranium). Aside from sheltering necessary organs such as the heart and lungs, the bones also protect themselves in that their hard outer covering protects the *hemopoietic tissues*, which are the red bone marrow where red blood cells are formed.

PREMATURE EPIPHISEAL CLOSURE

The growth stage of teenage life is by far one of the *most dangerous periods to take anabolic steroids.* Bones have not as yet achieved their full growth potential. In the early stages of growth, the bones have a large cartilage portion where certain enzymes are then secreted into the immediate intercellular environment to cause minerals to be deposited in the cartilage to make it become *calcified.* Calcification causes a variety of changes as the cartilage disintegrates and is replaced by osteoblasis (bone cells) which turns cartilage into bone. Now what was once the center of the cartilage is now replaced by bone, but the ends or *epiphyses* of the bone are still cartilage where cartilage continues to divide and makes the bone grow longer. Eventually, the bone replacement will catch up with the cartilage ends causing the epiphyseal cartilage to disappear, after which there would be no further increase in bone length.

If the epiphyses are caused to close early because of steroid abuse, one will not reach full growth potential. Anabolic steroids cause the cartilage in the epiphyses (bone ends) to close prematurely.

If you are interested in when bone growth is complete, it continues until quite late in life. For example, *ossification* is complete in the following bones at the corresponding ages.

bone	age at which fusion is complete
Clavical (bone in the front of your shoulder) You could end up with a misshaped, shallow chest if this necessary, supportive bone growth is cut short	23-31
Bones of leg, thigh, and foot If these bones are affected, full growth will be seriously endangered	18-22
Vertebrae (the supportive discs of the spinal column) This is the backbone (literally) for the whole skeletal structure	25
Sacrum (the lower end of the spinal column)	23-25
Sternum (the breast bone which comes down the center of the chest)	23
Manubrium (section on the sternum) Xiphoid (end tip of the sternum)	after 30

As can be seen from the chart, full bone growth is not achieved right after puberty or in the teens but much later in life. *Anabolic drugs, disrupting full bone growth, will seriously hamper true athletic potential.*

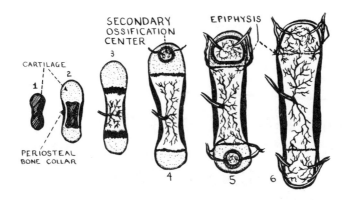

Some major events in the formation of a long bone organ by endochondral ossification. 1. hyaline cartilage model; hypertrophy of central chondrocytes; 2. hypertrophied chondrocytes begin to die due to initiation of matrix calcification; formation of the bone collar; 3. invasion of blood vessels and pluripotential osteoprogenitor cells; resorption of calcified cartilage matrix to form exposed surfaces for bone tissue apposition in primary center of ossification; 4. growth of bone organ and formation of marrow cavity via cartilage proliferation at epiphyseal ends, bone tissue apposition at calcified cartilage surfaces, and resorption in diaphyseal cavity; initiation of secondary center of ossification above; elongation of bone collar, 5-6. Further growth of bone organ; formation and development of secondary center of ossification above leaving cartilaginous epiphyseal plate separating epiphysis from diaphysis; appearance of additional secondary center of ossification below; growth in girth of bone organ by concomitant bone tissue opposition on outer diaphyseal surface and resorption from inner surface. Black, calcified cartilage: black arborizations, blood vessels.

Source: *Functional Histology* by M. Borysenko

19
TANNER STAGING SYSTEM OF NORMAL PHYSICAL GROWTH DEVELOPMENT

The following charts give a basic outline to normal development of physical growth in children. The Tanner Staging System is used by physicians to determine what stage of growth a child is at and can be utilized to determine abnormal or drug-induced growth patterns. The values are not absolute, since some children just normally develop faster than others.

These charts are from *Handbook of Endocrine Tests in Adults and Children*, by Alsever and Gotlin.

STAGES OF PUBERTY IN MALES WITH RELATION TO CHRONOLOGICAL AGE, BONE AGE, PHALLIC AND TESTICULAR SIZE

PUBERTAL STAGE	CHRONO-LOGICAL AGE†	BONE AGE	TESTICULAR LENGTH (CM)/TVI‡	LAX PENIS LENGTH (CM)	OTHER PHYSICAL CHANGES
I	4-12	5-12	1-3.7/ 0.7-5	2-8	No pubic hair, no axillary hair; testes, scrotum and penis unchanged from childhood
II	10-14	10.5-13.5	1-5.5/ 1.5-8.5	3-12	15-80% show sparse, long pubic hair at base of penis; skin of scrotum reddened and rugae form
III	13-15.5	12.5-15	2-5.5/ 4.5-12.5	3.5-12	80-100% show dark, coarse and curled pubic hair; 20-75% show pigmented axillary hair; scrotal pigment present; onset of beard growth; may be transient gynecomastia
IV	12-17	14-17	2.9-6/ 8-16	6-13	100% show adult type pubic hair, but no spread to medial thighs; 50-100% show axillary hair, but may not be adult type
V	⟩17	Adult	3.5-6/ 8-16	6-13	Adult; beard growth progresses

*Changes in androgen and gonadotropin levels are reviewed in previous chapters.
†Onset of puberty closely parallels that of other male family members.
‡TVI = testicular volume index = (length × width right testis) + (length × width left testis)/2.

Reproduced with permission from R. N. Alsever and R. W. Gotlin, *Handbook of Endocrine Tests in Adults and Children*, 2d Ed. Copyright © 1978 by Year Book Medical Publishers, Inc., Chicago.

FEMALE SECONDARY SEXUAL DEVELOPMENT

Tanner Stage	Description	Age (yr) (mean ± 2 SD)
Breast		
1	Prepubertal	
2	Subareolar breast budding (often begins unilaterally and with tenderness)	10.5 ± 2
3	Widening of breast tissue and areola without separation of contours	12 ± 1
4	Aerola and papilla project above the plane of enlarging breast	13 ± 2
5	Mature breast—areola and breast in same plane—papilla erect	15 ± 3
Pubic Hair		
1	Absence of pubic hair (downy fine body hairs may be present on mons at any age)	
2	A few long pigmented hairs develop over mons or on labia majora	11.7 ± 2.5
3	Hair curls and spreads over mons	12.4 ± 2.2
4	Abundant hair limited to mons	13 ± 2
5	Adult escutcheon with spread of hair to medial thighs	14.4 ± 2.2

PLASMA HORMONES IN FEMALES AND MALES

Plasma Hormones in Females				
Age//Tanner Stage	Testosterone (ng/100 ml)	Estradiol (pg/ml)	FSH (mlU/ml)	LH (mlU/ml)
Neonate	‹50	25	3	
0-3 mo	—	20	3	‹2
1 yr	—	‹20	2	‹2
2-8 yr	7-20	‹20	3	‹3
9-10//2	‹30	‹30	3	3
11-12//3-4	‹40	40	5	4
13-14//3-5	‹50	50	11	8
15//5	‹56	›50	12	9
16 and over//adult	‹56	›50	4-20	4-20

Plasma Hormones in Males				
Age//Tanner Stage	Testosterone (ng/100 ml)	Estradiol (pg/ml)	FSH (mlU/ml)	LH (mlU/ml)
Neonate	50	20		
0-3 mo	up to 200	‹20	‹2	—
1 yr	15	‹30	2	2
2-9 yr	10-15	‹30	4	2
10-11//2	25-100	‹30	4	6
12-13//3-4	50-300	‹40	6	9
14-15//4-5	100-500	‹40	8	14
16-21//adult	300-1100	14-36	2-15*	2-15*

*Occasional normal subjects have lower values.

The above two charts are from "Sexual Differentiation and Development," by Barbara Lippe, from Jeome M. Hershman, *Endocrine Pathology: A Patient-Oriented Approach*, 2nd ed. (Philadelphia: Lea & Febiger, 1982).

URINARY 17-KETOSTEROID (KS) FRACTIONS
BY GAS CHROMATOGRAPHY IN MALES° (SD)

AGE	E	A	DHEA	11-KETO E	11-OHE	11-OHA	KS TOTAL	MEAN E/A†	MEAN 11-OXO 11-DE-OXO‡
3-9	0-0.25	0-0.34	0-0.03	0.01-0.29	0.03-0.09	0.04-0.12	0.03-1.0	0.8	1.1
10-14	0.3-0.9	0.5-1.7	0-0.3	0.2-0.6	0.1-0.3	0.2-0.4	1.6-3.8	0.5	0.5
15-19	2.2-5.2	3.4-7.4	0-4.3	0.3-1.3	0.3-0.9	0.5-1.1	8.2-14.2	0.5	0.2
20-29	4.1-6.1	4.7-8.7	0-8.0	0.4-1.2	0.6-1.0	0.8-1.2	12.3-24.3	0.7	0.1
30-39	1.7-4.3	1.7-7.3	0-6.3	0.3-0.7	0.4-0.6	0.4-1.2	5.1-17.5	0.7	0.2
40-49	2.4-6.4	3.2-5.8	0-4.8	0.4-1.2	0.4-1.2	0.5-1.1	9.0-19.0	0.9	0.2
50-59	1.5-4.1	1.1-5.1	0-0.5	0.3-0.7	0.3-0.9	0.4-1.0	.4.4-11.2	0.9	0.3
⟩60	1.2-4.4	0.8-3.4	0-0.7	0.5-1.1	0.3-1.3	0.5-1.5	3.6-11.6	0.9	0.5

E = etiocholanolone; A = androsterone; DHEA = dehydroepiandrosterone; 11-Keto E = 11 ketoetiocholanolone; 11-OHE = 11-hydroxyetiocholanolone; 11-OHA = 11 hydroxyandrosterone.

°KS: mg/24 hours; range: 1 sp.

†E/A = etiocholanolone - androsterone ratio (increases with age).

‡11 Oxo/11 Deoxo = ratio of 11-oxygenated-17-ketosteroids (11-hydroxy and 11-keto E and A-adrenal in origin) to 11-deoxo-17-ketosteroids (adrenal and gonadal origin). Reflects a greater increase in gonadal contribution to total ketosteroid production in reproductive years.

WITH COMPLETE 24 HOUR URINE SAMPLE

URINARY 17-KETOSTEROIDS (KS) FRACTIONS (MG/24 HOURS) BY GAS
CHROMATOGRAPHY IN FEMALES° (RANGE OF 1 SD)

AGE	E	A	DHEA	11-KETO E	11-OHE	11-OHA	KS TOTAL	MEAN E/A†	MEAN 11-OXO 11-DE-OXO‡
2-9	0.02-0.16	0-0.2	0-.03	0.03-0.19	0.01-0.09	0.05-0.11	0.14-0.74	0.9	1.2
10-14	0.16-1.7	0.3-2.2	0-0.6	0.07-0.67	0.05-0.4	0.02-0.6	1.2-6.2	0.8	0.4
15-19	2.0-4.8	1.6-4.5	0-2.3	0.3-1.1	0.3-0.9	0.2-1.2	4.3-12.3	0.8	0.3
20-29	1.7-4.9	1.9-4.7	0.1-2.3	0-1.8	0.6-1.3	0.6-1.6	6.6-14.6	1.0	0.4
30-39	1.8-4.2	1.4-2.6	0.03-0.7	0.1-0.72	0.28-0.68	0.5-0.9	5.3-8.7	1.5	0.3
40-49	1.1-4.5	0.9-3.1	0-0.5	0.4-1.0	0.4-0.8	0.4-1.0	4.0-9.2	1.1	0.4
50-59	1.8-7.0	0.7-3.5	0-0.15	0.6-1.8	0-4.0	0.5-2.4	4.7-17.1	2.0	0.6
⟩60	1.4-1.7	0.5-0.9	0-1.3	0.8-1.2	0.3-0.9	0.5-0.7	3.5-6.1	2.0	0.9

E = etiocholanolone; A = androsterone; DHEA = dehydroepiandrosterone; 11-Keto E = 11 ketoetiocholanolone; 11-OHE = 11-hydroxyetiocholanolone; 11-OHA = 11 hydroxyandrosterone.

°KS: mg/24 hours; range: 1 SD.

†E/A = etiocholanolone - androsterone ratio (increases with age).

‡11 Oxo/11 Deoxo = ratio of 11-oxygenated-17-ketosteroids (11-hydroxy and 11-keto E and A-adrenal in origin) to 11-deoxo-17-ketosteroids (adrenal and gonadal origin). Reflects a greater increase in gonadal contribution to total ketosteroid production in reproductive years.

URINARY AND SERUM OR PLASMA
TESTOSTERONE LEVELS

PUBERTAL STAGE OR AGE	URINE TESTOSTERONE (μG/24 HR)		PLASMA TESTOSTERONE (NG/100 ML)	
	m	f	m	f
Newborn	—	—	10-50	10-50
2-8	—	—	3-10	5-10
I	0.25†	0.16	† 3-10	5-10
II	0.34†	0.16†	10-30	5-20
III	0.37†	0.16†	70-400	9-20
IV	0.49†	0.16†	250-900	20-60
20-50	50-135	2-12	350-1200	20-85
⟩50	40-60	2-8	160-950	—

†Expressed as μg/kg.

20
NORMAL BLOOD COMPOSITION

The following are the normal values for different parameters found in human blood.

NORMAL HEMATOLOGIC VALUES

Fetal hemoglobin	⟨2% of total
Methemoglobin	⟨3% of total
Carboxyhemoglobin	⟨5% of total
Haptoglobins	Adults; 100-300 mg/100 ml
	Age 1-6 months: gradual increase to 30 mg/100 ml
	Newborn: absent in 90%; 10 mg/100 ml in 10%
	Genetic absence in 1% of population
Osmotic fragility of RBC	Begins in 0.45-0.39% NaCl
	Complete in 0.33%-0.30% NaCl
Erythrocyte sedimentation rate	
Wintrobe	Males: 0-10 mm in 1 hour
	Females: 0-15 mm in 1 hour
Westergren	Males: 0-13 mm in 1 hour
	Females: 0-20 mm in 1 hour
Blood volume	Males: 75 ml/kg of body weight
	Females: 67 ml/kg of body weight (8.5-9.5% of body weight in kg)
Plasma volume	Males: 44 ml/kg of body weight
	Females: 43 ml/kg of body weight
Red blood cell volume	Males: 30 ml/kg of body weight
	Females: 24 ml/kg of body weight
RBC survival time (^{51}Cr)	Half-life: 25-35 days
Reticulocyte count	0.5-1.5% of erythrocytes
Plasma iron turnover rate	38 mg/24 hours (0.47 mg/kg)
Hemoglobin	Males 15 ($\pm$2)
	Females 13 ($\pm$2)
Hematocrit	Males 45 ($\pm$5)
	Females 42 ($\pm$5)

21
NORMAL HORMONAL LEVELS IN BLOOD AND URINE

The chart below (reprinted with permission from *Interpretation of Diagnostic Tests*, Jacques Wallach, M.D., 3d edition, Little, Brown & Co., Publishers) lists the normal levels for many hormones found in the blood and urine, determined through laboratory tests. Your physician will decide which of the parameters to focus on. The ones of importance are starred here.

BLOOD AND URINE HORMONE LEVELS

Measurement of Thyroid Function	*Blood*
T-3 (concentration)	50–210 ng/100 ml serum (radioimmunoassay)
T-4 (concentration)	4.8–13.2 µg/100 ml serum (mean = 8.6) (radioimmunoassay)
T-3/T-4 ratio	Average 1.3%
T-3 (resin sponge uptake)	24–36%
T-4 (resin sponge uptake)	4–11%
Free thyroxine index (T-3 uptake × T-4 uptake)	96–396
T-4 (thyroxine by column chromatography)	2.9–6.4 µg/100 ml
"Free thyroxine"	1.0–2.1 mµg/100 ml
Thyroxine-binding globulin (TBG)	10–26 µg/100 ml thyroxine
Thyroid-stimulating hormone (TSH)	≤ 0.2 µU/ml
Long-acting thyroid stimulator (LATS)	None detectable
Radioactive iodine uptake (RAIU)	9–19% in 1 hour 7–25% in 6 hours 10–50% in 24 hours
Radioactive iodine excretion	40–70% of administered dose in 24 hours
Protein-bound iodine (PBI)	3.6–8.8 µg/100 ml

Hormone	Blood	Urine
Pregnanediol		
Male		<1.5 mg/24 hours
Female		
Proliferative phase		0.5–1.5 mg/24 hours
Luteal phase		2–7 mg/24 hours
Postmeno-pausal		0.2–1.0 mg/24 hours
Pregnanetriol		<4 mg/24 hours
*Estrogens (total)		Male: 4–25 µg/24 hours
		Female: 4–60 µg/24 hours (marked increase during pregnancy)

Hormone	Blood	Urine
*Testosterone		
Male (adult)	0.30–1.0 µg/100 ml (average = 0.7)	47–156 µg/24 hours (average = 70)
Male (adoles-cent)	>0.10 µg/100 ml	
Female	0–0.1 µg/100 ml (average = 0.04)	0–15 µg/24 hours (average = <6)
*Pituitary gonado-tropins (FSH)		6–50 mouse uterine units/24 hours
*Chorionic gonadotro-pin		0
Prolactin	<20 ng/ml	
Progesterone	<1.0 ng/ml during follicular phase >2.0 ng/ml during luteal phase	
*Luteinizing hor-mone	<70 mIU/ml during follicular phase >70 mIU/ml during luteal phase	

*Growth hormone	≤6 ng/ml in men ≤10 ng/ml in women	
Aldosterone	0.015 μg/100 ml	3–32/24 hours

Catecholamines
  (adrenaline,
  noradrenaline)
		Epinephrine ‹10
		  μg/24 hours
		Norepinephrine
		  ‹100 μg/24 hours

Metanephrines, total		24–288 μg/24 hours
Metanephrine		24–95 μg/24 hours
Normetanephrine		72–288 μg/24 hours
Vanillylmandelic acid (VMA)		≤9 mg/24 hours
Homovanillic acid		‹15 mg/24 hours

Serotonin (as
  5-Hydroxyindole-
  acetic acid,
  5-HIAA)
	0.05–0.20 μg/ml	2–10 mg/24 hours
		  (qualitative = 0)

*17-Hydroxy-
  corticoids
	(cortisol)
	5–25 μg/100 ml at 8
	  A.M.
	‹10 μg/100 ml at 8
	  P.M.
	Falls to μ10 μg/100
	  ml by 9 P.M.
		3–8 mg/24 hours
		  (lower in women)

Glenn-Nelson		Males: 3–10 mg/24
		  hours
		Females: 2–6 mg/24
		  hours

Hormone	*Blood*	*Urine*
*17-Ketogenic steroids		Males: 5–23 mg/24 hours Females: 3–15 mg/24 hours

| *17-Ketosteroids | 25–125 µg/100 ml | |

Age (years)	Males (mg/24 hours)	Females (mg/24 hours)
10	1–4	1–4
20	6–21	4–16
30	8–26	4–14
50	5–18	3–9
70	2–10	1–7

*ACTH	9 A.M.: 5–95 pg/ml Midnight: 0–35 pg/ml	
*Insulin	6–26 µU/ml (fasting) ⟨20 µU/ml (during hypoglycemia) ⟨150 µU/ml (after glucose load	
Gastrin	0–200 pg/ml	
Calcitonin	Absent in normal (⟩100 pg/ml in medullary carcinoma)	

22
NORMS OF PRINCIPAL BLOOD-CHEMISTRY TESTS AND INTERPRETATION

The basic tests that an athlete should undergo are the SMAC (serum chemistry profile), CBC (complete blood count), UA (urinalysis), and, for males, a sperm count.

The following chart and analyses concentrate on the SMAC. First there is a printout for the SMAC, showing normal ranges in serum-chemistry values. This is followed by a list of differential diagnoses that need to be evaluated to determine the cause of the patient complaint. These diagnoses are from Jacques Wallach, *Interpretation of Diagnostic Tests* (Boston: Little, Brown, & Co.). These lab tests also serve as an early-warning system to pick up problems before they become critical.

SMAC (Serum Chemistry)

Name	Test abbrev.	Normals	Units
glucose	GLUH	70– 115	MG/DL
blood urinary nitrogen	*BUN	9– 22	MG/DL
creatinine	*CREA	0.7– 1.5	MG/DL
uric acid	*UA	3.9– 9.0	MG/DL
phosphate	PO4	2.5– 4.5	MG/DL
calcium	*CA	8.5–10.5	MG/DL
sodium	*NA	135– 145	MEQ/L
potassium	*K	3.5– 5.0	MEQ/L
chloride	CL	99– 110	MEQ/L
carbon dioxide	CO2	24– 30	MEQ/L
electrolyte balance	EBAL	5– 17	MEQ/L
triglycerides	*TRIG	0– 150	MG/DL
cholesterol	*CHOL	140– 270	MG/DL
total bilirubin	*TBIL	0.2– 1.2	MG/DL
direct bilirubin	DBIL	0.0– 0.4	MG/DL
indirect bilirubin	IBIL	0.0– 1.2	MG/DL
alkaline phosphatase	*ALK	30– 101	U/L
gamma-glutamyl transpeptidase	*GGT	9– 38	U/L
alanine aminotransferase	*SGPT (ALT)	0– 45	U/L
aspartate aminotransferase	*SGOT (AST)	0– 40	U/L
lactic dehydrogenase	*LDH	60– 230	U/L
creatinine phosphokinase	CK	0– 225	U/L

iron	IRON	35– 200	MCG/DL
protein	PRO	6.0– 8.0	G/DL
albumin	ALB	3.5– 5.5	G/DL
globulin	GLOB	2.0– 4.0	G/DL

The starred values are the ones to look for abnormalities in.

HEART	LIVER	ELECTROLYTE IMBALANCE
LDH	GGT	PO4
CK	SGPT	CA
	SGOT	NA
		K
		CL

The starred values (*) on the following diagnostic interpretations indicate symptoms to which particular attention should be paid.

All from: *Interpretation of Diagnostic Tests* by Jacques Wallach M.D. Pub. Little, Brown & Co.

SERUM UREA NITROGEN (BUN)
Increased In
*Impaired kidney function
Prerenal azotemia—any cause of reduced renal blood flow
    Congestive heart failure
    *Salt and water depletion (vomiting, diarrhea, diuresis, sweating)
    *Shock
    Etc.
Postrenal azotemia—any obstruction of urinary tract
    (ratio of BUN creatinine increases above normal of 10:1)
Increased protein catabolism (serum creatinine remains normal)
    Hemorrhage into gastrointestinal tract
    Acute myocardial infarction
    Stress

Decreased In
*Severe liver damage (liver failure)
    *Drugs
    Poisoning
    *Hepatitis
    Other
Increased utilization of protein for synthesis

Late pregnancy
Infancy
Acromegaly
Diet
Low-protein and high carbohydrate
IV feedings only
Impaired absorption (celiac disease)
Nephrotic syndrome (some patients)

A low BUN of 6–8 mg/100 ml is frequently associated with states of overhy-dration.
A BUN of 10–20 mg/100 ml almost always indicates normal glomerular function.
A BUN of 50–150 mg/100 ml implies serious impairment of renal function.
Markedly increased BUN (150–250 mg/100 mg) is virtually conclusive evi-dence of severely impaired glomerular function.
In chronic renal disease, BUN correlates better with symptoms of uremia than does the serum creatinine.

SERUM CREATININE
Increased In
Diet
Ingestion of creatinine (roast meat)
Muscle disease
Gigantism
Acromegaly
Prerenal azotemia
Postrenal azotemia
Impaired kidney function
Ratio of BUN: creatinine ⟩10:1

Excess intake of protein
Blood in small bowel
Excess tissue breakdown (cachexia, burns, high fever, cortiocosteroid therapy)
Urinary tract obstruction (postrenal)
Inadequate renal blood flow (e.g., prerenal congestive heart failure, dehydration, shock)
Urine reabsorption (e.g., ureterocolostomy)
Ratio of BUN: creatinine ⟨10:1
Low protein intake
Repeated dialysis
Severe diarrhea or vomiting
Hepatic insufficiency

Serum creatinine is a more specific and sensitive indicator of renal disease than BUN. Use of simultaneous BUN and creatinine determinations provides more information.

Decreased In
Not clinically significant

SERUM CREATINE

Increased In
High dietary intake (meat)
Destruction of muscle
Hyperthyroidism (this diagnosis almost excluded by normal serum creatine)
Active rheumatoid arthritis
Testosterone therapy

Decreased In
Not clinically significant

SERUM URIC ACID
Levels are very labile and show day-to-day and seasonal variation in same person; also increased by emotional stress, total fasting.

Increased In
Gout
25% of relatives of patients with gout
Renal failure (does not correlate with severity of kidney damage; urea and creatinine should be used)
Increased destruction of nucleoproteins
    Leukemia, multiole myeloma
    Polycythemia
    Lymphoma, especially postirradiation
    Other disseminated neoplasms
    Cancer chemotherapy (e.g., nitrogen mustards, vincristine, mercapto-purine)
    Hemolytic anemia
    Sickle cell anemia
    Resolving pneumonia
    Toxemia of pregnancy (serial determinations to follow therapeutic response and estimate prognosis)
    Psoriasis (one-third of patients)
Diet
    High-protein weight reduction diet
    Excess nucleoprotein (e.g., sweetbreads, liver)

Asymptomatic hyperuricemia (e.g., incidental finding with no evidence of gout; clinical significance not known but people so afflicted should be re-checked periodically for gout). The higher the level of serum uric acid, the greater the likelihood of an attack of acute gouty arthritis.

Miscellaneous

> Von Gierke's disease
> Lead poisoning
> Lesch-Nyham syndrome
> Maple syrup urine disease
> Down's syndrome
> Polycystic kidneys
> Calcinosis universalis and circumscripta
> *Some drugs (e.g., thiazides, furosemide, ethacrynic acid, small doses of salicylates)*
> Hypoparathyroidism
> Primary hyperparathyroidism
> Hypothyroidism
> Sarcoidosis
> Chronic berylliosis
> Some patients with alcoholism
> *Patients with arteriosclerosis and hypertension (Serum uric acid is increased in 80% of patients with elevated serum triglycerides.)*
> Certain population groups (e.g., Blackfoot and Pima Indians, Filipi-nos, New Zealand Maoris)

Decreased In

Administration of ACTH
Administration of uricosuric drugs (e.g., high does of salicylates, probene-cid, cortisone, allopurinol, coumarins)
Wilson's disease
Fanconi's syndrome
Acromegaly (some patients)
Celiac disease (slightly)
Pernicious anemia in relapse (some patients)
Xanthinuria
Administration of various other drugs (x-ray contrast agents, glyceryl guaiacolate)
Neoplasms (occasional cases) e.g., carcinomas, Hodgkin's disease
Healthy adults with isolated defect in tubular transport of uric acid (dalmation dog mutation)

Unchanged In

Colchicine administration

SERUM SODIUM
Increased In
Excess loss of water
    Conditions that cause loss via gastrointestinal tract (e.g., in vomiting), lung (hyperpnea), or skin (e.g., in excessive sweating)
    Conditions that cause diuresis
        Diabetes insipidus
        Nephrogenic diabetes insipidus
      Deabetes mellitus
      Diuretic drugs
      Diuretic phase of acute tubular necrosis
      Diuresis following relief of urinary tract obstruction
      Hypercalcemic nephropathy
      Hypokalemic nephropathy
Excess administration of sodium (iatrogenic), e.g., incorrect replacement following fluid loss
"Essential" hypernatremia due to hypothalamic lesions

Decreased In (serum osmolality is decreased)
    Dilutional (e.g., congestive heart failure, nephrosis, cirrhosis with ascites)
    Sodium depletion
      Loss of body fluids (e.g., vomiting, diarrhea, excessive sweating) with incorrect or no therapeutic replacement, diuretic drugs (e.g, thiazides)
      Adrenocortical insufficiency
      Salt-losing nephropathy
      Inappropriate secretion of antidiuretic hormone
    Spurious (serum osmolality is normal or increased)
      Hyperlipidemia
      Hyperglycemia (serum sodium decreases 3 mEq/L for every increase of serum glucose of 100 mg/100 ml)

SERUM POTASSIUM
Increased In
Renal failure
    Acute with oliguria or anuria
    Chronic end-stage with oliguria (glomerular filtration rate ⟨3–5 ml/minute)
    Chronic nonoliguric associated with dehydration, obstruction, trauma, or excess potassium
Decreased mineralocorticoid activity
    Addison's disease
    Hypofunction of renin-angiotensin-aldosterone system

Pseudohypoaldosteronism
Aldosterone antagonist (e.g., spironolactone)
Increased supply of potassium
Red blood cell hemolysis (transfusion reaction, hemolytic anemia)
Excess dietary intake or rapid potassium infusion
Striated muscle (status epilepticus, periodic paralysis)
Potassium-retaining drugs (e.g., triamterene)
Fluid-electrolyte imbalance (e.g., dehydration, acidosis)
Laboratory artifacts (e.g., hemolysis duing venipuncture, conditions associated with thrombocytosis, incomplete separation of serum and clot)

Decreased In
Renal and adrenal conditions with metabolic alkalosis
Administration of diuretics
Primary aldosteronism
Pseudoaldosteronism
Salt-losing nephropathy
Cushing's syndrome
Renal conditions associated with metabolic acidosis
Renal tubular acidosis
Diuretic phase of acute tubular necrosis
Chronic pyelonephritis
Diuresis following relief of urinary tract obstruction
Gastrointestinal conditions
Vomiting, gastric suctioning
Villous adenoma
Cancer of colon
Chronic laxative abuse
Zollinger-Ellison syndrome
Chronic diarrhea
Ureterosigmoidostomy

SERUM CHOLESTEROL
Increased In
Idiopathic hypercholesterolemia
Biliary obstruction
Stone, carcinoma, etc., of duct
Cholangiolitic cirrhosis
von Gierke's disease
Hypothyroidism
Nephrosis (due to chronic nephritis, renal vein thrombosis, amyloidosis, systemic lupus erythematosus, periarteritis, diabetic glomerulosclerosis
Pancreatic disease
Diabetes mellitus

Total pancreatectomy
Chronic pancreatitis (some patients)
Pregnancy

Decreased In
Severe liver cell damage (due to chemicals, drugs, hepatitis)
Hyperthyroidism
Malunitrition (e.g., starvation, terminal neoplasm, uremia, malabsorption
   in steatorrhea)
Chronic anemia
      Pernicious anemia in relapse
      Hemolytic anemias
      Marked hypochromic anemia
Cortisone and ACTH therapy
Hypo-beta- and a-beta-lipoproteinemia
Tangier disease

SERUM ALKALINE PHOSPHATASE
Increased In
Increased deposition of calcium in bone
      Osteitis fibrosa cystica(hyperparathyroidism)
      Paget's disease (osteitis deformans)
      Healing fractures (slightly)
      Osteoblastic bone tumors (osteogenic sarcoma, metastatic carcinoma)
      Osteogenesis imperfecta
      Familial osteoectasia
      Osteomalacia
      Rickets
      Polyostotic fibrous dysplasia
      Late pregnancy; reverts to normal level by 20th day postpartum
      Children
      Administration of erogosterol
Liver disease—any obstruction of biliary system
      *Nodules in liver (metastatic tumor, abscess, cyst, parasite, amyloid,
         tuberculosis, sarcoid, or leukemia)*
      Biliary duct obstruction (e.g., stone, carcinoma)
      Cholangiolar obstruction in hepatitis
      *Adverse reaction to therapeutic drug (e.g., chlorpropamide) (progres-
         sive elevation of serum alkaline phosphatase may be first indication
         that drug therapy should be halted)*
Marked hyperthyroidism
Hyperphosphatasia
Primary hypophosphatemia (often increased)
Intravenous injection of albumin; sometimes marked increase (e.g., 10

times normal level) lasting for several days

Some patients with myocardial or pulmonary infarction, usually during phase of organization

Decreased In
Excess vitamin D ingestion

Milk-alkali (Burnett's) syndrome

Scurvy

Hypophosphatasia

Hypothyroidism

Pernicious anemia in one-third of patients

Celiac disease

Malnutrition

Collection of blood in EDTA, fluoride, or oxalate anticoagulant

Alkaline phosphatase isoenzyme determinations are not clinically useful; heat inactivation may be more useful to distinguish bone from liver source of increased alkaline phosphatase.

SERUM GAMMA-GLUTAMYL TRANSPEPTIDASE
Increased In
Liver disease. Generally parallels changes in serum alkaline phosphatase, LAP, and 5'-nucleotidase but is more sensitive.

> *Acute hepatitis. Elevation is less marked than that of other liver enzymes, but it is the last to return to normal and therefore is useful to indicate recovery.*

> *Chronic hepatitis. Increased more than in acute hepatitis. More elevated than SGOT and SGPT. In dormant stage, may be the only enzyme elevated.*

> *Cirrhosis. In inactive cases, average values are lower than in chronic hepatitis. Increases greater than 10-20 times in cirrhotic patients suggest superimposed primary carcinoma of the liver.*

> Primary biliary cirrhosis. Elevation is marked.

> *Fatty liver. Elevation parallels that of SGOT and SGPT but is greater.*

> Obstructive jaundice. Increase is faster and greater than that of serum alkaline phosphatase and LAP.

> *Liver metastases. Parallels alkaline phosphatase; elevation precedes positive liver scans.*

Pancreatitis. Always elevated in acute pancreatitis. In chronic pancreatitis is increased when there is involvement of the biliary tract or active inflammation.

Renal disease. Increased in lipoid nephrosis and some cases of renal carcinoma.

Acute myocardial infarction. Increased in 50% of the patients. Elevation begins on fourth to fifth day, reaches maximum at 8-12 days. With shock or acute right heart failure, may have early peak within 48 hours, with rapid decline followed by later rise.

Heavy use of alcohol, barbiturates, or phenytoin sodium (Dilantin). Is the most sensitive indicator of alcoholism, since elevation exceeds that of other commonly assayed liver enzymes.

Normal In

Women during pregnancy (in contrast to serum alkaline phosphatase and LAP) and children over 3 months of age; therefore may aid in differential diagnosis of hepatobiliary disease occurring during pregnancy and childhood.

Bone disease or patients with increased bone growth (children and adolescents); therefore useful in distinguishing bone disease from liver disease as a cause of increased serum alkaline phosphatase.

Renal failure.

SERUM TRANSAMINASE (SGOT)
Increased In

Acute myocardial infarction
Liver diseases, with active necrosis of parenchymal cells
Musculoskeletal diseases, including trauma and intramuscular injections
Acute pancreatitis
Other
> Myoglobinuria
> Intestinal injury (e.g., surgery, infarction)
> Local irradiation injury
> Pulmonary infarction (relatively slight increase)
> Cerebral infarction (increased in following week in 50% of patients)
> Cerebral neoplasms (occasionally)
> Renal infarction (occasionally)

"Pseudomyocardial infarction" pattern. Administration of opiates to patients with diseased bliary tract or previous cholecystectomy causes increase in LDH and especially SGOT. SGOT increases by 2-4 hours, peaks in 5-8 hours, and increase may persist for 24 hours; elevation may be 2^1/$_2$-65 times normal.

Falsely Increased In (because enzymes are activated during test)
Therapy with Prostaphlin, Polycillin, opiates, erythromycin
Calcium dust in air (e.g., due to construction in laboratory)

Falsely Decreased In (because of increased serum lactate-consuming enzyme during test)
Diabetic ketoacidosis
Beriberi

Severe liver disease
Chronic hemodialysis (reason unknown)
Uremia (proportional to BUN level) (reason unknown)

Normal In
Angina pectoris
Coronary insufficiency
Pericarditis
Congestive heart failure without liver damage

Varies ⟨10 units/day in the same person.

SGPT generally parallels SGOT, but the increase is less marked in myocardial necrosis, chronic hepatitis, cirrhosis, hepatic metastases, and congestive changes in liver, and is more marked in liver necrosis and acute hepatitis.

SERUM LACTIC DEHYDROGENASE (LDH)
Increased In
Acute myocardial infarction
Serum LDH is almost always increased, beginning in 10-12 hours and reaching a peak (of about 3 times normal) in 48-72 hours. The prolonged elevation of 10-14 days is particularly useful for late diagnosis when the patient is first seen after sufficient time has elapsed for CPK and SGOT to become normal. Levels ⟩2000 units suggest a poorer prognosis. Because many other diseases may increase the LDH, isoenzyme studies should be performed. Increased serum LDH, with a ratio of LDH_1/LDH_2 ⟩1 ("flipped" LDH), occurs in acute renal infarction and hemolysis associated with hemolytic anemia or prosthetic heart valves as well as in acute myocardial infarction. In acute myocardial infarction, flipped LDH usually appears between 12 and 24 hours and is present within 48 hours in 80% of patients; after 1 week it is still present in ⟨50% of patients, even though total serum LDH may still be elevated; flipped LDH never appears before CPK MB isoenzyme. LDH_1 may remain elevated after total LDH has returned to normal; with small infarcts, LDH_1 may be increased when total LDH remains normal
Acute myocardial infarction with congestive heart failure. May show increase of LDH_1 and LDH_5.
Congestive heart failure alone. LDH isoenzymes are normal.
Insertion of intracardiac prosthetic valves consistently causes chronic hemolysis with increase of total LDH and of LDH_1 and LDH_2. This is also often present before surgery in patients with severe hemodynamic abnormalities of cardiac valves.
Cardiovascular surgery. LDH is increased up to 2 times normal without car-

diopulmonary bypass and returns to normal in 3-4 days; with extracorporeal circulation, it may increase up to 4-6 times normal; increase is more marked when transfused blood is older.

Hepatitis. Most marked increase is of LDH$_5$, which occurs during prodromal stage and is greatest at time of onset of jaundice. Total LDH is also increased in 50% of the cases. LDH$_5$ is also increased with other causes of liver damage (e.g., chlorpromazine hepatitis, carbon tetrachloride poisoning, exacerbation of cirrhosis, biliary obstruction) even when total LDH is normal.

Untreated pernicious anemia. Total LDH (chiefly LDH$_1$) is markedly increased, especially with hemoglobin ⟨8 gm/100 ml. Only slightly increased in severe hemolytic anemia. Normal in iron-deficiency anemia, even when very severe.

Malignant tumors. Increased in about 50% of patients with carcinoma, especially in advanced stages. Increased in ≅ 60% of patients with lymphomas and lymphomatic leukemias. Increased in ≅ 90% of patients with acute leukemia; degree of increase is not correlated with level of WBCs; relatively low levels in lymphatic type of leukemia. Increased in 95% of patients with myelogenous leukemia.

Diseases of muscle.
Pulmonary embolus and infarction.
Renal diseases. Occasional increase but to no clinically useful degree.
Other causes of hemolysis
> Artifactual (e.g., poor venipuncture, failure to separate clot from serum, heating of blood)
> Various hemolytic conditions in vivo (e.g., hemolytic anemias).

5'-NUCLEOTIDASE (5'-N)
This is a very sensitive test for liver problems.
Increased Only In
*Obstructive type of hepatobiliary disease

May be an early indication of liver metastases in the cancer patient, especially if jaundice is absent.

Normal In
Pregnancy and postpartum period (in contrast to serum LAP and alkaline phosphatase); therefore may aid in differential diagnosis of hepatobiliary disease occurring during pregnancy.

Whenever the alkaline phosphatase is elevated, a simultaneous elevation of 5'-N establishes biliary disease as the cause of the elevated alkaline phosphatase. If the 5'-N is not increased, the cause of the elevated alkaline posphatase must be found elsewhere, e.g., bone disease.

23
OVERVIEW OF TYPICAL SERIES OF DIAGNOSTIC PROCEDURES PHYSICIANS UTILIZE TO DETERMINE CAUSE AND ETIOLOGY OF AN INDIVIDUAL'S HEALTH COMPLAINTS

What follows is an overview explanation of some of the procedures used by physicians to diagnose patients' health problems. It is included here so that nonphysicians might gain a better understanding of why the tests are performed and what the physician is looking for.

RADIOLOGIC PROCEDURES

ABDOMINAL ROENTGENOGRAM Films of the upper abdomen and lower thorax rarely provide accurate estimates of liver size and shape, but gross hepatomegaly and hepatic masses that elevate or distort the diaphragm may be detected. However, the abdominal film is more accurate in determining the presence of splenomegaly and is often helpful in detecting minimal degrees of splenic enlargement. Plain films of the abdomen may reveal calcific densities in the gallbladder, biliary tree, pancreas, or liver (as echinococcal cysts, hemangioma, or, rarely, a metastatic tumor mass).

BARIUM STUDIES OF THE GASTROINTESTINAL TRACT An upper gastrointestinal series should be performed in suspected cases of portal hypertension, because esophagogastric varices can be demonstrated with about 70 to 90 percent accuracy when they are present. Enlargement of the left lobe of the liver (as with tumor, abscess, or cirrhosis) may displace the barium-filled stomach laterally and anteriorly. Tumors of the head of the pancreas often produce displacement or irregularity of the second portion of the duodenum. The radiologist can increase the diagnostic accuracy of a search for lesions involving the head of the pancreas or papilla of Vater by performing a hypotonic duodenogram. This involves injection of an anticholinergic drug or glucagon to inhibit motility: it often permits a better view of the mucosa and provides data concerning the distensibility of the duodenum.

CHOLECYSTOGRAPHY AND CHOLANGIOGRAPHY *Oral cholecystography* is useful primarily in the diagnosis of diseases of the gallbladder, especially gallstones. The dye tablets [iopanoic acid (Telepaque)] are given

293

the night before the study, absorbed from the intestine, and excreted by hepatocytes into the bile. Thus the test cannot be performed in the presence of hepatic excretory dysfunction or diarrhea (with decreased absorption of the dye). Nonvisualization of the gallbladder after a single dose of dye usually indicates gallbladder disease, but in some patients a second dose of the dye will show normal gallbladder opacification. A second dose study is required in at least 10 or 15 percent of patients who initially have inadequate visualization. This requirement limits the usefulness of oral cholecystography, especially in comparison to ultrasound which does not depend upon hepatic excretory functions.

Intravenous cholangiography requires the administration of dye as an intravenous bolus and, like oral cholecystography, requires hepatic excretion to visualize the bile ducts and gallbladder. Unfortunately even mild impairment of liver function may prevent adequate visualization of this technique, thus limiting its application in the evaluation of patients with serum bilirubin levels greater than 2.5 to 3 mg/dl.

Percutaneous transhepatic cholangiography with a very thin needle is sometimes used to distinguish between mechanical biliary obstruction and intrahepatic cholestasis. This approach is used when decreased liver function precludes the use of intravenous cholangiography. With experience and proper precautions, dilated major ducts proximal to an obstructing lesion can be cannulated and visualized in up to 90 percent of cases; the normal or small ducts associated with intrahepatic cholestasis are more difficult to demonstrate, but with modern techniques, they can be demonstrated in up to 75 percent of cases.

Endoscopic retrograde cholangiopancreatography (ERCP) with the fiberoptic duodenoscope is another method of demonstrating the bile ducts radiographically in jaundiced patients. The papilla of Vater is cannulated under direct vision, and contrast material is injected into the biliary and pancreatic ducts. ERCP is particularly useful in jaundiced patients with suspected lesions of the head of the pancreas or ampulla of Vater, since in addition to contrast studies one may also obtain washings or brushings for cytology, or biopsies of intraduodenal mass lesions. ERCP does not rely upon dilatation of the bile ducts for success, and since the liver itself is not punctured, there is no risk of bile peritonitis in patients with high-grade biliary obstruction. However, acute pancreatitis may result from injection of contrast material into the pancreatic duct.

ANGIOGRAPHY An increasingly useful and effective approach for visualizing the hepatic and portal circulation involves *selective angiography* of the celiac, superior mesenteric, and hepatic arteries. In most centers it has replaced splenoportography since by injection of these arteries one can visualize both the arterial (hepatic) and venous (hepatic and portal) systems. Selective arteriography is quite safe. It is useful (1) in demonstrating the hepatic arterial circulation which will be deranged in cirrhosis and in the diagnosis of primary and secondary liver tumor masses, and (2) in visualizing the portal circulation for evidence of a collateral circulation, venous obstruction, anomalous vessels, etc. In major medical centers, this angiographic method is increasingly used as a diagnostic tool for the study of chronic liver disease and portal hypertension.

RADIOISOTOPE LIVER SCANS (SCINTISCANS) Hepatic scintiscans are performed with gamma-emitting isotopes that are extracted selectively by the liver, followed by external radiation scanning of the upper abdomen. There are basically three types of liver scans: the colloidal scan which depends on uptake of labeled colloid by Kupffer cells, the HIDA or PIPIDA scans in which the dye is taken up and excreted by hepatocytes, and the gallium scan in which the radionuclide ^{67}Ga is concentrated in neoplastic and inflammatory cells to a greater degree than in hepatocytes. Hence, a hepatoma or liver abscess will produce an area of reduced uptake or "hole" using a colloid or HIDA or PIPIDA scans, but there will be an area of increased uptake or "hot spot" with gallium scan. The colloidal scan with ^{198}Au colloidal gold or ^{99m}Tc sulfur colloid is most commonly used. This technique can demonstrate filling defects greater than 2 to 3 cm in diameter; hence in metastatic liver disease with smaller diffuse deposits, the scan will be falsely negative. False-positive scans are frequently observed in cirrhosis, because the distorted lobular architecture will result in irregular uptake and sometimes produce filling defects. The gallium scan may be helpful in diagnosing neoplastic infiltration in the patient with cirrhosis since the tumor will show increased uptake, while fibrous bands will show decreased uptake. The HIDA or PIPIDA scans (^{99m}Tc-labeled-N-substituted iminoacetic acids) have been used as a method of differentiating intrahepatic cholestasis from extrahepatic obstruction. With complete biliary obstruction there is failure of the isotope to enter the duodenum, while in intrahepatic cholestasis some isotope will be seen in the lumen of the small bowel. However, a clear-cut distinction of these entities with the HIDA or PIPIDA scans is unusual, and in this situation they have limited clinical usefulness in differentiating intra- from extrahepatic cholestasis. The major application of HIDA or PIPIDA liver scans is in the diagnosis of acute cholecystitis, where failure of the nuclide to enter the gallbladder is considered evidence of cystic duct or common bile duct obstruction.

ULTRASONOGRAPHY Modern diagnostic ultrasound of the gallbladder is probably more accurate than oral cholecystography in detecting gallstones and has the added advantage of being independent of liver function. It can therefore be used to detect gallstones in the gallbladder or biliary tree in patients with jaundice. Ultrasound is also very useful in detecting mass lesions such as tumors, cysts, or liver abscess. Lesions as small as 1 to 2 cm can be visualized with this technique. Ultrasound of the upper abdomen is also quite useful in evaluating the possible causes of extrahepatic biliary obstruction. Abdominal computerized tomography (CT) scanning and ultrasound are approximately equal in their diagnostic sensitivity in evaluating patients with suspected mass lesions, gallstones, or obstructive jaundice. In general, ultrasound is the procedure of choice since it is less expensive than CT scanning and doses not expose the patient to radiation.

COMPUTERIZED TOMOGRAPHY (CT SCAN) The CT scan of the abdomen provides a visual image of the abdominal viscera without injection of contrast material. This technique is particularly useful in the diagnosis of mass lesions in the liver or pancreas, where it has an accuracy and sensitivity comparable to that obtained with ultrasound. The test is particularly useful in differentiating intrahepatic fluid collections such as cysts, abscesses, and hematomas, since the density of the fluid can be determined with relative accuracy. Dilatation of the gallbladder, extrahepatic bile ducts or portal vein can be diagnosed on the CT scan. The major advantage of CT scanning is the ability to obtain an excellent image of solid intraabdominal organs such as pancreas, liver, and spleen with modest doses of radiation, thus avoiding more invasive techniques such as angiography, cholangiography, or ERCP.

OTHER DIAGNOSTIC PROCEDURES

PORTAL AND HEPATIC VEIN MANOMETRY Estimation of the wedged hepatic venous pressure (WHVP, an approximation of the postsinusoidal intrahepatic venous pressure) by *hepatic vein catheterization* is useful in the study of patients with known or presumed portal hypertension. While demonstration of the WHVP is not a routine procedure, the demonstration of a normal or slightly elevated WHVP in a patient with clinical evidence of portal hypertension serves to localize the obstruction to the extrahepatic portion of the portal vein, the portal inflow system (as in schistosomiasis), or the presinusoidal vessels (as in some cases of fatty liver or portal fibrosis) rather than to the sinusoids or hepatic veins. Measurement of the splenic pulp pressure (a reliable reflection of the actual portal venous pressure) by *percutaneous portal manometry* is rarely performed. A WHVP greater than 10 mmHg above inferior vena cava pressure is indicative of portal hypertension.

PERCUTANEOUS NEEDLE BIOPSY OF THE LIVER Percutaneous needle biopsy is a safe, simple, and valuable method of diagnosing liver disease. Although the needle biopsy sample is small, *diffuse parenchymal disorders* such as cirrhosis, hepatitis, and drug reactions may be diagnosed with remarkable accuracy. In *disseminated focal diseases* (such as granulomas or tumor infiltrates) serial sections may demonstrate the lesion.

The biopsy is performed under local anesthesia, usually with the Menghini (aspiration), Klatskin, or Vim-Silverman (cutting) needle, by means of either the transpleural or subcostal approach. If the operator is skillful and the patient is carefully selected, morbidity should be low and limited to occasional postbiopsy pain or vasovagal reactions. The mortality of liver biopsy as reported in several large series is approximately 1 death in 5000 biopsies when the Menghini technique is used.

Some of the major indications for needle biopsy are (1) unexplained hepatomegaly or hepatosplenomegaly, (2) cholestasis of uncertain cause, (3) persistently abnormal liver function tests, (4) suspected systemic or infiltrative diseases such as sarcoidosis, military tuberculosis, or fever of unknown origin, and (5) suspected primary or metastatic liver tumor.

Needle biopsy should not be performed if (1) the patient is not able to cooperate; (2) clinical or laboratory evidence indicates impaired hemostasis (for example, the one-stage prothrombin time is prolonged by 3 s or more over control), thrombocytopenia (less than 80,000 to 100,000 platelets per cubic millimeters) or purpura is present, or the partial thromboplastin time or bleeding time is prolonged; (3) there is infection of the right pleural space or septic cholangitis; (4) profound anemia or tense ascites is present; or (5) compatible blood is not available for transfusion in case of hemorrhage. Amyloidosis and carcinoma of the liver may increase the hazard of postbiopsy hemorrhage. Although biopsy in mechanical biliary obstruction may lead occasionally to the escape of bile and localized bile peritonitis, this complication is uncommon. With the increasing use of CT and ultrasonography, it is possible to perform aspiration biopsies with very thin needles which can be "directed" to the site of the lesion with the aid of one of these imaging procedures. The aspirated material can then be used for cytology (tumors) and culture (abscesses).

PERITONEOSCOPY (LAPAROSCOPY) With this technique the serosal lining, liver, gallbladder, spleen, and other abdominal organs can be visualized with minimum discomfort and hazard. Diagnosis may be made by inspection or directed needle biopsy. Peritoneoscopy is useful in the study of patients with suspected intraabdominal malignancy since it may obviate the need for exploratory laparotomy to establish a diagnosis.

LAPAROTOMY When the most thorough clinical, laboratory, and biopsy studies fail to define the precise nature of hepatobiliary disease, exploratory laparotomy may be necessary. However, it must be reemphasized that when there is evidence of significant hepatocellular necrosis (e.g., markedly elevated SGOT levels), laparotomy will often be accompanied by an increased morbidity and mortality owing to postoperative liver decompensation.

When laparotomy is performed, the medico-surgical team should be prepared to obtain full benefit from this direct approach, using biopsy, culture, cholangiography, and angiography as required.

REFERENCES

H.L. Brensilver and M.M. Kaplan, "Significance of Elevated Liver Alkaline Phosphatase in Serum." *Gastroenterology,* 68 (1975):1556.

F. Lomas, et al, "Increased Specificity of Liver Scanning with the Use of ^{67}Gallium Citrate," *N. Engl. J. Med.,* 286 (1972):1323.

M.A. Mauro, et al, "Hepatobiliary Scanning with ^{99m}Tc-PIPIDA in Acute Cholecystitis," *Radiology,* 142 (1982):193.

K. Okuda, "Advances in Hepatobiliary Ultrasonography," *Hepatology,* 1 (1981):662.

R. Pereiras, *et al,* "Percutaneous Transhepatic Cholangiography with the 'Skinny' Needle," *Ann. Intern. Med.,* 86 (1977):562.

From Harrison's *Principles of Internal Medicine,* McGraw-Hill, 1982. Reprinted with permission.

24
LISTING OF COMMONLY USED ANABOLIC STEROIDS, WITH CHEMICAL STRUCTURES, NORMAL DOSAGES, AND TRADE NAMES

Please note that the dosages listed on the enclosed table are for sick patients; these are *far* below the quantities now being abused by normal, healthy athletes.

Testosterone, U.S.P.
 ANDROID-T
 ORETON
Aqueous suspension: 25, 50, and 100 mg/ml for i.m. use (50 mg three times weekly)
Pellets: 75 mg for s.c. use (300 mg every 4 to 6 months)

Testosterone Propionate, U.S.P.
 ORETON PROPIONATE
Tablets: 10 mg (buccal; 10 to 20 mg daily)
Oily solution: 25, 50, and 100 mg/ml for i.m. use (25 mg two to four times weekly)

Testosterone Enanthate, U.S.P.
 DELATESTRYL
Oily solution: 100 and 200 mg/ml for i.m. use (100 to 400 mg every 2 to 4 weeks)

Testosterone Cypionate, U.S.P.
 DEPO-TESTOSTERONE
Oily solution: 50,100, and 200 mg/ml for i.m. use (100 to 400 mg every 2 to 4 weeks)

Methyltestosterone, U.S.P.
 METANDREN
 ORETON METHYL
Tablets: 5, 10, and 25 mg (buccal: 5 to 25 mg daily)
Capsules: 10 mg (10 to 50 mg daily)

Fluoxymesterone, U.S.P.
  HALOTESTIN
  ORA-TESTRYL
Tablets: 2, 5, and 10 mg (2 to 30 mg daily)

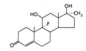

Danazol, U.S.P.
  DANOCRINE
Capsules: 200 mg (200 to 800 mg daily)

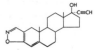

Calusterone
  METHOSARB
Tablets: 50 mg (200 mg daily for breast carcinoma)

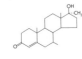

Dromostanolone Propionate, U.S.P.
  DROLBAN
Oily solution: 50 mg/ml for i.m. use (100 mg three times weekly for breast carcinoma)

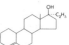

Ethylestrenol
  MAXIBOLIN
Elixir: 2 mg/5 ml
Tablets: 2 mg (4 to 8 mg daily)

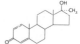

Methandriol
  ANABOL
Aqueous and oil solutions: 50 mg/ml for i.m. use (50 to 100 mg once or twice weekly)

Methandrostenolone, U.S.P.
  DIANABOL
Tablets: 2.5 and 5 mg (5 mg daiy)

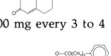

Nandrolone Decanoate, U.S.P.
  DECA-DURABOLIN
Oily solution: 50 and 100 mg/ml for i.m. use (50 to 100 mg every 3 to 4 weeks)

Nandrolone Phenpropionate, U.S.P.
  DURABOLIN
Oily solution: 25 and 50 mg/ml for i.m. use (25 to 50 mg weekly)

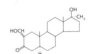

Oxandrolone, U.S.P.
  ANAVAR
Tablets: 2.5 mg (5 to 10 mg daily)

Listing 301

Oxymetholone, U.S.P.
ADROYD
ANADROL

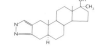

Tablets: 5, 10, and 50 mg (5 to 15 mg daily; as much as 50 to 100 mg daily for anemia)

Stanozolol, U.S.P.
WINSTROL
Tablets: 2 mg (6 mg daily)

Testolactone, U.S.P.
TESLAC
Tablets: 50 and 250 mg (150 mg daily)
Aqueous suspension: 100 mg/ml for i.m. use (100 mg three times weekly for breast carcinoma)

*Dosage schedules for breast carcinoma in females are generally two to three times those for androgen replacement.

From Goodman and Gilman's *Pharmalogical Basis of Therapeutics*, 6th ed. (New York: Mazcmillan Publishing Co., 1980).

From *Anabolic-Androgenic Steroids,* by Charles D. Kochakian (New York: Springer-Verlag, 1976) pp. 627-36.

25
STRUCTURES, NAMES, AND MANUFACTURERS OF ANABOLIC STEROIDS

Structure	Systematic name[a]	Trivial and/or generic name	Trade name	Manufacturer
1. Testosterone-derived protein anabolic steroids				
	17β-Hydroxyandrost-4-en-3-one	Testosterone	Geno-cristaux Malestrone Orquisteron Frosst Primotest Oreton	Gremy Kirk, N.Y. (Columbia) Schering A.G. Schering
		-acetate	Aceto-Sterandryl Aceto-Testoviron Perandrone A	Roussel Schering A.G. CIBA
		-propionate	Oreton Perandren Sterandryl Testoviron Anertan Enarmon	Schering Ciba-Geigy Roussel Schering Boehringer (M) Takeda (Japan)
		-(3-*p*-hexyloxiphenyl)-propionate	Androdurin	Leo. (Helsingborg)
		-heptanoate (enanthate)	Delatestryl Androtardyl Testoenant	Squibb Schering-Sepps Geymonod
		-cyclopentyl propionate	Depot testosterone cypionate	Upjohn
	4-Chloro-17β-hydroxy-androst-4-en-3-one	Chlorotestosterone	Steranabol	Farmitalia
		-acetate	Macrobin Turinabol Turinabol inj.	Teikoku Jenapharm Jenapharm
		-capronate	Macrobin-depot	Teikoku

Structure	Systematic name[a]	Trivial and/or generic name	Trade name	Manufacturer
	17β-Hydroxy-17-methyl-androst-4-en-3-one	Methyltestosterone	Metandren Anertan Oreton Android	Ciba Boehringer (M) Schering Brown
	9α-Fluoro-11β,17β-dihydroxy-17-methylandrost-4-en-3-one	Fluoxymesterone	Halotestin Ultandren Androfluorene Fluotestin Orateston	Upjohn Ciba Midy Roter Hoechst
	4,17β-Dihydroxy-17-methyl-androst-4-en-3-one	Oxymesterone, 4-Hydroxymethyltestosterone	Oranabol Sanaboral Theranabol	Farmitalia Kabi Lipfa May & Baker Ikapharm Theraplix
	11α,17β-Dihydroxy-17-methyl-androst-4-en-3-one	11α-Hydroxy-methyltestosterone	—	—
	17β-Hydroxy-17-methyl-androst-4-ene-3,11-dione	11-Oxomethyltestosterone	—	—

Structure	Systematic name[a]	Trivial and/or generic name	Trade name	Manufacturer
	4-Chloro-17β-hydroxy-17-methyl-androst-4-en-3-one	Chloromethyltestosterone	Turinabol tabl.	Jenapharm
	1α,7α-Bis(acetylthio)-17β-hydroxy-17-methyl-androst-4-en-3-one	Thiomesterone	Emdabol	Merck A. G.
	17β-Hydroxy-17-methyl-androsta-1,4-dien-3-one	Methandrostenolone Methandienone 1-Dehydromethyltestosterone	Dianabol Abirol Geabol Nabolin Nerobil Vanabol	Ciba Takeda Gea Eisai Richter Vitrum
		-cyclopentenyl ether (gen.) Quinbolon	Anabolicus	Vister
	4-Chloro-17β-hydroxy-17-methylandrosta-1,4-dien-3-one	Chloro-1-dehydromethyl-testosterone	Oral-Turinabol	Jenapharm
	17β-Hydroxy-7α,17α-dimethyl-androst-4-en-3-one	Bolasterone, Dimethyltestosterone Callusterone	Myagen Methosarb	Upjohn Upjohn

II. *19-Nortestosterone-derived protein anabolic steroids*

Structure	Systematic name[a]	Trivial and/or generic name	Trade name	Manufacturer
	17β-Hydroxyestr-4-en-3-one	19-Nortestosterone Nandrolone	Nerobolil Nortestonate	Medimpex Upjohn
		-n-capronate -propionate	Methybol-depot Norybol Anabolicus-Serono	Mepha Serono Ausonia
		-phenylpropionate	Activin Durabol Durabolin Nerobolil Neutrosteron	Aristegui Pharmacia Organon Richter Organon
		-furylpropionate -hexahydrobenzoate -hexyloxyphenylpropionate	Demolon Nor-Durandon Anadur	Mochida Ferring Leo-Lundbeck
		-laurate -undecylate	Laurabolin Dynabolon	Organon (Vet.) Theramex
		-decanoate	Abolon Deca-Durabol Deca-Durabolin Eubolin Nordecon Retabolil	Benzon Pharmacia Organon Futerapica IBSA Richter
		-hemisuccinate -cyclohexylpropionate	Menidrabol Fherbolico Sanabolicum	Menarini Fher Sanabo
		-cyclopentylpropionate	Sterocrinolo Depo-Nortestonate Pluropon	Orma Upjohn Boehringer
		-4-methylbicyclo[2.2.2]oct-2-ene-1-carboxylate	—	Syntex

Structure	Systematic name[a]	Trivial and/or generic name	Trade name	Manufacturer
	4,17β-Dihydroxyestr-4-en-3-one	Oxabolone 4-hydroxy-19-nortestosterone-cyclopentylpropionate	Steranabol-depot	Farmitalia
	4-Chloro-17β-hydroxyestr-4-en-3-one	Chloro-19-nortestosterone-acetate	Steranabol	Farmitalia
	17β-Hydroxy-17-methyl-estr-4-en-3-one	Methyl-19-nortestosterone	Methalutin Orgasteron	Syntex Organon
	17β-Hydroxy-19-nor-pregn-4-en-3-one	Norethandrolone Ethylnortestosterone -propionate	Nilevar Nor-Neutromone Pronabol Solevar	Searle ICI Isis Byla
	17β-Hydroxy-19-nor-pregna-4,9-dien-3-one	Ethyldienolone	—	—

Structure	Systematic name[a]	Trivial and/or generic name	Trade name	Manufacturer
	(dl)-17β-Hydroxy-13β,17α-diethylgon-4-en-3-one $\left(\begin{array}{l}(dl)\text{-13-Ethyl-17-}\\ \text{hydroxy-18,19-dinor-}\\ 17\alpha\text{-pregn-4-en-3-one}\end{array}\right)$	Norbolethone	Genabol	Wyeth

III. Androstane-derived protein anabolic steroids

Structure	Systematic name[a]	Trivial and/or generic name	Trade name	Manufacturer
	3β-Hydroxy-5α-androstan-17-one	Epiandrosterone Isoandrosterone	—	—
	17β-Hydroxy-5α-androstan-3-one	Androstanolone Stanolone Dihydrotestosterone -valerianate	Anaboleen Anabolex Androlone Proteina Protona Apeton Apeton depot	B.A.G. Uni Chemie Lloyd-Hamol Samil Orma Gremy Gremy Fujisawa Fujisawa
	3α-Hydroxy-5α-androstan-17-one	Androsterone	—	—

Structure	Systematic name[a]	Trivial and/or generic name	Trade name	Manufacturer
	17β-Hydroxy-2α-methyl-5α-androstan-3-one	Drostanolone 2α-Methylandrostanolone	Drolban Masterone Metorman Mastizol	Lilly Recovdati Sarva Syntex Latino Shionogi
	17β-Hydroxy-1α-methyl-5α-androstan-3-one	Mesterolone	Mestoran Proviron	Schering (Denmark) Schering A.G.
	5α-Androstane-3β,17β-diol-3-n-octyl-enol-ether	Androstanediol-3-n-octyl-enol ether	Ectovis Ectovister	Vister Drovyssa
	17β-Hydroxy-17-methyl-5α-androstan-3-one	Mestanolone Methylandrostanolone-enanthoyl-acetate	Ermalon Androstalone Notandron-depot	Roussel Roussel Boehringer (M)
	17β-Hydroxy-17-methyl-2-(hydroxy-methylene)-5α-androstan-3-one	Oxymetholone	Adroyd Anadrol Anadroyd Anapolon Anasterone Anasterona Nastenon Protanabol Synasterobe	Parke-Davis Sankyo Shionogi Syntex Parke-Davis ICI Syntex Latino Cassenne Recordati Sarva

IV. Heterocyclic protein anabolic steroids

Structure	Systematic name[a]	Trivial and/or generic name	Trade name	Manufacturer
	17-Methyl-5α-androstano-[3,2-c]-pyrazol-17β-ol	Stanozolol	Winstrol Stromba Tevabolin	Yamanouchi Winthrop Zambon Winthrop Teva
	17-Methyl-5α-androstano-[3,2-c]-isoxazol-17β-ol	Androisoxazole	Androxan Neo-Ponden Neo-Pondus	Leo-Lundbeck Serono Ausonia
	2',17-Dimethylandrost-5(10)-eno[3,2-d]-thiazol-17β-ol	—	—	—
	3-Azi-17-methyl-5α-androstan-17β-ol	Methyldiazirinol	—	—
	17β-Hydroxy-2α,17-dimethyl-5α-androstan-3,3'-azine	Dimethazine	Roxilon Dostalon	Richter Richter

Structure	Systematic name[a]	Trivial and/or generic name	Trade name	Manufacturer
	17β-Hydroxy-17-methyl-2-oxa-5α-androstan-3-one	Oxandrolone	Anavar	Searle

V. Miscellaneous structure protein anabolic steroids

Structure	Systematic name[a]	Trivial and/or generic name	Trade name	Manufacturer
	17β-Hydroxy-1-methyl-5α-androst-1-en-3-one	Methenolone -acetate -enanthate	Nibol Primobolan Primobolan-Acetate Primobolan-Depot	Squibb Schering A. G. Schering A. G. Schering A. G.
	17-Methyl-3-methylene-5α-androst-1-en-17β-ol	—	—	—
	17-Methyl-androst-5-ene-3β,17β-diol	Methylandrostenediol Methandriol	Crestabolic Diandrin Megabion Metilandrostendiol Neosteron Neutrormone Notandren Protandren Stenediol	Nutrition Control Products Astra Teikoku Schering A. G. Organon Pharmacia ISI Boehringer (M) Ciba Organon

Structure	Systematic name[a]	Trivial and/or generic name	Trade name	Manufacturer
		-3-propionate	Metilbisexovis	Vister
			Methilbisexovister	Drovyssa
			Metildiolo	Orma
		-dipropionate	Anabolin	Rafa
			Metandiol	Roussel
		-dienanthoylacetate	Notandren-depot	Boehringer (M)
	3β-Hydroxyandrost-5-en-17-one	Dehydroepiandrosterone	Psicosterone	ICI
		Dehydroisoandrosterone	Diandrone	Organon
		-acetate	17-Chetovis	Vister
	19-Norpregn-4-en-17β-ol	Ethylestrenol	Duraboral	Organon
			Maxibolin	Organon
			Orabolin	Organon
			Orgaboral	Organon
			Durabolin-0	Organon
			Orgabolin	Organon
	17α-Oxo-D-homo-androsta-1,4-diene-3,17-dione (1,2,3,4,4a,4b,7,9,10,10a-decahydro-2-hydroxy-2,4b-dimethyl-7-oxo-1-phenanthrene propionic acid)	Δ'-testololactone	Teslac	Squibb

[a] Chemical Abstracts Systematic Name, Collective Subject Indices, Chemical Abstract.

e. Prepared by Arnold, A., Potts, G. O., and Beyler, A. L.

26
DESCRIPTIVE BROCHURE INCLUDED WITH DIANABOL

Due to the abuse of their product, Ciba Pharmaceutical has discontinued the production and sale of Dianabol. The following is the information that was enclosed with each prescription.

CONTRAINDICATIONS
Hypersensitivity: male patients with carcinoma of the prostate or breast; carcinoma of the breast in some females; pregnancy, because of masculinization of the fetus; nephrosis or the nephrotic phase of nephritis.

PRECAUTIONS
Hypercalcemia may develop both spontaneously and as a result of hormonal therapy in women with disseminated breast carcinoma. If it develops while on this agent, the drug should be stopped.

Caution is required in administering these agents to patients with cardiac, renal, or hepatic disease. Edema may occur occasionally. Concomitant administration with adrenal steroids or ACTH may add to the edema.

If amenorrhea or menstrual irregularities develop, the drug should be discontinued until the etiology is determined.

Anabolic steroids may increase sensitivity to anticoagulants. Dosage of the anticoagulant may have to be decreased in order to maintain the prothrombin time at the desired therapeutic level.

Anabolic steroids have been shown to alter glucose tolerance tests. Diabetics should be followed carefully and the insulin or oral hypoglycemic dosage adjusted accordingly.

Since Dianabol contains a 17 alpha alkyl group, liver function should be checked at regular intervals in patients receiving this drug.

Anabolic steroids should be used with caution in patients with benign prostatic hypertrophy.

Serum cholesterol may increase during therapy. Therefore, caution is required in administering these agents to patients with a history of myocardial infarction or coronary artery disease. Serum determination of serus cholesterol should be made and therapy adjusted accordingly.

ADVERSE REACTIONS
In Males
Prepubertal: phallic enlargement; increased frequency of erections. Postpubertual: inhibition of testicular function; oligospermia; gynecomastia.

In Females

Hirsutism; male pattern baldness; deepening of the voice; clitoral enlargement. These changes are usually irreversible even after prompt discontinuance of therapy and are not prevented by concomitant use of estrogens. In addition, the following may occur: menstrual irregularities; masculinization of the fetus.

In Both Sexes

Nausea; fullness; loss of appetite; vomiting; burning of the tongue; increased or decreased libido; acne (especially in females and prepubertal males); inhibition of gonadotropin secretion; bleeding in patients on concomitant anticoagulant therapy, premature closure of epiphyses in children; jaundice. There have been rare reports of hepatocellular neoplasms and peliosis hepatis in association with long-term androgenic-anabolic steroid therapy.

Alterations may occur in the following clinical laboratory tests; metyrapone test; glucose tolerance test; thyroid function tests (decrease in protein bound iodine, thyroxine-binding capacity, and radioactive iodine uptake); electrolytes (retention of sodium, chloride, water, potassium, phosphates, and calcium); hepatic function tests (increased BSP, serum cholesterol, SGOT, serum bilirubin, and alkaline phosphatase); blood coagulation tests (suppression of clotting factors II, V, VII, and X); decreased 17-ketosteroid excretion.

REPRINTED WITH THE PERMISSION OF CIBA.

27
ADVICE TO PARENTS OF ATHLETES ON STEROIDS

Steroids are dangerous, far more dangerous than meets the eye of a young athlete bent on stacking as much muscle on his frame in as short a time as possible. Quite often, in fact, the athlete is not even aware of what he is taking as a matter of course in training. You, as a parent, will likely have to supply a little perspective that young athletes often cannot do for themselves in defining just how important winning is. When a young man or woman looks and feels great right now, it is difficult for him or her to realize the long-term harm he or she is doing by taking steroids; after all, "long-term" is just too far down the road for one bent on the next game or meet.

This final appendix is meant as an aid to parents and loved ones of athletes on steroids or suspected of being on steroids. Here are the warning signs to look for.

1. Drastic change in behavior patterns (very aggressive behavior not noted before; emotional rollercoaster, unexplained fits of anger).
2. Blood in the urine (make sure this is not a tumor that damages organ structures or trauma during very aggressive play).
3. Odd hair growth or patterns (men and women).
4. Breast-egg appearance on male athletes (gynecomastia) or tender or reddened nipples; small skin growths around or on nipple.
5. Drastic decrease in adipose (fat) tissue of female breast while muscle mass increases just as dramatically.
6. Exceptional change in voice is normal in boys but not as normal in postpubescent women.
7. Child complaining of upper-right-quadrant abdominal pains, after you've ruled out liver disease.
8. Pain on urination, after you've ruled out prostatic hypertrophy, prostatic infection, and bacterial infection (in males).
9. Testicular atrophy in males.
10. Absence of menses in females.
11. Postpubescent acne in young adults after they have outgrown it.
12. Cushinoid half-moon face; looks as though the person had cotton balls in his cheeks, puffing out.
13. Change in skin color, with yellow tinge on the skin or the white sclera of the eyes. This is an early indicator of jaundice.

314

14. Pain in the flank after you've ruled out kidney stone, kidney infection, or tumor if there is no history of trauma. This, combined with blood in the urine, is very important.
15. Empty drug bottles, syringes, and vials. Many times a child will leave a clue when he wants help and guidance.

Don't believe for a minute that "my child would never take these drugs. He's a scholar-athlete and straight as an arrow." This is what makes the situation so critical. The kids taking these drugs are the pride of our country.

BIBLIOGRAPHY

(1) Editorial, "Anabolic Steroids," *Journal of Sports Medicine*, 15, no. 1 (March 1975):1.

(2) "Anabolic Steroids: Doctors Denounce Them, But Athletes Aren't Listening," *Science*, 176 (June, 1972):1399.

(3) Sutton, Coleman, Casey, and Lazarus, "Androgen Responses during Physical Exercise." *British Medical Journal*, (March 3, 1973):520.

(4) Kochakian and Murlin, "The Effect of Large Doses of Male Hormone on Protein and Energy Metabolism of Castrated Dogs," *Nutrition* (1935)10:437.

(5) Torizuka, "The Effect of Anabolic Steroids upon Protein Metabolism Studies by Isotope Method,"*Metabolism* (1963)12:11.

(6) Morgan, W.P., *Erogogenic Aids and Muscular Performance.* New York: Academic Press, 1972.

(7) Kruskemper, H.L., *Anabolic Steroids*, translated by C.H. Doering, New York: Academic Press, 1968.

(8) Hermansen, Hultman, and Saltin, "Muscle Glycogen during Prolonged Severe Exercise." *Acta Physiol. Scand.*, 71 (1967):129.

(9) Johnson and O'Shea, "Anabolic Steroids: Effects on Strength Development," *Science*, 164 (1969):957.

(10) Johnson, L.C., Fisher, G., Silvester, L.J. and C.C. Hofheins, "Anabolic Steroid: Effects on Strength, Body Weight, Oxygen Uptake and Spermatogenesis upon Mature Males," *Medicine and Science in Sports*, 4 (1):43-45, 1972.

(11) Samuels, L.T., Henschel, A.F. and A. Keys, "Influence of Methyl-Testosterone on Muscular Work and Creative Metabolism in Normal Young Men," *Journal of Clinical Endrocrinology and Metabolism*, 2 (1942):649.

(12) Simonson, E., Kearns, W.M. and N. Enzer, "Effects of Methyltestosterone Treatment on Muscular Performance and the

Central Nervous System of Older Men," *Journal of Clinical Endocrinology and Metabolism*, 4 (1944):528-34.

(13) New Zealand Federation of Sports Medicine, "The Use of Anabolic Steroid Hormones in Sport," *The Australian Journal of Sports Medicine*, 3 (1971):26-28.

(14) Kochakian, C.D., "Mechanisms of Androgen Action," *Laboratory Investigation*, (1959):538.

(15) Kochakian, C.D., "The Protein Anabolic Effects of Steroid Hormones," *Vitamins and Hormones*, Ed. K.V. Thimann and R.S. Harris, 4 (1946):255.

(16) Kochakian, C.D., Humm, J.H., and M.N. Bartlett. "The Effect of Steroids on the Body Weight, Temporal Muscle, and Organs of the Guinea Pig," *American Journal of Physiology*, 155 (1948):242.

(17) Kochakian, C.D., Raut, V. and D.M. Nall, "The Metabolism of Testosterone by Guinea Pig Liver and Kidney Homogenates," *American Journal of Physiology*, 189 (1957):76-82.

(18) "Drugs in Sport," *Sports Illustrated* (May, 1969).

(19) Holloszy, J.O., "Biochemical Adaptions in Muscle: Effects of Exercise on Mitochondrial Oxygen Uptake and Respiratory Enzyme Activity in Skeletal Muscle," *Journal of Biological Chemistry*, 242(9) (1967):2278-82.

(20) Sanchez-Medal, L.A. Gomez-Leal, L. Duarte and M. Guadalupe Rico, "Anabolic Androgenic Steroids in Treatment of Acquired Aplastic Anemia," *Blood*, 34 (1969):283-300.

(21) Guyton, A.C., *Textbook of Medical Physiology*, 3rd ed., Philadelphia: W.B. Saunders Co., 1966.

(22) Sherlock S., *Diseases of the Liver and Binary System*. 4th Edition. Philadelphia: F.A. Davis Company.

(23) Rowell, L.B., Masoro, E.J. and M.J. Spencer, "Splanchnic Metabolism in Exercising Man," *Journal of Applied Physiology*, 20 (1965):1032-37.

(24) Tipton, C.M. and B.M. Taylor, "Influence of Atropine on Heart Rates of Rats," *American Journal of Physiology*, 208 (3) (1965):480-84.

(25) Shahidi, N.T., "Androgens and Erythropoiesis," *New England Journal of Medicine*, 289 (1973):72-79.

(26) Baghebi, S.A. and J.L. Boyer, "Peliosis Hepatis Associated with Androgenic-Anabolic Steroid Therapy," *Am. Int. Med.*, 81 (1974):610-18.

(27) Bernstein, M.S., R.L. Hunter, and S. Yachnin, "Hepatoma and Peliosis Hepatis Developing in a Patient with Fanconi's Anemia," *New England Journal of Medicine*, 284 (1971):1135-36.

(28) Farrell, G.C., D.E. Joshua, R.F. Uren, P.J. Baird, K.W. Perkins and

H. Kronenberg, "Androgen Induced Hepatoma," *Lancet* (22 February 1975):430-31.

(29) Gordon, B.S., J. Wolf, T. Krause, and F. Shal, "Peliosis Hepatis and Cholestasis following Administration of Norethandrolone," *American Journal of Clinical Pathology,* 33 (1960):156-65.

(30) Guy, J.T. and M.O. Auslander, "Androgenic Steroids and Hepatocellular Carcinoma," *Lancet* 1 (1973):148.

(31) Henderson, J.T., J. Richmond and M.D. Sumerling, "Androgenic-Anabolic Steroid Therapy and Hepatocellar Carcinoma," *Lancet,* 1 (1972):934.

(32) Johnson, F.L., J.R. Feagler, K.G. Lerner, P.W. Majerus, M. Siegle, J.R. Hartmann and E.D. Thomas, "Association of Androgenic-Anabolic Steroid Therapy with Development of Hepatocellular Carcinoma," *Lancet* 2 (1972):1273-76.

(33) Kintzen, W. and J. Silny, "Peliosis Hepatitis after Administration of Fluoxymesterone," *Canadian Medical Assoc. Journal,* 83 (1960):860-62.

(34) Meadows, A.T., J.L. Naiman, and M.V. Valdes-Dapena, "Hepatoma Associated with Androgen Therapy for Aplastic Anemia," *Journal of Pediatrics,* 84 (1974):109-10.

(35) Recant, L., and P. Lacy (editors), "Fanconi's Anemia and Hepatic Cirrhosis," Clinicopathologic Conference, *American Journal of Medicine,* 39 (1965):464-75.

(36) Zak, F.G., "Peliosis Hepatitis," *American Journal of Pathology,* 26 (1950):1-15.

(37) Ziegenfuss, J. and R. Carabasi, "Androgens and Hepatocellular Carcinoma," *Lancet,* 1 (1973):262.

(38) Johnson, F. Leonard, "The Association of Oral Androgenic-Anabolic Steroids and Life Threatening Disease," *Medicine and Science in Sports,* 7, No. 4 (1975):284-86.

(39) Landon, J., Wynn, V., Houghton, B.J., and J.N.C. Cooke, "Effects of Anabolic Steroid, Methandienone, on Carbohydrate Metabolism in Man." 11. "Effect of Methandienone on Response of Glucagon, Adrenalin, and Insulin in the Fasted Subject," *Metabolism,* 11(5) (1962):513.

(40) Weisenfield, S., and M.G. Goldner, "The Effect of Various Steroids on the Hyperglycemic Action of Glucagon," *Journal of Clinical Endocrinology,* 20 (1960):700-11.

(41) Weisenfield, S., "Effect of 17-Ethyl-19 Nortestosterone on Hyperglycemic Action of Glucagon in Humans," *Proceedings of the Society for Experimental Biology and Medicine,* 97 (1958):764-67.

(42) Kory, R.C., Bradley, M.H., Watson, R.N., Callahan, R., and Peters, B.J., "A Six Month Evaluation of an Anabolic Drug,

Norethandrolone, in Underweight Persons." 11. Bromsulphthalein (BSP) Retention and Liver Function, *American Journal of Medicine*, 26 (1959):243-48.

(43) Schaffner, F., Popper, H., and Chesrow, E., "Cholestasis Produced by the Administration of Norethandrolone," *American Journal of Medicine*, 26 (1959):243-48.

(44) Dubin, I.N., Professor of Pathology, Woman's Medical College of Pennsylvania, Personal Communication.

(45) Schrohe, T., "Telangiektasien der Leber." *Arch. Path. Anat.*, 156 (1899):37-61.

(46) Hendren, G., "Teleangiectasia Hepatis Disseminata und ihre Pathogenese," *Beitr. Path. Ant.*, 45 (1909):306-24.

(47) Mittasch, G., "Beitrage zur Patholigic der Leber." *Arch. Path. Anat.*, 251 (1924):638-48.

(48) Jaffe, R., "Angiomatosis Hepatis beim Mechschen," *Verhandl. Deutsch. Path. Gessellsch*, 19 (1923):202-14.

(49) Senf, H.W., "Uber die Enstehung der Verschi edenen formen miliarer leberblutungen (Peliosis Hepatitis)," *Ach. Path. Anat.*, 304 (1939):549-54.

(50) Geisler, W., "Uber die Sogenannte Peliosis der Leber," *Arch. Path. Anat.*, 280 (1931):565-78.

(51) Gratzer, G., Uber Sogennante "Peliosis Hepatitis," Frankfurt, *Ztschr. Path.*, 36 (1928):134-45.

(52) Peltason, F., "Uber multiple Leberbluntungen bei Miliartuberkulose," *Arch. Path. Anat.*, 230 (1921):230-59.

(53) Meyer, F.G.A., "Beitrage zur Pathologischen Anatomie des Leber." *Arch. Path. Anat.*, 194 (1908):212-55.

(54) Popper, H., Director of Laboratories, Mount Sinai Hospital, New York City, Personal Communication.

(55) Maurice Verdy, Leon Telreault, Walter Murphy, Louis Perron, "Effect of Methandrostenolone on Blood Lipids and Liver Function tests," *Canadian Medical Ass. Journal*, 98 (February 24, 1968).

(56) Berger, R.A. and P.M. Marcuse, "Peliosis Hepatitis, Report of a Case," *American Journal of Clinical Pathology*, 22 (1952):569-73.

(57) Kintzen, W. and J. Silny, "Peliosis Hepatitis after Administration of Fluoxymesterone," *Canadian Medical Assoc. Journal*, 83 (1960):860-62.

(58) Albanese, Lorenze, Orto, and Wein, "Nutritional and Metabolic Effects of Some Newer Steroids," *New York State Journal of Medicine* (September 15, 1968):2392-406.

(59) James, Landon, and Wynn, "Effect of an Anabolic Steroid (Methandienone) on the Metabolism of Cortisol in the Human," *Journal of Endocrinology*, 25 (1962):211-20.

(60) Landau, Barbara R., *Essential Human Anatomy and Physiology.* Chicago: Scott, Foresman & Co., 1976.

(61) Eisenberg, E., G. Gordon and H. Elliott, "Testosterone and Tissue Respiration of the Castrate Male Rat with a Possible Test for Myotrophic Activity," *Endocrinology,* 45 (1949):113-19.

(62) Gordan, G., H. Evans and M. Simpson, "Effects of Testosterone Propionate on Body Weight and Urinary Nitrogen Excretion of Normal and Hypophysectomized Rats," *Endocrinology,* 40 (1937):375-80.

(63) Kochakian, C., "Mechanism of Androgen Actions," *Laboratory Investigation,* 8 (1959):538-56.

(64) Korner, A., "The Influence of Methylandrostenediol on the Protein Fractions and Adenosinetriphosphatase Activity of Muscles of the Rat," *Journal of Endocrinology,* 13 (1955):90-93.

(65) Johnson, L. and J.P. O'Shea, "Anabolic Steroid: Effects on Strength Development," *Science,* 164 (1969):957.

(66) O'Shea, J.P. and William Winkler Jr., "Biochemical and Physical Effects of Anabolic Steroid in Competitive Swimmers and Weightlifters," *Nutritional Reports International,* 2 (1970):351.

(67) O'Shea, John P., "The Effects of an Anabolic Steroid on the Dynamic Strength Levels of Weightlifters," *Nutritional Reports International,* 4, No. 6 (December 1971):363.

(68) Ward, M., "The Effects of Anabolic Steroids Used in the Training of Athletes," unpublished masters thesis, Chapman College, 1968.

(69) O'Shea, J.P., "Steroids: The Effects on Growth and Development," research paper, OAHPER Convention, Salem, Oregon, 1970.

(70) Murray, Elizabeth P., "Exercise, Anabolic Steroids and Castration: the Effect of Engergy Mobilization," unpublished masters thesis, Ohio University, June, 1973.

(71) Fahey, T.D., and C.H. Brown, "The Effects of an Anabolic Steroid on the Strength, Body Composition, and Endurance of College Males When Accompanied by a Weight Training Program," *Medicine and Science in Sports,* 5, No. 4 (1973):272-76.

(72) Kruskemper, H.L., *Anabolic Steroids.* New York: Academic Press, 1968.

(73) Ward, P., "Physiological Effects of Anabolic Steroids," *Track Technique,* 41 (1970):1312-14.

(74) Johnson, L.C., E.S. Roundy, P.E. Allsen, A.G. Fisher and L.J. Silvester, "Effect of Anabolic Steroid Treatment on Endurance," *Medicine and Science in Sports,* 7, No. 4 (1975):287-89.

(75) Stromme, S.B., H.D. Meen, and A. Aakvaag, "Effects of an Androgenic-Anabolic Steroid on Strength Development and Plasma Testosterone Levels in Normal Males," *Medicine and Science in Sports,* 6, No. 3 (1974):203-8.

(76) Fowler, W.H., Gardner, G.W., Egstrom, G.H., "Effect of an Anabolic Steroid on Physical Performance of Young Men," *Journal of Applied Physiology*, 20 (1965):1038-40.

(77) Casner, S.W., Early, R.G., Carlson, B.R., "Anabolic Steroid Effects on Body Composition in Normal Young Men," *Journal of Sports Medicine and Physical Fitness*, 11 (1971):98-103.

(78) Golding, L.A., Freydinger, Sandra, and Fishel, "Weight, Size, and Strength-Unchanged with Steroids," *The Physician and Sports Medicine*, (June 1974):39-43.

(79) Homburger and Pettengill, "The Protein Anabolic and Other Effects of Testosterone Propionate in Mice: Effects of Nutrition and Interrelationship of Biologic Activities of the Hormone," *Endocrinology*, 57 (September 1955):296-301.

(80) Bartlett, P.D. and A. Stevenson, "Effects of Protein Anabolic Hormones on Rates of Protein Degradation and Protein Loss in the Fasting Dog," *Endocrinology* 55 (August 1954):200-204.

(81) Scales, F.M., and Harrison, A.P., "Boric Acid Modification of the Kjeldahl Method for Crop and Soil Analysis," *J. Industrial Engineering Chem.*, 12 (1920):350.

(82) Dowben, R.M., "Treatment of Muscular Dystrophy with Steroids," *New England Journal of Medicine*, 268, No. 7, (April 25, 1963):912-16.

(83) Lihenthal, J.L., Jr. and Zierler, K.L., "Diseases of Muscle," *Biochemical Disorders in Human Disease*, edited by R.H.S. Thompson and E.J. King, New York: Academic Press, 1957, p.483.

(84) James, V.H.T. & Jong, M., "The Use of Tetramethylammonium Hydroxide in the Zimmermann Reaction," *Journal of Clinical Pathology*, 14 (1961):425.

(85) Bartter, F.C., Forbes, A.P., Jefferies, W.M., Carroll, E.L. & Albright, F., "Mechanism of Action of Testosterone in the Therapy of Cushing's Syndrome," *Journal of Clinical Endocrinology*, 9 (1949):663.

(86) Braunsberg, H. & James, V.H.T., "The Determination of Adrenocortical Steroids in Blood: Results in Normal Individuals and Adrenal Hyper-function," *Journal of Endocrinology*, 21 (1960):327.

(87) Moor, P. de, Steeno, O., Raskin, M. & Hendrikx, A., "Fluorimetric Determination of Free Plasma 11-Hydroxycorticosteroids in Man," *Acta Endocr.*, Copenhagen, 33 (1960):297.

(88) Braunsberg, H. & James, V.H.T., "The Determination of Adrenocortical Steroids in Blood. Observations on the Reliability of a Simple Fluorimetric Method for Cortisol," *Journal of Endocrinology*, 25 (1962).

(89) Aakvaag, A. and S.B. Stromme, "The Effects of Mesterolone

Administration to Normal Men on the Pituitary-Testicular Function," *Acta Endocrinol*, Copenhagen (1974).

(90) *Muscle Training Illustrated* (October 1978).

(91) Holloszy, J.O., Oscai, L.B., Mole, P.A. and I.J. Don, "Biochemical Adaptions to Endurance Exercise in Skeletal Muscle," ed. B. Pernow and B. Saltin, *Advances in Experimental Medicine and Biology*. New York: Plenum Press, 1971.

(92) Karlsson, J. and B. Saltin, "Lactate, Adenosine Triphosphate, and Creatine-Phosphate in the Working Muscles during Exhaustive Exercise in Man, *Journal of Applied Physiology*. 29 (1971):596-602.

(93) Astrand, P.O., "Interrelation between Physical Activity and Metabolism of Carbohydrate, Fat, and Protein," *Symposium of the Swedish Nutrition Foundation*, V.G. Blix, Ed., Uppsala, Sweden: Almquist and Wicksell, 1967.

(94) Knuttgen, H.G., "Lactate and Oxygen Debt: An Introduction," *Advances in Experimental Medicine and Biology*, ed. B. Pernow and B. Saltin, New York: Plenum Press, 1971.

(95) Jervell, O., "Investigation of the Concentration of Lactic Acid in Blood and Urine," *Acta Medica Scandinavinca Supplement*, 24 (1928):1-135.

(96) Johnson, R.E. and H.T. Edwards, Lactate and Pyruvate in Blood and Urine after Exercise," *Journal of Biological Chemistry*, 118 (1937):427-32.

(97) Hawk, P.B., Oser, B.L. and Summerson, W.H., *Practical Physiological Chemistry*, 12th ed. Philadelphia: The Blakiston Company 1949, p. 559, 839.

(98) Rowell, L.B., Kraning, K.K., II, Evans, T.O., Kennedy, J.W., Blackman, J.R. and F. Kusumi, "Splanchnic Removal of Lactate and Pyruvate during Prolonged Exercise in Man," *Journal of Applied Physiology*, 21 (1966):1773-83.

(99) Hermansen, L., Pruett, E.D.R., Osnes, J.B. and F.A. Giere, "Blood Glucose and Plasma Insulin in Response to Maximal Exercise and Glucose Infusion," *Journal of Applied Physiology*, 29 (1879):13-16.

(100) Wallace, W.M., Holliday, M., Cushman, M., and Elkinton, J.R., "Application of Internal Standard Flame Photometer to Analysis of Biologic Materials," *Journal of Lab. & Clinical Medicine*, 37 (1951):621.

(101) Saifer, A., and Kornblum, M., "Determination of Chlorides in Biologic Fluids by the Use of Absorption Indicators. Use of Dichlorofinorescein for Volumetric Micro Determination of Chlorides in Cerebrospinal Fluids and Blood Serum," *Journal of Biology and Chemistry*, 112 (1935):117.

(102) Wintrobe, M.M., and Landsberg, J.W., "A Standardized Technique for the Blood Sedimentation Test," *American Journal of Medical*

Science, 189 (1935):102.

(103) Delory, G.E., *Photoelectric Methods in Clinical Biochemistry.* London, Hilger & Watts, 1949, p. 37.

(104) Maclagan, N.E., "The Thymol Turbidity Test as an Indicator of Liver Dysfunction," *British Journal of Experimental Pathology,* 25 (1944):234.

(105) Albanese, A.A., and Irby, V., "Determination of Amino Nitrogen of Blood Filtrates by the Copper Method," *Journal of Lab. & Clinical Medicine,* 30 (1945):718.

(106) Albanese, A.A., and Orto, L.A., "Protein and Amino Acids," in Albanese, A.A., ed., *Newer Methods of Nutritional Biochemistry,* New York: Academic Press, Inc., 1963, p. 1.

(107) Albanese, A.A., Higgens, R.A., Vestal, B., and Stephanson, L., "Photo-Chromatographic Analysis of Amino Acids in Body Fluids," *Journal of Lab. & Clinical Medicine,* 37 (1951):885.

(108) Reitman, S., and Frankel, S., "A Colorimetric Method for the Determination of Serum Glutamic Oxalacetic and Glutamic Pyruvic Transaminases," *American Journal of Clinical Pathology,* 28 (1957):56.

(109) Delamore, I.W. and C.G. Geary, "Aplastic Anemia, Oxymetholone and Acute Myeloid Leukemia," *British Medical Journal,* 2 (1971):743-45.

(110) King, J.B. and D.G. Burns, "Aplastic Anemia, Oxymetholone and Acute Myeloid Leukemia," *South African Medical Journal,* 46 (1972):1622-23.

(111) Deca-Durabolin (Organon) Inc. & Dianabol, Ciba Pharmaceutical Company.

(112) Furth, J., and Sobel, H., "Hypervolemia Secondary to Grafted Granulosacell Tumor," *Journal of National Cancer Institute,* 7 (1946):103-13.

(113) Hamilton, F.T., and Lubitz, J.M., "Peliosis Hepatitis: a Report of 3 Cases, with Discussion of Pathogenesis," *AMA Arch. Path.,* 54 (1952):564-72.

(114) Kracht, J., "Beitrage zur Peliosis Hepatis," *Beitr. Klin. Tuberk,* 105 (1951):172.

(115) Walton, J.N., and Nattrass, F.J., "On Classification, Natural History, and Treatment of Myopathies," *Brain,* 77 (1954):169-231.

(116) Dowben, R.M., "Prolonged Survival of Dystrophic Mice Treated with 17 Ethyl-19-Nortestosterone," *Nature* (London), 184, Supp. 25 (1959):1966.

(117) Dowben, R.M., "Prolonged Survival of Dystrophic Mice Treated with 17$\propto$-Ethyl-19-Nortestosterone," *Nature* (London) 184, Suppl. 25 (1966).

(118) Dowben, R.M., Unpublished data.

(119) Horvah, B., Berg, L., Cummings, D.J., and Shy, G.M., "Muscular Dystrophy: Cation Concentrations in Residual Muscle," *Journal of Applied Physiology*, 8 (1955):22-30.

(120) Dreyfus, J.C., Schapira, G., and Schapira, F., "Biochemical Study of Muscle in Progressive Muscular Dystrophy," *Journal of Clinical Investigation*, 33 (1954):794-97.

(121) Simon, E.J., Gross, C.S. and Lessell, I.M., "Turnover of Muscle and Liver Proteins in Mice with Hereditary Muscular Dystrophy," *Arch. Biochem.*, 96 (1962):41-46.

(122) Dowben, R.M., "Treatment of Muscular Dystrophy with Steroids," *New England Journal of Medicine*, 268, No. 17 (April 1963):912-16.

(123) Jose, A.D. and Mitchell, A.S., *Lancet*, 1 (1964):473.

(124) Werner, M., et al, *Klin. Wscher.*, 39 (1961):1006.

(125) Thomas, C.B., Holljes, H.W.D. and Eisenberg, F.F., *Ann. Intern. Med.*, 54 (1961):413.

(126) Gherondache, C.N., Dowling, W.J., and Pincus, "Metabolic Changes Induced in Elderly Patients with an Anabolic Steroid (Oxandrolone)," *Journal Gerontol.*, 22 (July 1967):290.

(127) Eilert, M.L., *Amer. Heart F.*, 38 (1949):1942.

(128) Barr, D.P., *Circulation*, 8 (1953):641.

(129) Orver, M.F., Boyd, G.S., *Circulation*, 13 (1956):82.

(130) Coogan, W.D., Higano, N., Robinson, R.W., le Beau, R.J., *Pharmacology* (1961):1208.

(131) Ouver, M.F., *Lancet* (1962):1321.

(132) Bradlow, H.L., Zumoff, B., Fukushima, D.K., *Journal of Clinical Endocr.*, 19 (1959):936.

(133) Landon, J., Wynn, V., Cooke, J.N.C., and Kennedy, A., "Effects of Anabolic Steroid Methandienone on Carbohydrate Metabolism in Man," *Metabolism*, 2 (1962):501.

(134) Landon, J., Victor Wynn and E. Samols, "The Effect of Anabolic Steroids on Blood Sugar and Plasma Insulin Levels in Man," *Metabolism* (1963):924-35.

(135) Hoffman, W.S., "Rapid Photoelectric Method for Determination of Glucose in Blood and Urine," *Journal Biological Chemistry*, 120 (1937):51.

(136) Yalow, R.S., and Berson, S.A., "Immunoassay of Endogenous Plasma Insulin in Man," *Journal of Clinical Investigation*, 39 (1960):1157.

(137) Sirek, O.V., and Best, C.H., "The Protein Anabolic Effect of Testosterone," *Endocrinology*, 52 (1953):390.

(138) Talaat, M., Habib, Y.A., and Habib, M., "The Effect of Testosterone on the Carbohydrate Metabolism of Normal

Subjects," *Arch. Int. Pharmacodyn.*, 3 (1957):215.

(139) Hazelwood, R.L., and O'Brien, K.D., "Modification of Glucagon Induced Hyperglycemia in Rats by 17-Ethyl-19-Nortesterone," *Proc. Soc. Exper. Biol. & Med.*, 106 (1961):851.

(140) Weisenfeld, S., and Goldner, M.G., "Effect of Various Steroids on the Hyperglycaemic Action of Glucagon," *Journal of Clinical Endocrinology and Metab.* 20 (1960):700.

(141) Weisenfield, S., "Effect of 17 Ethyl 19-Nortestosterone on the Hyperglycaemic Action of Glucagon in Humans." *Proc. Soc. Exper. Biol. & Med.*, 97 (1958):764.

(142) Kinsell, L.W., Margin, S., and Michaels, G.D., "Evaluation of the effect of Testosterone Propionate upon Ketone, Carbohydrate and Protein Metabolism in Diabetes Mellitus Complicated by Thyrotoxicosis," *Journal of Clin. Invest.*, 30 (1951):1486.

(143) Myhre, L.A., "A Comparison of Body Density and Potassium-40 Measurements of Body Composition," Doctoral Dissertation, Indiana University, Bloomington, Indiana, 1964.

(144) Katch, F.E., Michael and S. Horvath, "Estimation of Body Volume by Underwater Weighting: Description of a Simple Method," *Journal of Applied Physiology*, 23 (1967):811-13.

(145) Wilmore, J. and A. Behnke, "An Anthropometric Estimation of Body Density and Lean Body Weight in Young Men," *Journal of Applied Physiology*, 27 (1969):25-31.

(146) Wilmore, J. and A. Behnke, "Predictability of Lean Body Weight through Anthropometric Assessment in College Men," *Journal of Applied Physiology*, 25 (1968):349-55.

(147) Lumex, Inc., *The Cybex II System Handbook*, New York.

(148) Brozek, J.F. Grande, J.T. Anderson and A. Keys, "Densitometric Analysis of Body Composition: Revision of Some Quantitative Assumptions," *Ann. New York Acad. Sci.*, 110 (1963):492-502.

(149) Laron, Z. and A. Kowadlo-Silbergeld, "Further Evidence for Fat Mobilizing Effect of Androgens," *Acta. Endocrin.*, 45 (1964):427-36.

(150) Kimeldorf, D.J. and S.F. Baum, "Alternations in Organ and Body Growth of Rats following Daily Exhaustive Exercise, X-Irradiation, and Post-Irradiation Exercise," *Growth*, 18 (1954):79-96.

(151) Selye, H., "Studies on Adaptation," *Endocrinology*, 21 (1937):169-88.

(152) Steinhaus, A.H., Hoyt, L.A., and H.A. Rice, "Studies in the Physiology of Exercise X: The Effects of Running and Swimming on the Organ Weights of Growing Dogs," *American Journal of Physiology*, 99 (1931):12-520.

(153) Hati, S., "On the Influence of Exercise on the Growth of Organs in the Albino Rat," *Anatomical Record*, 9 (1915):647-65.

(154) Hearn, G.R. and W.W. Wainio, "Succinic Dehydrogenase Activity of the Heart and Skeletal Muscle of Exercised Rats," *American Journal of Physiology*, 185 (1956):349-50.

(155) O'Shea, J.P., "The Effects of Anabolic Steroid on Blood Chemistry Profile, Oxygen Uptake, Static Strength and Performance in Competitive Swimmers," Doctoral Dissertation, University of Utah, Salt Lake City, 1970.

(156) Cournand, A.E.D. Baldwin, R.C. Darling and D.W. Richards, Jr., "Studies on the Intra-Pulmonary Mixture of Gases, IV: Significance of Pulmonary Emptying Rate and Simplified Open Circuit Management of Residual Air," *Journal of Clinical Invest.*, 20 (1941):681.

(157) Darling, R.C.A., Cournand and D.W. Richards, Jr., "Studies on the Intra-Pulmonary Mixture of Gases, III: An Open Circuit Method for Measuring Residual Air," *Journal of Clinical Invest.*, 19 (1940):609.

(158) Ward, P., "The Effect of an Anabolic Steroid on Strength and Lean Body Mass," *Medicine and Science in Sports*, 5, No. 4 (1973):277-82.

(159) Wilmore, J.A. Girandola and D. Moody, "Validity of Skinfold and Girth Assessments for Predicting Alterations in Body Composition," *Journal of Applied Physiology*, 29 (1970):313.

(160) Wilmore, J.A., "Simplified Method for Obtaining Aliquots of Respiratory Air," *Res. Quart.*, 39 (1968):824-28.

(161) Hermiston, R. and J. Faulkner, "Prediction of Maximal Oxygen Uptake by a Stepwise Regression Technique," *Journal of Applied Physiology*, 30 (1971):833-37.

(162) Rowell, L.B., H.L. Taylor and Y. Wang, "Limitations to the Prediction of Maximal Oxygen Uptake," *Journal of Applied Physiology*, 19 (1964):919-27.

(163) Wiley J. and L. Shaver, "Prediction of Maximum Oxygen Intake from Running Performances of Untrained Young Men," *Res. Quart.*, 43 (1972):89-93.

(164) Bowers, R. and J. Reardon, "Effects of Methandrostenolone (Dianabol) on Strength Development and Aerobic Capacity," *Medical Science in Sports*, 4 (1972):54.

(165) Astrand, I., "Aerobic Work Capacity in Men and Women with Special Reference to Age," *Acta Physiol. Scand.*, 49, suppl. 169, (1960).

(166) Johnson, R.E., P.A. Mole, "Disclosure by Dietary Modification of an Exercise-Induced Protein Catabolism in Man," *Journal of Applied Physiology*, 31, No. 2 (August 1971):186.

(167) Mathews, D.K., Fox, E.L., *The Physiological Basis of Physical Education and Athletics*. Philadelphia: W.B. Saunders, 1971.

(168) Scholander, P.F., "Analyzer for Accurate Estimation of Respiratory Gases in One-Half Cubic Centimeter Samples," *Journal of Biology and Chemistry*, 167 (1947):235.

(169) *Weightlifting: AAU Official Rules*. New York: A.A.U. House, 1970.

(170) Ariel, G. and W. Saville, "Anabolic Steroids: The Physiological Effects of Placebos," *Medical Science in Sports*, 4 (1972):124-26.

(171) Byerly, H., "Explaining and Exploiting Placebo Effects," *Prosp. Biol. Medicine*, 19 (1976):423.

(172) Nathan, D.G., Cahill, G.F., Jr., and Gardner, F.H., "The Effect of Large Doses of Testosterone on the Body Fat of Elderly Men," *Metabolism*, 12 (1963):850.

(173) Ingle, D., "The Time For the Work Capacity of the Adrenalectomized Rats Treated with Cortin," *American Journal of Physiology*, 116 (1934):622-25.

(174) Ingle, D., "The Time for the Occurrence of Corticadrenal Hypertrophy in Rats during Continual Work," *American Journal of Physiology*, 124 (1938):627-30.

(175) Ingle, D. and F. Lukens, "Reversal of Fatigue in the Adrenalectomized Rat by Glucose and Other Agents," *Endocrinology*, 29 (1941):443-52.

(176) Ingle, D., "The Quantitative Assay of Adrenal Cortical Hormones by the Muscle Test in the Adrenalectomized Nephrectomized Rat," *Endocrinology*, 34 (1944):191-202.

(177) Ingle, D., J. Nezamis and E. Morely, "Effect of Cortisone upon the Work Output of the Adrenalectomized Rat," *American Journal of Physiology*, 166 (1951):504-8.

(178) Ingle, D., E. Morely and J. Nezamis, "The Work Performance of Normal Rats Given Continuous Intravenous Injections of Cortisone and Corticotropin," *Endocrinology*, 51 (1952):487-91.

(179) Ingle, D., J. Nezamis and E. Morely, "The Comparative Value of Cortisone, 17-Hydroxycorticosteroids and Adrenal Cortical Extract Given by Continuous Intravenous Injection in Sustaining the Ability of the Adrenalectomized Rat to Work," *Endocrinology*. 50 (1952):1-4.

(180) Eagle, E.S. Britton and R. Kline, "The Influence of Cortico-Adrenal Extract on Energy Output," *American Journal of Physiology*, 102 (1932):707-13.

(181) Berdanier, C. and P. Moser, "Metabolic responses of Adrenalectomized Rats to Exercise," *Proc. Soc. Experimental Biology Medicine*, 141 (1972):490-93.

(182) Bellet, S.L. Roman and F. Barham, "Effect of Physical Exercise on Adrenocortical Excretion," *Metabolism Clinical Experimentation*, 18 (1969):484-97.

(183) Bunyatyan, A. and V. Erez, "Effect of Physical Exertion on Transcortin Binding of Corticosteroids in the Plasma," *Probl. Endok.* 18 (1972):13-17.

(184) Crabbe, J., A. Rionel and E. Mach, "Modification du taux des 17-OH Corticosteroides Plasmatiques a la Suite d'un Effort Physique (Competition d'Aviron)," *Acta Endocrinology*, 22 (1956):119-24.

(185) Davies, C. and J. Few, "Adrenocortical Activity in Exercise," *Journal of Physiology*, 213 (1971):35P-36P.

(186) Gogi, Y., K. Aoki and T. Tsutsumi, "Effect of Muscular Exercise on the Urinary Excretion of Adrenocorticortal Hormone in Man," *Bull. Phys. Fitness. Res. Inst.* 15 (1968):9-18.

(187) Hartley, L.J. Mason, R. Hogan, L. Jones, T. Kotchen, K. Mougey, F. Wherry, L. Pennington and P. Ricketts, "Multiple Hormonal Responses to Graded Exercise in Relation to Physical Training," *Journal of Applied Physiology*. 33 (1972):602-6.

(188) Hartley, L., J. Mason, R. Hogan, L. Jones, T. Kotchen, E. Mougey, F. Wherry, L. Pennington and P. Ricketts, "Multiple Hormone Responses to Prolonged Exercise in Relation to Physical Training," *Journal of Applied Physiology*, 33 (1972):607-10.

(189) Kagi, H. "Deer Einfluss von Muskerlarbeit auf die Blutkonzentration der Nervennierenrinden Hormone," *Helvetica Med. Acta.*, 22 (1955):258-67.

(190) Korenskaya, E., "Fatigue in Physical Exercise and the Adrenal Cortex Function," *Prob. Endocrinology*. 13 (1967):65-68.

(191) Nazar, K. "Changes in 17-Hydroxycorticosteroid Levels in Blood Plasma under the Influence of Muscular Exercise," *Acta Physiol. Polon.*, 2 (1965):176-85.

(192) Nazar, K. "Relation between Total Amount of Muscular Work Performed and Changes in 17-Hydroxysteroid Level in the Blood," *Acta Physiol. Polon.* 17 (1966):767-73.

(193) Chin, A. and E. Evonuk, "Changes in Plasma Catecholamines and Corticosterone Levels after Muscular Exercise," *Journal of Applied Physiology*, 30 (1971):205-7.

(194) Dlusskaya, I. and I. Balakhovskii, "Variational Character of Glucocorticoid Reactions in Rats in Response to ACTH Administration and Other Stimuli," *Probl. Endok.* 18 (1972):79.

(195) Federspil, G. "Effects of Continuous Muscular Exercise on Levels of Blood Glucose and Plasma Free Fatty Acids, Insulin and Corticosterone," *Arch. Int. Physiol. Biochem.* 77 (1969):778-86.

(196) Foss, M.R. Barnard and C. Tipton, "Free 11-Hydroxycorticosteroid Levels in Working Dogs as Affected by Exercise Training," *Endocrinology*. 89 (1971):96-104.

(197) Korge, P. and A. Viru. "Water and Electrolyte Metabolism in

Skeletal Muscle of Exercising Rat," *Journal of Applied Physiology*, 31 (1971):1-4.

(198) Maling, H., D. Stern, P. Altland, B. Highman and B. Brodie, "The Physiologic Role of the Sympathic Nervous System in Exercise," *Journal Pharamcol. Exp. Therapy*, 154 (1966):35-45.

(199) Hill, S., F. Goetz, H. Fox, B. Murawski, L. Krakauer, R. Reifenstein, S. Gray, W. Reddy, S. Hedberg, J. St. Marc and G. Thorn, "Studies on Adrenocortical and Pshychological Responses to Stress in Man," *Arch. Int. Med.* 97 (1956):269-98.

(200) Connell, A., J. Copper and J. Redrearn, "The Contrasting Effects of Emotional Tension and Physical Exercise on the Excretion of 17-Ketogenic Steroids and 17-Ketosteroids," *Acta Endocrinol*, 27 (1958):179-94.

(201) Cornil, A., A. Decoster, G. Copinschi and J. Franckson, "Effect of Muscular Exercise on the Plasma Level of Cortisol in Man," *Acta Endocrinol*, 48 (1965):163-68.

(202) Tharp, G.D., "The Role of Glucocorticoids in Exercise," *Medicine and Science in Sports*, 7, No. 1 (1975):6-11.

(203) Boris, A., R.H. Stevenson, and T. Timal. "Comparative Androgenic, Myotrophic and Antigonadotrophic Properties of Some Anabolic Steroids," *Steroids*, (January 1970):61-71.

(204) Taylor, A.W., Thayer, R. and S. Rao. "Human Skeletal Muscle Glycogen Synthatase Activities with Exercise and Training," *Canadian Journal of Physiology and Pharmacology*, 50 (1972):411-15.

(205) Mitchell, H.H., and Hamilton, T.S. *The Biochemistry of the Amino Acids*. New York: J. Little & Ives, 1929. p. 487.

(206) Allison, J.B., "The Efficiency of Utilization of Dietary Proteins," in Albanese, A.A., ed. *Protein and Amino Acid Nutrition*. New York: Academic Press, Inc., 1959. p. 96.

(207) Albanese, A.A. *Criteria of Protein Nutrition in Protein and Amino Acid Nutrition*. New York Academic Press, 1959. p. 297.

(208) Kochakian, C.D. and J.R. Murlin. "Effect of the Male Hormone on the Protein and Energy Metabolism of Castrate Dogs." *Journal of Nutrition*. 10 (1935):437.

(209) Kochakian, C.D. "Effect of the Male Hormone on Protein Metabolism of Castrate Dogs," *Proceedings of the Society for Experimental Biology and Medicine*. 32 (1935):1064.

(210) Stafford, R.O., Bowman, B.J. and K.J. Olson, "The Influence of 19-Northesterone Cyclopentyl Propionate on Urinary Nitrogen of Castrated Male Rats." *Proceedings of the Society for Experimental Biology*, 86 (1954):322-29.

(211) Forsyth, B.T. "The Effect of Testosterone Propionate at Various Protein and Caloric Intakes in Malnutrition after Trauma," *Journal*

of *Laboratory and Clinical Medicine*, 43 (1954):732.

(212) Spencer, H., Burger, E., Charles, M.L., Gottesman, E.D., and Laszlo, D., "The Metabolic Effects of 17-Ethyl-10-Nortestosterone in Man," *Journal of Clinical Endocrinology*. 17 (1957):975.

(213) Whedon, G.D., and Shorr, E., "Metabolic Studies in Paralytic Acute Anterior Poliomyelitis. IV. Effects of Testosterone Propionate and Estradiolbenzoate on Calcium, Phosphorous, Nitrogen, Creatine, and Electrolyte Metabolism," *Journal of Clinical Investigation*, 36 (1957):995.

(214) McSwinny, P.R., and Prunty, F.T.G., "Metabolic Effects of Three Testosterone Derivatives including 17-Alpha-Ethyl-19 Nortestosterone," *Journal of Endocrinology*, 16 (1957):28.

(215) Peden, J.C., Jr., Ohin, A., and Williams, P.T., "Influence of Anabolic Agents on Nitrogen Balance of Patients with Major Extremity Fractures," *Arch. Surg.*, 80 (1960):1036.

(216) Stokes, P.E., Horwith, M. Pennington, T.G., and Clarkson, B., "17-Alpha-Ethyl-19-Nortestosterone as an Anabolic Agent and Its Effect on Creatine Metabolism and Vaginal Cytology in Humans," *Metabolism*, 8 (1959):709.

(217) Metcalf, W. and H.G. Greene, "A Quantitative Expression for Nitrogen Retention with Anabolic Steroids. I. Norethandrolone," *Metabolism*, 12, No. 10 (1963):899-909.

(218) Ariel G., and W. Saville, "The Effect of Anabolic Steroids on Reflex Components," *Medicine and Science in Sports*, 4, No. 2 (1972):120-23.

(219) Kroll, W. Patellar, "Reflex Time and Latency under Jendrassik and Crossed Extensor Facilitation," *American Journal Phys. Med.*, 47 (1968):292-301.

(220) Astrand, "Diet and Athletic Performance," *Federal Proceedings*, 26 (December 1967):1772-77.

(221) Krogh, A., and J. Lindhard, *Biochem. Journal.* 14 (1920):290.

(222) Christensen, E.H., and O. Hansen, *Skand. Arch. Physiol.* 81 (1939):137.

(223) Watts, J.H., B. Tolbert and W.L. Ruff, "Nitrogen Balances for Young Adult Males Fed Two Sources of Non-Essential Nitrogen at Two Levels of Total Nitrogen Intake," *Metabolism*, 13 (1964):172.

(224) Swendseid, M.E., J.H. Watts, C.L. Harris and S.G. Tuttle, "An Evaluation of the FAO Amino Acid Reference Pattern in Human Nutrition. I. Studies with Young Men," *Journal of Nutrition*, 75 (1961):295.

(225) Swendseid, M.E., C.L. Harris and S.G. Tuttle, "An Evaluation of the FAO Amino Acid Reference Pattern in Human Nutrition. II. Studies with Young Women," *Journal of Nutrition*, 77 (1962):391.

(226) Kurk, M.C.N. Mecheny and M.S. Reynolds, "Nitrogen Balances of

Young Women Fed Amino Acids in the FAO Reference Pattern, the Milk Pattern and the Peanut Pattern," *Journal of Nutrition*, 77 (1962):998.

(227) Levenson, R.M. and D. Snell, "Nitrogen Balances of Young Women Fed the FAO Amino Acids and the Oat Pattern," *Journal of Nutrition*, 78 (1962):10.

(228) Albanese, A.A., "Newer Methodology in the Clinical Investigation of Anabolic Steroids," *New York Journal of Medicine* (June 1965).

(229) Kochakian, C.D. and G. Costa, "The Effect of Testosterone Propionate on the Protein and Carbohydrate Metabolism in the De-Pancreatized-Castrated Dog," *Endocrinology*, 65 (1959):298.

(230) Paulsen, C.A., "Production, Metabolism, Actions, and Clinical Effects of Testosterone," in *Textbook of Endocrinology*, ed. R.H. Williams, 4th ed. Philadelphia: W. B. Saunders, 1968, p. 414.

(231) Howard, R.P. and P.R. Furman, "Metabolic and Serum Lipid Effects of Methylandrostane and Methylandrostene Pyrazoles," *Journal of Clinical Endocrinology*, 22 (1962):43-51.

(232) Gaebler, O.H., S.M. Tarnowski, *Endocrinology*, 33 (1943):299.

(233) Sirek, O.V., C.H. Best, *Endocrinology*, 52 (1952):390.

(234) Cavallero, C.B. Malandra, *Boll. Soc. Ital. Biol. Sper.*, 32 (1956):748.

(235) Kochakian, C.D., G. Costa, *Endocrinology*, 65 (1959):298.

(236) Manchester, K.L., F.G. Young, *Biochem. J.*, 70 (1958):353.

(237) Wool, I.G., K.L. Manchester, *Nature* (London) 193 (1962):345.

(238) Necheles, T., *Fed. Proc.*, 20 (1961):67.

(239) Krahl, M.E., J.C. Penhos, *Fed. Proc.* 20 (1961):193.

(240) Chance, B., in *Amino Acids, Proteins and Cancer Biochemistry*, ed. J.T. Edsall, New York, 1960.

(241) Novak, A., *Amer. J. Physiol.*, 191 (1957):306.

(242) Bernelli-Zazzera, A.M. Bassi, R. Comolli, P. Lucchelli, *Nature* (London) 182 (1958):663.

(243) Bernelli-Zazzera, A.M. Bassi, *Sperimentale*, 108 (1958):291.

(244) Freiden, E.H., M.R. Laby, F. Bates, N. Layman, *Endocrinology*, 60 (1957):290.

(245) Indovina, I., C. Pattavina, *Arch. Stud. Fisiopat*, 22 (1958):551.

(246) Kruskemper, H.L. *Anabolic Steroids*, New York: Academic Press, 1968.

(247) Kowalewski, K., R.T. Morrison, *Canad. J. Biochem. Physiol.*, 35 (1957):771.

(248) Sciapiades, E. *Proc. Soc. Exp. Biol.* (New York) 37 (1937):242.

(249) Kruskemper, H.L., F.J. Kessler, S.H. Hassan, *Klin. Wschr.*, 39 (1961):1013.

(250) Kassenaar, A., A. Kouwenhoven, A. Querido, *Acta Endocrin.* (Copenhagen) 39 (1962):233.

(251) Kochakian, C.D., D.G. Harrison, *Endocrinology,* 70 (1962):99.

(252) Burt, F.B., R.V. Finney, W.W. Scott, *Cancer,* 10 (1957):825.

(253) Brendler, H.W.E. Chase, W.W. Scott, *Arch. Surg.,* 61 (1950):433.

(254) Lesser, M.A., S.N. Vose, G.M. Dixey, *J. Clin. Endocrinology,* 15 (1955):297.

(255) Kochakian, C.D., *American Journal Physiol,* 160 (1950):53.

(256) Stafford, R.O., B.J. Bowman, K.J. Olsen, *Proc. Soc. Exp. Biol.,* (New York) 86 (1954):322.

(257) Kochakian, C.D., *Macy Conf. Metab. Aspects Convalesc.,* 7 (1944):97.

(258) Kochakian, C.D., *Endocrinology,* 66 (1960):786.

(259) Kochakian, C.D., J. Dolphin, *Amer. Journal of Physiol.,* 180 (1955):317.

(260) Bourliere, F.H. Cendron, B. Tenniere. *C.R. Soc. Biol.,* (Paris) 152 (1958):1636.

(261) Kochakian, C.D., in *Protein Metabolism, Hormones and Growth.* Rutgers Univ. Press, 1953.

(262) Kochakian, C.D.J., R. Merlin, *Journal of Nutrition,* 10 (1935):437.

(263) Knowlton, K., A.T. Kenyon, I. Sandiford, G. Lotwin, L. Fricker, *J. Clinical Endocrinology,* 2 (1942):671.

(264) Porloff, W.H., E. Rose, W.F. Sunderman, *Arch. Int. Med.,* 72 (1943):494.

(265) Bassett, S.H., E.H. Keutmann, C.D. Keutmann, C.D. Kochakian, *J. Clinical Endocrinology,* 3 (1943):267.

(266) Talbot, N.B., A.M. Butler, E.L. Pratt, E.A. McLachlan, *Amer. J. Dis. Children,* 69 (1945):267.

(267) Weller, O., *Arzneimittelforsch.,* 12 (1962):234.

(268) Wayjen, Van, R.G.A., *Helv. Med. Acta.,* 27 (1960):523.

(269) Almqvist, S., D. Ikkos, R. Luft, *Acta Endocrin* (Copenhagen) 38 (1961):413.

(270) Werner, M., Hitz, H. Tholen, H. Staub., *Helv. Med. Acta.,* 27 (1960):543.

(271) Lachnit, V., C. Eberhartinger, *Wien. Z. Inn. Med.,* 34 (1953):379.

(272) Poulsen, H., Winkler K., "Liver Disease with Periportal Sinusoidal Dilation," *Digestion,* 8 (1973):441-42.

(273) Irey, N.S., Manion, W.C., Taylor, H.B., "Vascular Lesions in Women Taking Oral Contraceptives," *Arch. Pathol.,* 89 (1970):1-8.

(274) Crain, J.M., "The Pathology of Birth Control," *Arch. Pathol.* 99 (1975):233-36.

(275) Contostavlos, D.L., "Benign Hepatomas and Oral Contraceptives,"

Lancet, 2 (1973):1200.

(276) Knapp, W.A., Ruebner, B.H., "Hepatomas and Oral Contraceptives," *Lancet,* 1 (1974):270.

(277) O'Sullivan, J.P., Wilding, R.P., "Liver Hamartomas in Patients on Oral Contraceptives," *British Medical Journal,* 3 (1974):7-10.

(278) Wexler, B.C., "Pathophysiologic Changes Induced in Arterioscleroitic and Monarteriosclerotic Rats by Methylandrostenediol," *Lab. Invest.* 25 (1971):158-68.

(279) Foss, G.L., *British Medical Journal,* 2 (1939):11.

(280) Werner, S.C., *American Journal of Medicine,* 3 (1954):52.

(281) Brick, I.B., H. Kyle, *New England Journal of Medicine,* 246 (1952):176.

(282) Wood, J.C., *Journal of the American Medical Assn.,* 150 (1952):1484.

(283) Peters, J.H., A.H. Randall, J. Mendeloff, R. Peace, J.C. Coberly, M.B. Hurley, *Journal of Clinical Endocrinology,* 18 (1958):114.

(284) Gordon, B.J., J. Wolf, T. Krause, F. Shai, *American Journal of Clinical Pathology,* 33 (1959):249.

(285) Gilbert, E.F., A.Q. DaSilva, D.M. Queen, *Journal of American Medical Assn.,* 185 (1963):411.

(286) Rhoads, Dobriner, *Science,* 95 (1942):534.

(287) Lipschutz, *Texas Rep. Biol. Med.,* 6 (1948):3.

(288) Gardner, W.U., *Hormones and Carcinogenesis: Report of the Second Canadian Cancer Conference.* New York: Academic Press, 1957.

(289) Huggins, C., "Steroids, Growth and Cancer," in *Biological Activities of Steroids in Relation to Cancer,* Pincus, G., and Vollmer, E.P. New York: Academic Press, p. 1-8, 1960.

(290) Lockhart-Department of Physical Education, University of Southern California, Unpublished Paper, (1959).

(291) Delorme, T.L., "Restoration of Muscle Power by Heavy Resistance Exercises," *Journal of Bone Journal Surgery.* 37 A. (1945):645-67.

(292) Morgan, R.E., Adamson, G.T., *Circuit Training.* London: G. Bell and Sons, 1957.

(293) Walters, C.E., "The Effects of Therapeutic Agents on Muscular Strength and Endurance," *Physical Therapy Rev.* 40 (1960):266-70.

(294) Hettinger, T., Muller, E.A., "Muskelleistung und Muskeltraining," *Arb. Physiol.,* 15 (1953):111-26.

(295) Perrine, J.J., "Isokinetic Exercise and the Mechanical Energy Potentials of Muscle," *Journal of Health and Physical Education,* Rec. 39 (1968):40-44.

(296) Chang, J.C., Slutzker, B., Lindsay, N., "Remission of Pure Red

Cell Aplasia following Oxymetholone Therapy," *Am. J. Med. Sci.* 275, No. 3 (May-June 1978):345-51.

(297) Kounis, N.G., Evans, W.H., "Treatment of Chronic Thromboembolism with Arvin, Oral Fibrinolytics and Standard Anticoagulants," *Vasc. Surg.*, 11, No. 2 (March-April 1977):68-72.

(298) Galbraith, H., Watson, H.B., "Performance, Blood and Carcase Characteristics of Finishing Steers Treated with Trenbolone Acetate and Hexoestrol," *Vet. Rec.* 103, No. 2 (8 July 1978):28-31.

(299) Corkery, J. Bern, M.M., Tullis, J.L., "Resolution of Amyloidosis and Plasma-Cell Dyscrasia with Combination Chemotherapy Letter," *Lancet*, 2, No. 8086 (19 August 1978):425-26.

(300) Jacqueson, A., Thevenin, M., Wanet, J.M., Claude, J.R., Truhaut, R., "Comparative Study of the Protective Effect of an Anabolic Steroid. The 19-Nortestosterone-Phenylpropionate (19·NTPP), on Liver Steatosis Induced by Amanita Phalloides and White Phosphorus in Rats," *Arch. Toxicol.*, Suppl. 1 (1978):193-96.

(301) Gangitano, J.L., Foster, S.H., Contro, R.M., "Nonfatal Methazolamide-Induced Aplastic Anemia," *Am. J. Ophthalmol.*, 86, No. 1 (July 1978):138-39.

(302) Robinson, C.P., Smith, P.W., Endecott, B.R., "Depression of Cholinesterase Activity by Ethylestrenol in Toxicol," *Appl. Pharmacol.*, 44, No. 1 (April 1978):207-11.

(303) Romero, C.H., Claflin, W., Frank, F., Chang, T.S., Purchase, H.G., "Vaccination Immunity to Selected Diseases in Chickens Fed the Androgen Analog Mibolerone," *Poult. Sci.*, 57, No. 1 (January 1978):74-79.

(304) Deslauriers, R. Hasan, F., Lodge, B.A., Smith, I.C., "Assignment by 13-C-NMR Spectroscopy of Configuration at C-5 in 17 Alpha-Ethylestran-17 Beta-01, an Impurity in the Anabolic Steroid Ethylestrenol," *J. Pharm. Sci.*, 67, No. 8 (August 1978):1187-89.

(305) Krzeminski, L.F., Cox, B.L., Dunn, G.H., "3D Determination of 17 Beta-Hydroxy-7 Alpha, 17-Dimethylestr-4-En-3-One (Mibolerone) in Canned Dog Food by High-Performance Liquid Chromatography," *J. Agric. Food Chem.*, 26, No. 4 (July-Aug. 1978):891-93.

(306) Fortt, G., Calabresi, E., Giannotti, P., Borrelli, D., Gonnelli, P. Barbieri, U., Serio, M., "Measurement of 5-Androsten-3-Beta, 17-Beta-Diol in Spermatic and Peripheral Venous Blood Samples from the Same Human Subjects by a Radioimmunoassay Method," *Horm. Res.* 9, No. 4 (1978):194-200.

(307) Stoj, Cevski, T., Nedelkoski, J., Jovanovski, M., "Bone Marrow Histology before and after the Treatment of Idiopatic Aplastic Anaemia with Oxymetholone," *God ZB Med. Fak Skopje*, 23 (1977):389-96.

(308) Hast, R., Engstedt, L. Jameson, S., Killander, A., Lundh, B.,

Reizenstein, P., Sk Arberg Ko, Ud En Am, Wadman, B., "Oxymetholone Treatment in Myelofibrosis," *Blut.* 37, No. 1, (14 July 1978):19-26.

(309) Shimizu, K., "Formation of 5-17 Beta-2H Androstene-3 Beta, 17 Alpha-Diol from 3-Beta-Hydroxy-5-17, 21, 21, 21-2H Pregnen-20-One by the Microsomal Fraction of Boar Testis," *J. Biol. Chem.*, 253, No. 12 (25 June 1978):4237-41.

(310) Taxy, J.B., "Peliosis: A Morphologic Curiosity Becomes an Iatrogenic Problem," *Hum. Pathol.* 9, No. 3 (May 1978):331-40.

(311) Ban, T.A., "The Treatment of Depressed Geriatric Patients," *Am. J. Psychother.*, 32, No.1 (January 1978):93-104.

(312) Amin, M.I., Koshy, K.T., Bryan, J.T., "Stability of Aqueous Solutions of Mibolerone," *J. Pharm. Sci.* 65, No. 12 (December 1976): 1777-79.

(313) Browse, N.L., Burnand, K.G., "The Postphlebitic Syndrome: A New Look," pp. 395-404, in Bergan, J.J., Yao, J.S., ed., *Venous Problems.* Chicago, Year Book Medical Publ., 1978.

(314) Fisher, J.W., Moriyama, Y., Modder, B., "Effects of Steroids on in Vitro Erythroid Colony Growth and Erythropoietin Production," pp. 65-79, in Hibino, S., et al., ed., *Aplastic Anemia.* Baltimore, Univ. Park Press, 1978.

(315) Whang, K.S., "Aplastic Anemia in Korea: A Clinical Study of 309 Cases," pp. 225-42, in Hibino, S., et al., ed., *Aplastic Anemia.* Baltimore, Univ. Park Press, 1978.

(316) Lusch, C.J., Ramsey, H.E., Katayama, I., "Leukemic Reticuloendotheliosis: Report of a Case with Peripheral Blood Remission on Androgen Therapy," *Cancer.* 41, No. 5 (May 1978):1964-66.

(317) Romero, C.H., Purchase, HG., Frank, F.R., Chang. T.S., "Absence of B Stem Cells in Spleens of Chickens Fed the Androgen Analog Mibolerone," *Avian Dis.*, 22, No. 1 (January-March 1978):53-60.

(318) Vuorenkoski, V., Lenko, H.L., Tjernlund, P., Vuorenkoski, L., Perheentupa, J., "Fundamental Voice Frequence during Normal and Abnormal Growth, and after Androgen Treatment," *Arch Dis Child.*, 53, No. 3 (March 1978):201-9.

(319) Aynsley-Green, A., Zachmann, M., Werder, E.A., Illig, R., Prader, A., "Endocrine Studies in Fanconi's Anaemia. Report of 4 Cases," *Arch Dis Child.*, 53, No. 2 (February 1978):126-31.

(320) Krzeminski, L.F., Sokolowski, J.H., Dunn, G.H., Vanravenswaay, F., Pineda, M., "Serum Concentrations of Mibolerone in Beagle Bitches as Influenced by Time, Dosage Form, and Geographic Location," *Am. J. Vet. Res.*, 39, No. 4 (April 1978):567-72.

(321) Jondorf, W.R., Moss, M.S., "Radioimmunoassay Technique for Detecting Urinary Excretion Products after Administration of Synthetic Anabolic Steroids to the Horse," *Xenobiotica*, 8, No. 8 (April 1978):197-206.

(322) Atkins, P., Brown, I.K., Downie, R.J., Haggart, B.G., Littler, J., Robb, P.M., Santer, G.J., Jones, I., "The Value of Phenformin and Ethyloestrenol in the Prevention of Deep Venous Thrombosis in Patients Undergoing Surgery," *Thromb. Haemostas.*, 39, No. 1 (28 February 1978):89-96.

(323) Gould, D.J., Cunliffe, W.J., Smiddy, F.G., "Anabolic Steroids in Hereditary Angiooedema Letter," *Lancet*, 1, No. 8067 (8 April 1978):770-71.

(324) Stanczyk, F.Z., Goebelsmann, U., Nakamura, R.M., "Further in Vitro Steroid Metabolic Studies of Testicular 17 Beta-Reduction Deficiency," *J. Steroid Biochem.*, 9, No. 2 (February 1978):153-57.

(325) Yadav, R.N., Teare, F.W., "Determination of Fluoxymesterone, Norethandrolone, Prednisolone, and Prednisone in Tablets by Differential Pulse Polarography," *J. Pharm. Sci.*, 67, No. 3 (March 1978):436-38.

(326) Franks, C.R., Williams, Y., "The Effect of Sex Hormones on Peripheral Immunity in Patients with Advanced Breast Cancer," *Clin. Oncol.*, 4, No. 1 (March 1978):19-24.

(327) Robinson, C.P., Smith, P.W., Crane, C.R., McConnell, J.K., Allen, L.V., Endecott, B.R., "The Protective Effects of Ethylestrenol against Acute Poisoning by Organophosphorus Cholinesterase Inhibitors in Rats," *Arch. Int. Pharmacodyn. Ther.*, 231, No. 1 (January 1978):168-76.

(328) Steele, P., Ellis, J., Jr., Genton, E., "Effects of Platelet Suppressant, Anticoagulant and Fibrinolytic Therapy in Patients with Recurrent Venous Thrombosis," *Am. J. Med.*, 64, No. 3 (March 1978):441-45.

(329) Cattran, D.C., Fenton, S.S., Wilson, D.R., Oreopoulos, D., Shimizu, A., Richardson, R.M., "A Controlled Trial of Nondrolone decandate in the Treatment of Uremic Anemia," *Kidney Int.*, 12, No. 6 (December 1977):430-37.

(330) Foreman, M.I., Clanachan, I., Kelly, I.P., "The Diffusion of Nandrolone through Occluded and Non-Occluded Human Skin," *J. Pharm. Pharmacol.*, 30, No. 3 (March 1978):152-57.

(331) Acchiardo, S.R., Black, W.D., "Fluoxymesterone Therapy in Anemia of Patients on Maintenance Hemodialysis: Comparison between Patients with Kidneys and Anephric Patients," *J. Dial.*, 1, No. 4 (1977):357-66.

(332) "2 Alpha, 3 Alpha-Epithio-5 Alpha-Androstan-17 Beta-Y1

1-Methoxycyclopentyl Ether in the Treatment of Advanced Breast Cancer: Japanese Cooperative Group of Hormonal Treatment for Breast Cancer," *Cancer,* 41, No. 2 (February, 1978):758-60.

(333) Heitzman, R.J., Harwood, D.J., "Residue Levels of Trenbolone and Oestradiol-17 Beta in Plasma and Tissues of Steers Implanted with Anabolic Steroid Preparations," *Br. Vet. J.,* 133, No. 6 (November-December 1977):564-71.

(334) Rao, A.N., Brown, A.K., Rieder, R.F., Clegg, J.B., Marsh, W.L., "Aplastic Anemia with Fetallike Erythropoiesis following Androgen Therapy," *Blood,* 51, No. 4 (April 1978):711-19.

(335) Houghton, E., Oxley, G.A., Moss, M.S., Evans, S., "Studies Related to the Metabolism of Anabolic Steroids in the Horse: A Gas Chromatographic Mass Spectrometric Method to Confirm the Administration of 19-Nortestosterone or its Esters to Horses," *Biomed. Mass. Spectrom.,* 5, No. 2 (February 1978):170-73.

(336) Sato, S., Chen, J.N., Maruyama, S., "A histochemical Study of the Effects of 19-Nortestosterone on the RNA in the Secretory Tubules of the Submandibular Glands of Castrated-Adrenalectomized Mice," *Arch. Oral. Biol.,* 22, Nos. 10-11 (1977):563-69.

(337) Benjamin, D.R., Shunk, B., "A Fatal Case of Peliosis of the Liver and Spleen," *Am. J. Dis. Child,* 132, No. 2 (February 1978):207-8.

(338) Bank, J.I., Lykkebo, D.H., Agerstrand, I., "Peliosis Hepatis in a Child," *Acta. Paediatr. Scand.,* 67, No. 1 (January 1978):105-7.

(339) Dawson, H.A., Gersten, K.E., "Use of an Anabolic Steroid in Racetrack Practice," *Mod. Vet. Pract.,* 59, No. 2 (February 1978):129-30.

(340) Vose, G.P., Keele, D.K., Milner, A.M., Rawley, R., Roach, T.L., Sprinkle, E.E., "3D Effect of Sodium Fluoride, Inorganic Phosphate, and Oxymetholone Therapies in Osteoporosis: A Six-Year Progress Report," *J. Gerontol.,* 33, No. 2 (March 1978):204-12.

(341) Asihan, E.M., Warin, R.P., "Treatment of Hereditary Angioneurotic Oedema with Methandienone Letter," *Br. Med. J.,* 1, No. 6109 (11 February 1978):367.

(342) Bhathal, P.S., Fone, D.J., Hurley, T.H., Sullivan, J.R., Wall, A.J., Young, G.P., "Drug-Induced Hepatic Injury Letter," *Aust. Nz. J. Med.,* 7, No. 5 (October 1977):539-40.

(343) Leong, A.S., Sage, R.E., "Drug-Induced Hepatic Injury Letter," *Aust. Nz. J. Med.,* 7, No. 5 (October 1977):537-39.

(344) Raich, P.C., Korst, D.R., "Plasma Erythropoietin Levels in

Patients Undergoing Long-Term Hemodialysis," *Arch. Pathol. Lab. Med.*, 102, No. 2 (February 1978):73-75.

(345) Amaku, E.O., "A Study of the Effect of Anabolic Steroids on Nitrogen Balance," *West Afr. J. Pharmacol. Drug Res.*, 4, No. 1 (June 1977):1-5.

(346) Bricolo, A., "The Medical Therapy of the Apalltic Syndrome," *Monogr. Gesamtgeb. Psychiatr.* (Berlin), 14, (1977):182-88.

(347) Laitem, L., Gaspar, P., Bello, I., "Detection of Trenbolone Residues in Meat and Organs of Slaughtered Animals by Thin-Layer Chromatography," *J. Chromatogr.*, 147 (11 January 1978):538-39.

(348) Charny, C.W., Gordon, J.A., "Testosterone Rebound Therapy: A Neglected Modality," *Fertil. Steril.* 29, No. 1 (January 1978):64-68.

(349) Ghanadian, R., Smith, C.B., Williams, G., Chisholm, G.D., "The Effect of Antiandrogens and Stilboestrol on the Cytosol Receptor in Rat Prostate," *Br. J. Urol.*, 49, No. 7 (1977):695-700.

(350) Schwarz, L.R., Schwenk, M., Pfaff, E., Greim, H., "Cholestatic Steroid Hormones Inhibit Taurocholate Uptake into Isolated Rat Hepatocytes," *Biochem. Pharmacol.*, 26, No. 24 (15 December 1977):2433-37.

(351) Rico, A.G., Benard, P., Braun, J.P., Burgat-Sacaze, V., "Metabolism of 19 Nortestosterone-14C Associated with Oestradiol in Mice and Calves," *Ann. Rech. Vet.*, 8, No. 8 (1977):135-41.

(352) Lye, M.D., Ritch, A.E., "Long-Term Anabolic Therapy in the Elderly," *Age Ageing*, 6, No. 4 (November 1977):221-27.

(353) Haak, H.L., Hartgrink-Groeneveld, C.A., Guiot, H.F., Speck, B., Eernisse, J.G., Von Rood, J.J., "Acquired Aplastic Anaemia in Adults. II. Conventional Treatment: Retrospective Study in 40 Patients," *Acta Haematol* (Basel), 58, No. 6 (1977):339-52.

(354) Remes, K., Vuopio, P., J. Arvinen, M., H. Ark Onen, M., Adlercreutz, H., "Effect of Short-Term Treatment with an Anabolic Steroid (Methandienone) and Dehydroepiandrosterone Sulphate on Plasma Hormones, Red Cell Volume and 2,3-Diphosphoglycerate in Athletes," *Scand. J. Clin. Lab. Invest.*, 37, No. 7 (November 1977):577-86.

(355) Andriesse, R., Thussen, J.H., Donker, G.H., "The Influence of Nandrolone Decanoate (Deca-Durabolin) on the Peripheral Conversion of Androstenedione to Oestrone," *J. Steroid Biochem.*, 8, No. 12 (December 1977):1271-72.

(356) Saure, A., Ter Av Ainen, T., Karjalainen, O., "The Effect of Synthetic Gestagens on Progesterone Formation in Vitro in Human Placenta of Early Pregnancy," *J. Reprod. Fertil.*, 51, No.

2 (November 1977):369-73.

(357) Malmendier, C.L., Van Den Bergen, C.J., Emplit, G., Delcroix, C., "A Long-Term Study of the Efficacy of Oxandrolone in Hyperlipoproteinemias," *J. Clin. Pharmacol.*, 18, No. 1 (January 1978):42-53.

(358) Dunn, C.D., Napier, J.A., Ford, T.W., Price, V.A., "Oxymetholone and Erythropoiesis: Failure to Detect an Effect in Fetal Mouse Liver Cell," *Cultures. Exp. Hematol.*, 5, No. 6 (November 1977):546-50.

(359) Houhton, E., "Studies Related to the Metabolism of Anabolic Steroids in the Horse: 19-Nortestosterone," *Xenobiotica*, 7, No. 11 (November 1977):683-93.

(360) Jondorf, W.R., "19-Nortestosterone, A Model for the Use of Anabolic Steroid Conjugates in Raising Antibodies for Radioimmunoassay," *Xenobiotica*, 7, No. 11 (November 1977):671-81.

(361) Wildt, D.E., Seager, S.W., "Reproduction Control in Dogs," *Vet. Clin. North Am.*, 7, No. 4 (November 1977):775-87.

(362) Burke, T.J., "Fertility Control in the Cat," *Vet. Clin. North Am.*, 7, No. 4 (November 1977):699-703.

(363) Agmo, A., "The Comparative Actions of Fluoxymesterone and Testosterone on Sexual Behavior and Accessory Sexual Glands in Castrated Rabbits," *Horm. Behav.*, 9, No. 2 (October 1977): 112-19.

(364) Matsuzawa, A., Yamamoto, T., "Antitumor Effect of Two Oral Steroids, Mepitiostane and Fluoxymesterone, on a Pregnancy-Dependent Mouse Mammary Tumor (TPDMT-4)," *Cancer Res.*, 37, No. 12 (December 1977):4408-15.

(365) Sokolowski, J.H., Geng, S., "Biological Evaluation of Mibolerone in the Female Beagle," *Am. J. Vet. Res.*, 38, No. 9 (September 1977):1371-76.

(366) Romero, C.H., Frank, F.R., "Immune Responses and Prevention of Lymphoid Leukosis Tumors in Chickens Fed an Androgen Analog.," *Adv. Exp. Med. Biol.*, 88, (1977):355-62.

(367) Pirke, K.M., "A Radioimmunoassay for the Measurement of 5-Androstene-3 Beta, 17 Beta-Diol in Plasma," *Steroids*, 30, No. 1 (July 1977):53-60.

(368) Young, M., Crookshank, H.R., Ponder, L., "Effects of an Anabolic Steroid on Selected Parameters in Male Albino Rats," *Res. Q. Am. Assoc. Health Phys. Educ.*, 48, 3 (October 1977):653-56.

(369) Henningsen, B., "Clinical Experiences with Tamoxifen for Estrogen Receptor Blocking Therapy in Metastatic Breast Cancer," *Prog. Clin. Biol. Res.*, 12 (1977):479-82.

(370) Nesterin, M.F., "Dependence of Hormonal Effects from Nutrients Supply," *Nutr. Metab. 21 Suppl.*, 1 (1977):249-53.

(371) Ward, R.J., Lawson, A.M., Shackleton, C.H., "Metabolism of Anabolic Steroid Drugs in Man and the Marmoset Monkey (Dallithrix Jacchus)—I. Nilevar and Orabolin," *J. Steroid Biochem.*, 8, No. 10 (October 1977):1057-63.

(372) Takatani, O., Kumaoka, S., "Inhibitory Effect of Mepitiostane on the Growth of Mammary Tumor of a Rat," *Gan.* 68, No. 3 (June 1977):337-41.

(373) Maynard, P.V., Pike, A.W., Weston, A., Griffiths, K., "Analysis of Dehydroepiandrosterone and Androstenediol in Human Breast Tissue using High Resolution Gas Chromatography—Mass Spectrometry," *Eur. J. Cancer*, 13, No. 9 (September 1977):971-75.

(374) Bandhauer, K., Meili, H.U., "Combined Mesterolon-Clomiphene Citrate Therapy for Treatment of Oligospermia," *Eur. Urol.*, 3, No.5 (1977):292-94.

(375) De Kretser, D.M., "The Management of the Infertile Male," *Clin. Obstet. Gynaecol.*, 1, No. 2 (August 1974):409-27.

(376) Templeton, J.F., Kim, R.S., "Metabolism of 17 Beta-Hydroxy-2 Alpha-Methyl-5 Alpha-Androstan-3-One in the Rabbit," *Steroids*, 29, No. 3 (March 1977):371-81.

(377) Rep Cekov, A.D., Mijulaj, L., "Plasma Testosterone Response to HCG in Normal Men without and after Administration of Anabolic Drug," *Endokrinologie*, 69, No. 1 (February 1977): 115-18.

(378) Jarrett, P.E., Morland, M., Browse, N.L., "Idiopathic Recurrent Superficial Thrombophlebitis: Treatment with Fibrinolytic Enhancement," *Br. Med. J.*, 1, No. 6066 (9 April 1977):933-34.

(379) Picton, W., Clark, C., "The Effect of Various Treatments on the Size of Sebaceous Glands of Hairless Mice and Hairless Hamsters," *Br. J. Dermatol.*, 96, No. 3 (March 1977):277-82.

(380) Clark, M.A., Picton, W., "The Effect of Intracutaneous Injections of Micronized Crystalline Suspensions of Nandrolone Phenyl-Propionate in the Skin of Female Hairless Hamsters," *Br. J. Dermatol.*, 96, No. 3 (March 1977):271-76.

(381) Shapiro, P., Ikeda, R.M., Ruebner, B.H., Connors, M.H., Halsted, C.C., Abildgaard, C.F., "Multiple Hepatic Tumors and Peliosis Hepatis in Fanconi's Anemia Treated with Androgens," *Am. J. Dis. Child.*, 131, No. 10 (October 1977):1104-6.

(382) Persson, L., "Evidence of Decarboxylation of Lysine by Mammalian Ornithine Decarboxylase," *Acta Physiol. Scand.*, 100, No. 4 (August 1977):424-29.

(383) Pirke, K.M., Doerr, P., Sintermann, R., Vogt, H.J., "Age

Dependence of Testosterone Precursors in Plasma of Normal Adult Males," *Acta Endocrinol.* (Copenhagen), 86, No. 2 (October 1977):415-29.

(384) Choudhury, S., Kundu, S., Ghosh, S., Hazra, S., "Anabolic Steroid as an Adjuvant in the Treatment of Chronic Lepra Reaction and Enl under Corticosteroid Therapy," *Lepr. Rev.* 48, No. 3 (September 1977):181-84.

(385) Check, J.H., Rakoff, A.E., "Androgen Therapy of a Varicocele," *J. Urol.*, 118, No. 3 (September 1977):494.

(386) Rosenfield, R.L., Lucky, A.W., "Oxandrolone Therapy for Children with Turner Syndrome Letter," *J. Pediatr.*, 91, No. 5 (November 1977):854-56.

(387) Sengupta, P., Sarkar, S.K., "Role of Anabolic Steroid on Hepatic Regeneration following Partial Hepatectomy," *J. Indian Med. Assoc.*, 68, No. 3 (1 February 1977):47-49.

(388) Labrie, F., Ferland, L., Lagace, L., Drouin, J., Asselin, J., Azadian-Boulanger, G., Raynaud, J.P., "High Inhibitory Activity of R 5020, A Pure Progestin, at the Hypothalamic-Adenohypophyseal Level on Gonadotropin Secretion," *Fertil. Steril.*, 28, No. 10 (October 1977):1104-12.

(389) Teller, M.N., Stock, C.C., Hellman, L., Mountain, I.M., Bowie, M., Rosenberg, B.J., Boyar, R.M., Budinger, J.M., "Comparative Effects of a Series of Prolactin Inhibitors, 17 Beta-Estradiol and 2 Alpha-Methyldihydrotestosterone Propionate, on Growth of 7, 12-Dimethylbenz (A) Anthracene-Induced Rat Mammary Carcinomas," *Cancer Res.*, 37, No. 11 (November 1977):3932-38.

(390) Broxmeyer, H.E., Ralph, P., "In Vitro Regulation of a Mouse Myelomonocytic Leukemia Line Adapted to Cluture," *Cancer Res.*, 37, No. 10 (October 1977):3578-84.

(391) Hernandez-Nieto, L., Bruguera, M., Bombi, J., Camacho, L., Rozman, C., "Benign Liver-Cell Adenoma Associated with Long-Term Administration of an Androgenic-Anabolic Steroid (Methandienone)," *Cancer,* 40, No. 4 (October 1977):1761-64.

(392) Scotti De Carolis, A., Longo, V.G., "Effect of Sexual Steroid Hormones and of Clomiphene on the Behavioral Response to L-Dopa in Mice," *Arch. Int. Pharmacodyn. Ther.*, 227, No. 1 (May 1977):93-97.

(393) Kozaryn, I., W. Ojciakowa, Z., Chodera, A. Szczawi Nska, K., Cenajek, D., "Pharmacodynamics and Pharmacokinetics of Psycholeptic Drugs in the Course of Radiation Disease," *Acta Physiol. Pol.*, 28, No. 3 (May-June 1977):263-70.

(394) Szczawi Nska, Cenajek, D., Chodera, A., W. Ojciakowa, Z. Okulicz-Kizaryn, I., "Pharmacodynamics and Pharmacokinetics of Psycholeptic Drugs in the Course of Radiation Disease: Effect of Premedication with Metanabol on Dynamics and Kinetics of

Nitrazepam," *Acta Physiol. Pol.*, 28, No. 3 (May-June 1977): 255-61.

(395) Krieg, M., Voigt, K.D., "Biochemical Substrate of Androgenic Actions at a Cellular Level in Prostate, Bulbocavernosus/Levator Ani and in Skeletal Muscle," *Acta Endocrinol. Suppl.* (Copenhagen), 85, No. 214 (1977):43-89.

(396) P. Erez, A.E., Beyer, C., Larsson, K., P. Erez-Palacios, G., "In Vitro Conversion of 5-Androstenediol to Testosterone by the Central Nervous System and Pituitary of the Male Rat," *Steroids*, 29, No. 5 (May 1977):627-33.

(397) Freedman, M.H., Saunders, E.F., "Factors Affecting Erythroid Colony Growth (CFU-E) from Human Marrow," *Exp. Hematol.*, 5, No. 4 (1977):250-53.

(398) Browse, N.L., Jarrett P.E., Morland, M., Burnand, K., "Treatment of Liposclerosis of the Leg by Fibrinolytic Enhancement: A Preliminary Report," *Br. Med. J.*, 2, No. 6084 (13 August 1977):434-35.

(399) Skovby, F., Mckusick, V.A., "Estrogen Treatment of Tall Stature in Girls with the Marfan Syndrome," *Birth Defects*, 13, No. 30 (1977):155-61.

(400) Francis, G.E., Berney, J.J., Bateman, S.M., Hoffbrand, A.V., "The Effect of Androstanes on Granulopoiesis in Vitro and in Vivo," *Br. J. Haematol.*, 36, No. 4 (August 1977):501-10.

(401) Kovary, P.M., Lenau, H., Niermann, H., Zierden, E., Wagner, H., "Testosterone Levels and Gonadotrophins in Klinefelter Patients Treated with Injections of Mesterolone Cipionate," *Arch. Dermatol. Res.*, 258, No. 3 (27 May 1977):289-94.

(402) Azen, E.A., Shahidi, N.T., "Androgen Dependency in Acquired Aplastic Anemia," *A.M. J. Med.*, 63, No. 2 (August 1977):320-24

(403) Monteleone, M., Albo, G., Papalta, M., Rispoli, R., Scafidi, G., Vernale C., "Effect of the Administration of an Anabolic Drug on the Evolution of the Bone Callus after Diaphyseal Osteotomy of Rabbit Femur," *Acta Orthop. Belg.* 43, No. 1 (January-February 1977):5-18.

(404) Jondorf, W.R., MacDougall, D.F., "Application of Radioimmunoassay Method for Detecting 19-Nortestosterone (Nandrolone) in Equine and Canine Plasma," *Vet. Rec.*, 100, No. 26 (25 June 1977):560-62.

(405) Milewich, L., Winters, A.J., Stephens, P., MacDonald, P.C., "Metabolism of Dehydroisoandrosterone and Androstenedione by the Human Lung in Vitro," *J. Steroid Biochem.*, 8, No. 4 (April 1977):277-84.

(406) Loriaux, D.L., Vigersky, R.A., Marynick, S.P., Janick, J.J., Sherins R.J., "Androgen and Estrogen Effects in the Regulation

of LH in Man," in Troen, P., Nankin, H.R., ed., *The Testis in Normal and Infertile Men.* New York: Raven Press, 1977.

(407) Alippi, R., Giglio, J., Bozzoni, C.E., "Erythrocyte Volume and Body Composition in Oxymetholone treated Hypophysectomized Rats," *Horm. Metab. Res.*, 9, No. 3 (May 1977):246-47.

(408) Bicikov, A.M., Hampl, R., Starka, L., "Binding of Synthetic Anabolic Steroids to Testosterone-Estradiol Binding Globulin and to Rat Prostate Cytosol," *Endocrinol Exp.* (Bratislava), 11, No. 2 (1977):85-90.

(409) Behrendt, H., Boffin, H., "Myocardial Cell Lesions Caused by an Anabolic Hormone," *Cell Tissue Res.*, 181, No. 3 (15 July 1977):423-26.

(410) Jondorf, W.R., Moss, M.S., "On the Detectability of Anabolic Steroids in Horse Urine Proceedings," *Br. J. Pharmacol.*, 60, No. 2 (June 1977):297P-98P.

(411) Liao, S., Hung, S.C., Tymoczko, J.L., Liang, T., "Active Forms and Biodynamics of the Androgen-Receptor in Various Target Tissues," *Curr. Top Mol. Endocrinol.*, 4, (1976):139-51.

(412) Garrett, M.J., Das, S., Smith, J.D., Freedman, L.S., "Long Term Experience with Combination Chemotherapy in Advanced Hodgkin's Disease," *Clin. Oncol.*, 3, No. 2 (June 1977):145-54.

(413) Jackaman, F.R., Ansell, I.D., Ghanadian, R., McLoughlin, P.V., Lewis, J.G., Chisholm, G.D., "The Hormone Response to a Synthetic Androgen (Mesterolone) in Oligospermia," *Clin. Endorcrinol (Oxf)*, 6, No. 5 (May 1977):339-45.

(414) Behrendt, H., "Effect of Anabolic Steroids on Rat Heart Muscle Cells. I. Intermediate Filaments," *Cell Tissue Res.*, 180, No. 3 (31 May 1977):303-15.

(415) Howard, C.W., Hanson, S.G., Wahed, M.A., "Anabolic Steroids and Anticoagulants Letter," *Br. Med. J.*, 1, No. 6077 (25 June 1977):1659-60.

(416) Kakuk, T.J., Frank, F.R., Weddon, T.E., "Avian Lymphoid Leukosis Prophylaxis with Mibolerone," *Avian Dis.*, 21, No. 2 (April-June 1977):280-89.

(417) Romero, C.H., Purchase, H.G., Frank, F., Burmester, B.R., Kakuk, T.J., Chang, T.S., "Immune Responses of Chickens Fed the Androgen Analog Mibolerone," *Avian Dis.*, 21, No. 2 (April-June 1977):264-79.

(418) Young, G.P., Bhathal, P.S., Sullivan, J.R., Wall, A.J., Fone, D.J., Hurley, T.H., "Fatal Hepatic Coma Complicating Oxymetholone Therapy in Multiple Myeloma," *Aust. NZ J. Med.*, 7, No. 1 (February 1977):47-51.

(419) Lev-Ran, A., "Androgens, Estrogens, and the Ultimate Height in XO Gonadal Dysgenesis," *Am. J. Dis. Child*, 131, No. 6 (June 1977):648-49.

(420) Heitzman, R.J., "The Response of Sheep with Pregnancy Toxaemia to Trenbolone Acetate," *Vet. Rec.*, 100, No. 15 (9 April 1977):317-18.

(421) Mayer, M., Shafrir, E., "Skeletal Muscle Protease and Glucocorticoid Hormone Receptors in Muscle Wasting Conditions and Muscular Dytrophy," *Isr. J. Med. Sci.*, 13, No. 2 (February 1977):139-46.

(422) "Iarc Monographs on the Evaluation of the Carcinogenic Risk of Chemicals to Man: Some Miscellaneous Pharmaceutical Substances," *Iarc Monogr. Eval. Carcinog. Risk Chem. Man.*, 13, No. 1 (1977):1-255.

(423) Eneroth, P., Gustafsson, J.A., Skett, P., Stenberg, A., "The Effects on Hepatic Steroid Metabolism of an Ectopic Pituitary Graft: A Time Study," *Mol. Cell. Endocrinol*, 7, No. 2 (April 1977):167-75.

(424) Gelli, D., Vignati, E., "Metabolic Studies with Formebolone (2-Formyl-17 (Alpha) Methyl-Androsta-1, 4-Diene-11 (Alpha), 17 (Beta) Diol-3-One) in Humans," *J. Int. Med. Res.*, 4, No. 2 (1976):96-105.

(425) Kawashima,K., Nakaura, S., Nagao, S., Tanaka, S., Kuwamura, T., "Virilizing Activities of Various Steroids in Female Rate Fetuses," *Endocrinol JPN*, 24, No. 1 (February 1977):77-81.

(426) Pertzelan, A., Blum, I., Grunebaum, M., Laron, Z., "The Combined Effect of Growth Hormone and Methandrostenolone on the Linear Growth of Patients with multiple Pituitary Hormone Deficiences," *Clin. Endocrinol.* (Oxf) 6, No. 4 (April 1977):271-76.

(427) Steele, R.E., Didato, F., Steinetz, B.G., "Relative Importance of 5 Alpha Reduction for the Androgenic and LH-Inhibiting Activities of Delta-4-3-Ketosteroids," *Steroids*, 29, No. 3 (March 1977):331-46.

(428) Buchwald, D., Argyres, S., Easterling, R.E., Oelshlegel, F.J. J.R., Brewer, G.J., Schoomaker, E.B., Abbrecht, P.H., Williams, G.W., Weller, J.M., "Effect of Nandrolone Decandate on the Anemia of Chronic Hemodialysis Patients," *Nephron*, 18, No. 4 (1977):232-38.

(429) Mokrohisky, S.T., Ambroso, D.R., Hathaway, W.E., "Fulminant Hepatic Neoplasia after Androgen Therapy Letter," *N. Engl. J. Med.*, 296, No. 24 (16 June 1977):1411-12.

(430) Krieg, M., Voigt, K.D., "In Vitro Binding and Metabolism of Androgens in Various Organs: A Comparative Study," *J. Steroid Biochem.*, 7, Nos. 11-12 (November-December 1976):1005-12.

(431) Vermorken, A.J., Van de Ven, W.J., Gielen, W.H., Bloemendal, H., Ketelaars, H.C., "Metabolism of Dehydroepiandrosterone in the Eye Lens Epithelium," *Exp. Eye Res.*, 24, No. 3 (March 1977):263-70.

(432) Trams, G., "Effect of Drostanolone Propionate on the Binding of Oestradiol and Dihydrotestosterone by Normal and Malignant Target Tissues," *Eur. J. Cancer,* 13, No. 2 (February 1977):149-53.

(433) Edelstyn, G.A., Macrae, K.D., "Concommittant Androgen Therapy in the Management of Advanced Breast Cancer by Cyclical Combined Chemotherapy Letter," *Clin. Oncol.,* 2, No. 4 (December 1976):403-5.

(434) Antunes, C.M., Stolley, P.D., "Cancer Induction by Exogenous Hormones: Possible Androgen-Induced Cancer," *Cancer,* 39, No. 4 Suppl. (April 1977):1896-98.

(435) Burke, T.J., Reynolds, H.A., Sokolowski, J.H., "A 280-Days Tolerance-Efficacy Study Mibolerone for Suppression of Estrus in the Cat," *Am. J. Vet. Res.,* 38, No. 4 (April 1977):469-77.

(436) Hopwood, N.J., Kelch, R.P., "Hormonal Therapy in Delayed Adolescence," in Hafez, E.S., Peluso, J.J., ed., *Sexual Maturity.* Ann Arbor: Ann Arbor Science, 1976.

(437) Pruszewicz, A., Obrebozski, A., Gr. Adzki, J., "Postmedicamentous Voice Virilisation. X-Ray Examination of the Larynx," in Loebell, E., ed., *XVI International Congress of Logopedics and Phoniatrics.* Basel: Karger, 1976.

(438) Lunenfeld, B., Epstein, Y., Kraiem, Z., "Regulation of Hypothalamic-Pituitary Axis by Testicular Secretion," in Hubinont, P.O., et al., ed., *Sperm Action.* Basel: Karger, 1976.

(439) Eliasson, R., "Pharmacological Actions on the Production and Physiology of Mammalian Spermatozoa," in Hubinont, P.O., et al., ed., *Sperm Action.* Basel: Karger, 1976.

(440) Itil, T.M., "Neurophysiological Effects of Hormones in Humans: Computer EEG Profiles of Sex and Hypothalamic Hormones," in Sachar, E.J., ed., *Hormones, Behavior, and Psychopathology.* New York: Raven Press, 1976.

(441) Nissen-Meyer, R., "Ovarian Suppression and its Supplement by Additive Hormonal Treatment," in Namer, M., Lalanne, C.M., ed., *Hormones and Breast Cancer.* Paris: Inserm, 1976.

(442) Hunt, T.K., "Control of Wound Healing with Cortisone and Vitamin A," in Longacre, J.J., ed., *The Ultrastructure of Collagen.* Springfield, Ill.: Thomas, 1976.

(443) Buselmeier, T.J., "The Aggressive Approach to Patients with Acute Renal Failure in the Postoperative Critical Care Period," in Shoemaker, W.C., Tavares, B.M., ed., *Current Topics in Critical Care Medicine.* Basel: Karger, 1976.

(444) Glendinning, E.S., "Anabolic Steroids and Drug Clearance in the Racehorse Letter," *Vet. Rec.,* 100, No. 8 (February 1977):164.

(445) Lye, M.D., Ritch, A.E., "A Double-Blind Trial of an Anabolic Steroid (Stanozolol) in the Disabled Elderly," *Rheumatol Rehabil.,* 16, No. 1 (February 1977):62-69.

(446) Bartsch, G., Frick, J., Rohr, H.P., "Stereology: A New Morphological Method of Study Prostatic Function and Disease," *Prog. Clin. Biol. Res.*, 6 (1976):123-41.

(447) Foreman, M.I., Kelly, I., Lukowiecki, G.A., "A Method for the Measurement of Diffusion Constants Suitable for Studies of Non-Occluded Skin," *J. Pharm. Pharmacol*, 29, No. 2 (February 1977):108-9.

(448) Chayvialle, J.A., Courpron, P., Mikaelian, S., Lambert, R., "Serum Alpha-Fetroprotein Concentration in Adult Patients under Corticoid, Estroprogestative or Androgen Therapy," *Digestion*, 15, No. 3 (1977):223-26.

(449) Tormey, D.C., Simon, R.M., Lippman, M.E., Bull, J.M., Myers, C.E., "Evaluation of Tamoxifen Dose in Advanced Breast Cancer: A Progress Report," *Cancer Treat Rep.*, 60, No. 10 (October 1976):1451-59.

(450) Rosse, W.F., Logues, G.L., Silberman, H.R., Frank, M.M., "The Effect of Synthetic Androgens in Hereditary Angioneurotic Edema: Alteration of CI Inhibitor and C4 Levels," *Trans. Assoc. Am. Physicians*, 89 (1976):122-32.

(451) Moore, D.C., Tattoni, D.S., Ruvalcaba, R.H., Limbeck, G.A., Kelley, V.C., "Studies of Anabolic Steroids. VI. Effect of Prolonged Administration of Oxandrolone on Growth in Children and Adolescents with Gonadal Dysgenesis," *J. Pediatr.*, 90, No. 3 (March 1977):462-66.

(452) Holma, P.K., "Effects of an Anabolic Steroid (Metandienone) on Spermatogenesis," *Contraception*, 15, No. 2 (February 1977):151-62.

(453) Heitzman, R.J., Chan, K.H., Hart, I.C., "Liveweight Gains, Blood Levels of Metabolites, Proteins and Hormones following Implantation of Anabolic Agents in Steers," *Br. Vet. J.*, 133, No. 1 (January-February 1977):62-70.

(454) Chesnut, C.H. 3d, Nelp, W.B., Baylink, D.J., Denney, J.D., "Effect of Methandrostenolone on Postmenopausal Bone Wasting as Assessed by Changes in Total Bone Mineral Mass," *Metabolism*, 26, No. 3 (March 1977):267-77.

(455) Jones, T.M., Fang, V.S., Landau, R.L., Rosenfield, R.L., "The Effects of Fluoxymesterone Administration on Testicular Function," *J. Clin. Endocrinol Metab.*, 44, No. 1 (January 1977):121-29.

(456) Glick, B., Rao, D.S., McDuffie, F.C., "Identifying Lympholytic and Androgenic Effects of Androgenic Steroids," *Gen. Comp. Endocrinol*, 31, No. 1 (January 1977):133-37.

(457) Huys, J., Van Vaerenbergh, P.M., "The Effect of Nandrolone Decanoate on Bone Marrow Suppression Induced by Cytostatic Agents," *Clin. Oncol.*, 2, No. 3 (September 1976):207-14.

(458) Chowdhury, M.S., Banks, A.J., Bond, W.H., Ward, H.W., "A Comparison of Drostanolone Propionate (Masteril) and Nandrolone Decanoate (Deca-Durabolin) in the Treatment of Breast Carcinoma," *Clin. Oncol.*, 2, No. 3 (September 1976):203-6.

(459) Napier, J.A., Cavill, I., Dunn, C.D., May, A., Ricketts, C., "Oxymetholone Treatment in Aplastic Anaemia: Changes in and Serum Erythropoietin," *Br. Med. J.*, 2, No. 6049 (11 December 1976):1426.

(460) Usherwood, M.M., Halim, A., Evans, P.R., "Artificial Insemination (A.I.H.) for Sperm Antibodies and Oligozoospermia," *Br. J. Urol*, 48, No. 6 (December 1976):499-503.

(461) Vernon, B.G., Buttery, P.J., "Protein Turnover in Rats Treated with Trienbolone Acetate," *Br. J. Nutr.*, 36, No. 3 (November 1976):575-79.

(462) Wexler, B.C., "Comparative Effects of Cortisone, Dianabol and Enovid on Isoprenaline-Induced Myocardial Infaction in Arteriosclerotic VS Nonarteriosclerotic Rats," *Br. J. Exp. Pathol.*, 57, No. 6 (December 1976):663-85.

(463) Aertgeerts, J., Aussems, J., Put, H., "Double-Blind Investigation of Two Corticoid Preparations for the Treatment of Eczematous Skin Disorders," Short Communication, *Arzneim Forsch*, 26, No. 8 (1976):1617-18.

(464) Branda, R.F., Amsden, T.W., Jacob, H.S., "Randomized Study of Nandrolone Therapy for Anemias Due to Bone Marrow Failure," *Arch. Intern Med.*, 137, No. 1 (January 1977):65-69.

(465) Nilsson, A., Broom, E., Karlsson, A., "Influence of Steroid Hormones on the Carcinogenicity of 90SR," *Acta Rariol. Ther.* (Stockholm), 15, No. 5 (October 1976):417-26.

(466) Kumada, T., Abiko, Y., "Enhancement of Fibrinolytic and Thrombolytic Potential in the Rat by Treatment with an Anabolic Steroid, Furazabol," *Thromb. Haemostas.*, 36, No. 2 (30 November 1976):451-64.

(467) James, K.C., "Free Energies of Solution in Water, of some Androstanolone, Nandrolone and Testosterone Esters," *J. Pharm. Pharmacol*, 28, No. 12 (December 1976):929-31.

(468) Chaudry, M.A., James, K.C., Nicholls, P.J., "Anabolic and Androgenic Activities, in Rat, of some Nandrolone and Androstanolone Esters," *J. Pharm. Pharmacol.*, 28, No. 12 (December 1976):882-85.

(469) Perzanowski, A., Bielawiec, M., Mysliwiec, M., "The Influence of Long-Term Therapy with Phenformin plus Metanabol on Blood Fibrinolytic Acticity, Platelet Adhesiveness and Lipid Metabolism in Patients with Arteriosclerosis," *Folia Haematol.*,

(Leipzig), 103, No. 3 (1976):381-88.

(470) Hedner, U., Nilsson, I.M., Isacson, S., "Phenformin and Ethyloestrenol in Recurrent Deep Venous Thrombosis (DVT)" *Folia Haematol.*, (Leipz), 103, No. 3 (1976):372-80.

(471) Singer, J.W., Adamson, J.W., "Steroids and Hematopoiesis. III. The Response of Granulocytic and Erythroid Colony-Forming Cells to Steroids of Different Classes," *Blood*, 48, No. 6 (December 1976):855-64.

(472) Cerutt, S., Forlani, A., Galimberti, E., "Anticatabolic Action of Formebolone in the Castrated Rat Treated with Dexamethasone," *Arzneim Forsch*, 26, No. 9 (1976):1673-77.

(473) Henningsson, S., Persson, L., Rosengren, E., "Biosynthesis of Cadaverine in Mice under the Influence of an Anabolic Steroid," *Acta Physiol. Scand.*, 98, No. 4 (December 1976):445-49.

(474) Holma, P., Adlercreutz, H., "Effect of an Anabolic Steroid (Metandienon) on Plasma LH-FSH, and Testosterone and on the Response to Intravenous Administration of LRH," *Acta Endocrinol.*, (Copenhagen), 83, No. 4 (December 1976):856-64.

(475) Herrmann, W.M., Beach, R.C., "Psychotropic Effects of Androgens: A Review of Clinical Observations and New Human Experimental Findings," *Pharmakopsychiatr. Neuropsychopharmakol*, 9, No. 5 (September 1976):205-19.

(476) De Peretti, E., Forest, M.G., "Unconjugated Dehydroepiandrosterone Plasma Levels in Normal Subjects from Birth to Adolescence in Human: The Use of a Sensitive Radioimmunoassay," *J. Clin. Endocrinol Metab.*, 43, No. 5 (November 1976):982-91.

(477) Geller, J., Albert, J., Geller, S., Lopez, D., Cantor, T., Yen, S., "Effect of Megestrol Acetate (Megace) on Steroid Metabolism and Steroid-Protein Binding in the Human Prostate," *J. Clin. Endocrinol Metab.*, 43, No. 5 (November 1976):1000-1008.

(478) Alpert, L.I., "Veno-Occlusive Disease of the Liver Associated with Oral Contraceptives: Case Report and Review of Literature," *Hum. Pathol.*, 7, No. 6 (November 1976):709-18.

(479) Henningsson, S., Rosengren, E., "The Effect of Nandrolone, an Anabolic Steroid on Putrescine Metabolism in the Mouse," *Br. J. Pharmacol.*, 58, No. 3 (November 1976):401-6.

(480) Howsden, S.M., Hodge, S.J., Herndon, J.H., Freeman, R.G., "Malignant Atrophic Papulosis of Degos. Report of a Patient who Failed to Respond to Fibrinolytic Therapy," *Arch. Dermatol.*, 112, No. 1 (November 1976):1582-88.

(481) Stepan, J., "The Study of Calcium, Phosphorus, Hydroxyproline, and Nitrogen in Decompensated Coxarthroses and Gonarthroses," *Zrheumatol*, 35, Nos. 9-10, (September-October 1976):363-76.

(482) Fether, T., Sarfy, E.H., "A Simple Gas Chromatographic Method for the Determination of Methandienone in Human Urine," *J. Sports Med. Phys. Fitness*, 16, No. 3 (September 1976):165-70.

(483) Sharp, F., Hay, J.B., Hodgins, M.B., "Metabolism of Androgens in Vitro by Human Foetal Skin," *J. Endocrinol*, 70, No. 3 (September 1976):491-99.

(484) Eckstein, B., Lerner, N., Yehud, S., "Pre-Ovulatory Changes in Steroidogenesis in Ovaries from Immature Rats Treated with Pregnant Mare Serum Gonadotrophin," *J. Endocrinol*, 70, No. 3 (September 1976):485-90.

(485) Krieg, M., Dennis, M., Voigt, K.D., "Comparison between the Binding of 19-Nortestosterone, 5 Alpha-Dihydrotestosterone and Testosterone in Rat Prostate and Bulbocavernosus/Levator Ani Muscle," *J. Endocrinol*, 70, No. 3 (September 1976):379-87.

(486) Sharma, K.K., Chowdhury, N.K., Sharma, A.L., "Effect of Phenformin and Ethyloestrenol on Blood Fibrinolytic Activity on Rabbits Maintained on High Cholesterol Diet," *Indian J. Med. Res.*, 64,. No. 6 (June 1976):915-22.

(487) Dunn, C.D., Napier, J.A., "The Influence of Steroids on Erythropoiesis in Mouse Fetal Liver Cell Cultures: Relevance of Cell Cycle State," *Exp. Hematol.*, 4, No. 5 (September 1976):289-300.

(488) Popovic, V., Schaffer, R., Popovic, P., "Techniques for Induction of Neutropenia and Granulocytosis in Rats," *Exp. Hematol.*, 4, No. 5 (September 1976):285-88.

(489) Hickson, R.C., Heusner, W.W., Van Huss, W.D., Taylor, J.F., Carrow, R.E., "Effects of an Anabolic Steroid and Sprint Training on Selected Histochemical and Morphological Observations in Rat Skeletal Muscle Types," *Eur. J. Appl. Physiol.*, 35, No. 4 (23 September 1976):251-59.

(490) Ebbesen, F., Holck, F., Mygind, K.I., "Treatment of Cystinosis by a Cystine — and Methionine — Poor Diet plus Anabolic Steroid: Treatment of Two Children and Survey of Previous Treatment Results," *Dan. Med. Bull.*, 23, No. 5 (October 1976):210-16.

(491) Dericks-Tan, J.S., Taubert, H.D., "Elevation of Serum Prolactin during Application of Oral Contraceptives," *Contraception*, 14, No. 1 (July 1976):1-8.

(492) Hedner, U., Nilsson, I.M., Isacson, S., "Effect of Ethyloestrenol on Fibrinolysis in the Vessel Wall," *Br. Med. J.*, 2, No. 6038 (25 September 1976):729-31.

(493) Davis, P.J., Davis, F.B., Charache, P., "Hereditary Angioedema: Modification of Clinical Manifestations with Androgens," *Birth Defects*, 12, No. 6 (1976):283-87.

(494) Foreman, M.I., Kelly, I., "The Diffusion of Nandrolone through

Hydrated Human Cadaver Skin," *Br. J. Dermatol*, 95, No. 3 (September 1976):265-70.

(495) Batzold, F.H., Benson, A.M., Covey, D.F., Robinson, C.H., Talalay, P., "The Delta 5-3-Ketosteroid Isomerase Reaction: Catalytic Mechanism, Specificity and Inhibition," *Adv. Enzyme Regul.*, 14, (1976):243-67.

(496) Kew, M.C., Van Coller, B., Prowse, C.M., Skikne, B., Wolfsdorf, J.I., Isdale, J., Krawitz, S., Altman, H., Levin, S.E., Bothwell, T.H., "Occurrence of Primary Hepatocellur Cancer and Peliosis Hepatis after Treatment with Androgenic Steroids," *S. Afr. Med. J.*, 50, No. 32 (24 July 1976):1233-37.

(497) Sinha, A.K., "Anabolic Steroid (Methandienone) in Corneal Ulcers," *J. Indian Med. Assoc.*, 66, No. 9 (1 May 1976):202-3.

(498) Gallus, A.S., Hirsh, J., "Antithrombotic Drugs: Part II," *Drugs*, 12, No. 2, (1976):132-57.

(499) Kritchevsky, D., Tepper, S.A., Story, J.A., "Influence of Four Agents (Tibric Acid, DH 990, Oxandrolone and SCH 9122) on Aspects of Lipid Metabolism in Rats," *Arzneim Forsch*, 26, No. 5 (1976):862-64.

(500) Jyv Asjarvi, S., Hopsu-Havu, V.K., "A Model for Studies of Dermal Surface Epithelization: with Observations on the Effects of Dexamethasone and Nandrolone Decanoate," *Arzneim Forsch*, 26, No. 3 (1976):443-47.

(501) Oakley, J.R., Else, P., Asplin, P., Taitz, L.S., "Balanced Translocation, Impaired Sperm Mutility, and Offspring Anomaly," *Arch. Dis. Child*, 51, No. 8, (August 1976):638-40.

(502) Holzbach, R.T., "Jaundice in Pregnancy-1976," *Am. J. Med.*, 61, No. 3 (September 1976):367-76.

(503) Lees, R.S., Lees, A.M., "Therapy of the Hyperlipidemias," *Postgrad Med.*, 60, No. 3 (September 1976):99-107.

(504) Moore, D.C., Tattoni, D.S., Limbeck, G.A., Ruvelcaba, R.H., Lindner, D.S., Gareis, F.J., Al-Agba, S., Kelley, V.C., "Studies of Anabolic Steroids: V. Effect of Prolonged Oxandrolone Administration on Growth in Children and Adolescents with Uncomplicated Short Stature," *Pediatrics*, 58, No. 3 (September 1976):412-22.

(505) Pierson, R.E., Jensen, R., Braddy, P.M., Horton, D.P., Christie, R.M., "Bulling among Yearling Feedlot Steers," *J. Am. Vet. Med. Assoc.*, 169, No. 5 (1 September 1976):521-23.

(506) Abou Akkada, A.R., El-Shazly, K., "Application of Synthetic Estrogen in Sheep," *Environ. Qual. Saf. Suppl.*, 5 (1976):99-108.

(507) Heitzman, R.J., "The Effectiveness of Anabolic Agent in Increasing Rate of Growth in Farm Animals: Report on Experiments in Cattle," *Environ. Qual. Saf. Suppl.*, 5 (1976):89-98.

(508) Trenkle, A., "The Anabolic Effect of Estrogens on Nitrogen Metabolism of Growing and Finishing Cattle and Sheep," *Enviro. Qual. Saf. Suppl.*, 5 (1976):79-88.

(509) Vanderwal, P., "General Aspects of the Effectiveness of Anabolic Agents in Increasing Protein Production in Farm Animals, in Particular in Bull Calves," *Environ. Qual. Saf. Suppl.*, 5 (1976):60-78.

(510) Michel, G., Baulieu, E.E., "An Approach to the Anabolic of Androgens by an Experimental System," *Environ. Qual. Saf. Suppl.*, 5 (1976):54-59.

(511) Nesterin, M.F., "Experimental Observations on Evaluation of Products from Anabolic Agents-Stimulated Farm Animals," *Environ. Qual. Saf. Suppl.*, 5 (1976):265-73..

(512) Neumann, F., "Pharmacological and Endocrinological Studies on Anabolic Agents," *Environ. Qual. Saf. Suppl.*, 5 (1976):253-64.

(513) Coulston, F., Wills, J.H., "Epidemiological Studies Related to the Use of Hormonal Agents in Animal Production," *Environ. Qual. Saf. Suppl.*, 5 (1976):238-52.

(514) Rose, F.J., "Carcinogenicity Studies in Animals Relevant to the Use of Anabolic Agents in Animal Production," *Environ. Qual. Saf. Suppl.*, 5 (1976):227-37.

(515) Kolbye, A.C., Perez, M.K., "Human Safety Considerations from the Use of Anabolic Agents in Foodproducing Animals," *Environ. Qual. Saf. Suppl.*, 5 (1976):212-18.

(516) Calvert, C.C., Smith, L.W., "Recycling and Degradation of Anabolic Agents in Animal Excreta," *Environ. Qual. Saf. Suppl.*, 5 (1976):203-11.

(517) Kroes, R., Huis In't Veld, L.G., Schuller, P.L., Stephany, R.W., "Methods for Controlling the Application of Anabolics in Farm Animals," *Environ. Qual. Saf. Suppl.*, 5 (1976):192-202.

(518) Hoffman, B., Karg, H., "Metabolic Fate of Anabolic Agents in Treated Animals and Residue Levels in their Meat," *Environ. Qual. Saf. Suppl.*, 5 (1976):181-91.

(519) Shamberev, Y.N., "The Metabolic and Growth Effects of Anabolic Agents," *Environ. Qual. Saf. Suppl.*, 5 (1976):142.

(520) Gropp, J., Herlyn, D., Boehncke, E., Schulz, V., Sandersleben, J.V., Hanichen, T., Geisel, O., "Physiological Data Including Evaluation of Immuno-Response in Relation to Anabolic Effects on Veal Calves," *Environ. Qual. Saf. Suppl.*, 5 (1976):131-41.

(521) Verbeke, R., Debackere, M., Hicquet, R., Lauwers, H., Pottie, G., Stevens, J., Van Moer, D., Van Hoof, J., Vermeersch, G., "Quality of the Meat after the Application of Anabolic Agents in Young Calves," *Environ. Qual. Saf. Suppl.*, 5 (1976):123-30.

(522) Van Weerden, E.J., Grandadam, J.A., "The Effect of an Anabolic

Agent on N Deposition, Growth, and Slaughter Quality in Growing Castrated Male Pigs," *Environ. Qual. Saf. Suppl.*, 5 (1976):115-22.

(523) Nesheim, M.C., "Some Observations on the Effectiveness of Anabolic Agents in Increasing the Growth Rate of Poultry," *Environ. Qual. Saf. Suppl.*, 5 (1976):110-4.

(524) Fowler, V.R., "Some Aspects of the Use of Anabolic Steroids in Pigs," *Environ. Qual. Saf. Suppl.*, 5 (1976):109.

(525) Miller, W.R., Shivas, A.A., Forrest, A.P., "Steroid Interconversions by Metastatic Deposits of a Human Bronchogenic Carcinoma," *Clin. Oncol.*, 2, No. 2 (June 1976):127-30.

(526) Heitzman, R.J., Oettel, G., Hoffmann, B., "Proceedings: The Determination by Radioimmunoassay of Residues of an Anabolic Steroid in Tissues of Calves Treated with a Combined Preparation of Trenbolone Acetate and Oestradiol-17 Beta," *J. Endocrinol*, 69, No. 3 (June 1976):10P-11P.

(527) Anthony, L.E., Jones, A.L., "Lack of Enhanced Microsomal Enzyme Activity by Oxandrolone, an Inducer of Hepatic Smooth Endoplasmic Retuculum," *Biochem. Pharmacol.*, 25, No. 13 (1 July 1976):1549-51.

(528) Wynne, K.N., Renwick, A.G.C., "16 Beta-Hydroxylation of Dehydroepiandrosterone Sulphate by Homogenates of Human Foetal Liver," *Biochem. J.*, 156, No. 2 (15 May 1976):419-25.

(529) Gorshein, D., Gardner, F.H., Tyree, W., Oski, F., Delivoria-Papadopoulos, M., "Effect of Hyperoxia and Androgen on Red Cell 2, 3-Diphosphoglycerate and Oxygen Affinity," *Acta Haemator* (Basel), 55, No. 5-2 (1976):306-12.

(530) Ribas-Mundo, M., San Miguel, J.G., Rozman, C., "Oxymetholone Effect of Acute Myeloblastic Leukemia Cells in Vitro," *Acta Haematol* (Basel), 55, No. 5-2 (1976):277-81.

(531) Delespess, G., Vassart, G., Sternon, J., "Hereditary Angioneurotic Oedema Successful Treatment of One Case with Metandienone," *Acta Clin. Belg.*, 31, No. 3 (1976):158-61.

(532) Victor, A., Weiner, E., Johansson, E.D., "Sex Hormone Binding Globulin: The Carrier Protein for D-Norgestrel," *J. Clin. Endocrinol. Metab.*, 43, No. 1 (July 1976):244-47.

(533) Vigersky, R.A., Easley, R.B., Loriaux, D.L., "Effect of Flooxymesterone on the Pituitary-Gonadal Axis: the Role of Testosterone-Estradiol-Binding Globulin," *J. Clin. Endocrinol. Metabl.*, 43, No. 1 (July 1976):1-9.

(534) Ganguly, M., Cheo, K.L., Brodie, H.J., "Estrogen Biosynthesis and 1 Beta-Hydroxylation Using C19 and 19-NOR Steroid Precursors," *Biochem. Biophys. Acta.*, 431, No. 2 (27 May 1976):326-34.

(535) Shreiner, D.P., "Spontaneous Hematologic Remission in Agnogenic Myeloid Metaplasia," *Am. J. Med.*, 60, No. 7 (June 1976):1014-18.

(536) Abiko, Y., Kumada, T., "Enhancement of Fibrinolytic and Thrombolytic Potential in the Rat by an Anabolic Steroid, Furazabol," *Thromb. Res.*, 8 (2 Suppl.) (May 1976):107-14.

(537) Reeves, R.D., Morris, M.D., Barbour, G.L., "Hyperlipidemia due to Oxymetholone Therapy. Occurrence in a Long-Term Hemodialysis Patient," *Jama*, 236, No. 5 (2 August 1976):469-72.

(538) Urry, R.L., Cockett, A.T., "Treating the Subfertile Male Patient: Improvement Semen Characteristics after Low Dose Androgen Therapy," *J. Urol.*, 116, No. 1 (July 1976):54-55.

(539) Ambrus, J.L., Ambrus, C.M., Mirand, E.A., "Erythroid and Myeloid Regeneration after Nitrogen Mustard Therapy, Autologous Bone Marrow Transplantation, and Treatment with an Anabolic Steroid," *J. Med.*, 7, No. 1 (1976):47-62.

(540) Seneca, H., Grant, J.P., "Urologic Sepsis/Shock," *J. Am. Geriatr. Soc.*, 24, No. 7 (July 1976):292-300.

(541) Knock, F.E., Galt, R.M., Oester, Y.T., Sylvester, R., Haefliger, R., "Coordinated Surgical and Drug Treatment of Cancer," *Int. Surg.*, 61, No. 5 (May 1976):287-92.

(542) Black, M.M., "Malignant Atrophic Papulosis (Degos' Disease)," *Int. J. Dermatol.*, 15, No. 6 (July-August 1976):405-11.

(543) Spona, J., "Action of Steroids on LH-RH Provoked Gonadotropin Release," *Endocrinol. Exp.* (Bratislava), 10, No. 2 (June 1976):91-100.

(544) Rendina, G.M., Patrono, D., "The Use of a Biological Preparation in the Treatment of Some Gynaecological Disease," *Curr. Med. Res. Opin.*, 4, No. 2 (1976):151-57.

(545) Goldfarb, S., "Sex Hormones and Hepatic Neoplasia," *Cancer Res.*, 36, No. 7, Pt. 2, (July 1976):2584-88.

(546) Guinan, P.D., Sadoughi, W., Alsheik, H., Ablin, R.J., Alrenga, D., Bush, I.M., "Impotence Therapy and Cancer of the Prostate," *Am. J. Surg.*, 131, No. 5 (May 1976):599-600.

(547) Hoffman, B., Oettel, G., "Radioimmunoassays for Free and Conjugated Trienbolone and for Trienbolone Acetate in Bovine Tissue and Plasma Samples," *Steroids*, 27, No. 4 (April 1976):509-23.

(548) Slater, S.D., Davidson, J.F., Patrick, R.S., "Jaundice Induced by Stanozolol Hypersensitivity," *Postgrad Med. J.*, 52, No. 606 (April 1976):229-32.

(549) Armitage, J.O., Leighton, M., Ware, F., "The Effective Use of Nandrolone Decanoate in the Management of the Anemia of Uremia: a Prospective Study," *Nebr. Med. J.*, 61, No. 6 (June 1976):202-6.

(550) Glueck, C.J., Gartside, P., Fallat, R.W., Mendoza, S., "Effect of Sex Hormones on Protamine Inactivated and Resistant Postheparin Plasma Lipases," *Metabolism*, 25, No.6 (June 1976):625-32.

(551) Robinson, C.P., Smith, P.W., McConnell, J.K., Endecott, B.R., "Comparison of Protective Effects of Ethylestrenol, Norbolethone, and Spironolactone against Lethality from Acute Doses of Parathion and Paraoxon in Female Rats," *J. Pharm. Sci.*, 65, No. 4 (April 1976):595-96.

(552) Singer, J.W., Adamson, J.W., "Steroids and Hematopoiesis. II. The Effect of Steroids on In Vitro Erythroid Colony Growth: Evidence for Different Target Cells for Different Classes of Steroids," *J. Cell. Physiol.*, 88, No. 2 (June 1976):135-43.

(553) Cunliffe, W.J., "Dowling Operation, 1975. Fibrinolysis and Vasculitis," *Clin. Exp. Dermatol*, 1, No. 1 (March 1976):1-16.

(554) Wilson, C.M., Ward, P.E., Erdos, E.G., Gecse, A., "Studies on Membrane-Bound Renin in the Mouse and Rat," *Circ. Res.*, 38, No. 6, Suppl. 2, pp. 95-98.

(555) Riis, P.M., Suresh, T.P., "The Effect of a Synthetic Steroid (Trienbolone) on the Rate of Release and Excretion of Subcutaneously Administered Estradiol in Calves," *Steroids*, 27, No. 1 (January 1976):5-15.

(556) Farrell, G.C., "Fanconi's Familial Hypoplastic Anaemia with Some Unusual Features," *Med. J. Aust.*, 1, No. 5 (31 January 1976):16-18.

(557) Lesna, M., Spencer, I., Walker, W., "Letter: Liver Nodules and Androgens," *Lancet*, 1, No. 7969 (22 May 1976):1124.

(558) Conner, E.A., Blake, D.A., Parmley, T.H., Burnett, L.S., King, T.M., "Efficacy of Various Locally Applied Chemicals as Contragestational Agents in Rats," *Contraception*, 13, No. 5 (May 1976):571-82.

(559) Falkson, G., Falkson, H.C., "Letter: Calusterone in Advanced Breast Cancer," *Cancer Treat. Rep.*, 60, No. 3 (March 1976):220-21.

(560) Ohgo, S., Kato, Y., Chihara, K., Imura, H., "Plasma Prolactin Responses to Thyrotropin-Releasing Hormone in Patients with Breast Cancer," *Cancer*, 37, No. 3 (March 1976):1412-16.

(561) Fitzgerald, T.J., Morse, S.A., "Alteration of Growth, Infectivity, and Viability of Neisseria Gonorrhoeae by Gonadal Steroids," *Can. J. Microbiol.*, 22, No. 2 (February 1976):286-94.

(562) Morley, A., Remes, J., Trainor, K., "A Controlled Trial of Androgen Therapy in Experimental Chronic Hypoplastic Marrow Failure," *Br. J. Haematol*, 32, No. 4 (April 1976):533-36.

(563) Yeshurun, D., Gotto, A.M. J.R., "Drug Treatment of Hyperlipidemia," *Am. J. Med.*, 60, No. 3 (March 1976):379-96.

(564) Alexander, M.R., "Use of Androgens in Chronic Renal Failure Patients on Maintenance Hemodialysis," *Am. J. Hosp. Pharm.*, 33, No. 3 (March 1976):242-48.

(565) Diding, E., Sandstrom, H., Ostelius, J., Karlen, B., Bogentoft, C., "Studies on the Application of Integrated Gas Chromatography-Mass Spectrometry in Drug Purity Control. Impurities in Clofibrate, Norethindrone, Methandienone, Haloperidol and Meladrazine," *Acta Pharm. Suec.*, 13, No. 1 (1976):55-64.

(566) Bellmann, O., Duhme, H.J., Gerhards, E., "In Vitro Studies on Enzymatic Cleavage of Steroid Esters in the Female Organism," *Acta Endocrinol*, (Copenhagen), 1, No. 4 (April 1976):839-53.

(567) Hast, R., Skarberg, K.O., Engstedt, L., Jameson, S., Killander, A., Lundh, B., Reizenstein, P., Uden, A.M., Wadman, B., "Oxymetholone Treatment in Aregenerative Anaemia. II. Remission and Survival - A Prospective Study," *Scand. J. Haematol.*, 16, No. 2 (February 1976):90-100.

(568) Williams, J.R., Griffin, J.P., Parkins, A., "Effect of Concomitantly Administered Drugs on the Control of Long Term Anticoagulant Therapy," *Q.J. Med.*, 45, No. 177 (January 1976):63-73.

(569) Vannie, R., Hilgers, J., "Genetic Analysis of Mammary Tumor Induction and Expression of Mammary Tumor Virus Antigen in Hormone-Treated Ovariectomized GR Mice," *J. Natl. Cancer Inst.*, 56, No. 1 (January 1976):27-32.

(570) Vincent, F., Weintraub, H., Alfsen, A., Baulieu, E.E., " 'Half-of-the-Sites' Reactivity of Steroid Isomerase," *Febs Lett.*, 62, No. 2 (15 February 1976):124-31.

(571) Boyer, J.L., Preisig, R, Sbinden, G., De Kretser, D.M., Wang, C., Paulsen, C.A., "Guidelines for Assessment of Potential Hepatotoxic Effects of Synthetic Androgens, Anobolic Agents and Progestagens in their Use in Males as Antifertility Agents," *Contraception*, 13, No. 4 (April 1976):461-68.

(572) Gravanis, M.D., Majmudar, B.N., "Clinicopathologic Conference: A case of Multiple Myeloma Followed up for 15 Years," *South Med. J.*, 69, No. 2 (February 1976):233-38.

(573) Janda, J., Mrhov, A.O., Urbanov, A.D., Linhart, J., "The Effect of Anabolic Hormone 19-Nortestosterone Propionate on the Metabolism of Striated Muscle during Experimental Ischaemia," *Pfluegers Arch.*, 361, No. 2 (30 January 1976):159-63.

(574) Low-Beer, T.S., Scott, G.L., "Polycythaemia in Androgen-Dependent Aplastic Anaemia," *Br. Med. J.*, 1, No. 6003 (24 January 1976):197-98.

(575) Gribbin, H.R., Matts, S.G., "Mode of Action and Use of Anabolic Steroids," *Br. J. Clin. Pract.*, 30, No. 1 (January 1976):3-5.

(576) Ruvalcaba, R.H., Limbeck, G.A., Tattoni, D.S., Moore, D.C., Kelley, V.C., "Studies of Anabolic Steroids. VIII. Adult Stature of Males with Down Syndrome Treated with Oxandrolone during Childhood," *J. Pediatr.*, 88, No. 3 (March 1976):504-45.

(577) Crocker, S.G., Milton, P.J., King, R.J., "Uptake of (6, 7-3H) Oestradiol-17 Beta by Normal and Abnormal Human Endometrium," *J. Endocrinol*, 62, No. 1 (July 1974):145-52.

(578) Gabb, R.G., Stone, G.M., "Uptake and Metabolism of Tritiated Oestradiol and Oestrone by Human Endometrial and Myometrial Tissue in Vitro," *J. Endocrinol.*, 62, No. 1 (July 1974):109-23.

(579) Briggs, M., "Tetracycline and Steroid Hormone Binding to Human Spermatozoa," *Acta Endocrinol*, (Copenhagen), 75, No. 4 (April 1974):785-92.

(580) Papadimitriou, G., Razis, D., Zis, J., Dracopoulou, I., "Preoperative Hormonal Treatment in Endometrial Carcinoma," *Int. Surg.*, 59, No. 8 (August 1974):397-99.

(581) Mirkin, Gabe, *The Sportsmedicine Book.* Boston: Little, Brown, 1978

(582) Gambrell, R.D., Jr., "Postmenopausal Bleeding," *J. Am. Geriatr. Soc.*, 22, No. 8 (August 1974):337-43.

(583) Koos, E.B., de, "Oestrogen-induced Endometrial Hyperplasia in Gonadal Dysgenesis," *Proc. R. Soc. Med.*, 67, No. 7 (June 1974):590-91.

(584) Danillescu-Goldinberg, D., Branchaud, C., Arato, J., Giroud, C.J., "Metabolism of 14C-Cortisol and 3H-6 Beta Hydroxycortisol during the Neonatal Period. A Case Report," *Steroids Lipids Res.*, 4, No. 5 (1973):351-60.

(585) Kesser u-Ko os, E., Larra naga-Legufa, A., Hurtado-Koo, H., Scharff, II.J., "Fertility Control with Norethindrone Enanthate, a Long-Acting Parenteral Progestogen," *Acta Eur. Fertil.*, 4, No. 4 (December 1973):203-21.

(586) Brook, C.G., Zachmann, M., Prader, A., Murset, G., "Experience with Long-Term Therapy in Congenital Adrenal Hyperplasia," *J. Pediatr.*, 85, No. 1 (July 1974):12-19.

(587) Papaioannou, A.N., "Etiologic Factors in Cancer of the Breast in Humans," *Surg. Gynecol. Obstet.*, 138, No. 2 (February 1974):257-87.

(588) Dewald, G., Spurbeck, J.L., Vitek, H.A., "Chromosomes in a Patient with the Sezary Syndrome," *Mayo Clin. Proc.*, 49, No. 8 (August 1974):553-57.

(589) Dabancens, A., Prado, R., Larraguibel, R., Za nartu, J., "Intraepithelial Cervical Neoplasia in Women using Intrauterine Devices and Long-Acting Injectable Progestogens as Contraceptives," *Am. J. Obstet. Gynecol.*, 119, No. 8 (15

August 1974):1052-56.

(590) Ventura, W.P., Freund, M.J., "The Cross-species Spasmogenic Effects of Semen and Prostatic Gland Fluids on the Motility of the Female Reproductive Tract, in Vitro," *Acta. Eur. Fertil.*, 5, No. 1 (March 1974):73-89.

(591) Bramble, F.J., Houghton, A.L., Eccles, S., O'Shea, A., Jacobs, H.S., "Reproductive and Endocrine Function after Surgical Treatment of Bilateral Crytorchidism," *Lancet*, 2, No. 876 (10 August 1974):311-14.

(592) Gray, L.A., "Some Newer Developments in Gynecologic Cancer," *J. Arkansas Med. Soc.*, 71, No. 3 (August 1974):109-12.

(593) Board, J.A., "When to Discontinue Oral Contraceptives," *Va. Med. Mon.*, 97, No. 10 (October 1970):623-27.

(594) Reiter, E.O., Kulin, H.E., Hamwood, S.M., "The Absence of Positive Feedback between Estrogen and Luteinizing Hormone in Sexually Immature Girls," *Pediatr. Res.*, 8, No. 8 (August 1974):740-45.

(595) Pinsky, L., Kaufman, M., Straisfeld, C., Shanfield, B., "Lack of Difference in Tetosterone Metabolism between Cultured Skin Fibroblasts of Human Adult Males and Females," *J. Clin. Endocrinol. Metab.*, 39, No. 2 (August 1974):395-98.

(596) Novak, E.R., "The Endometrium," *Clin. Obstet. Gynecol.*, 17, No. 2 (June 1974):31-49.

(597) Wilcox, C.S., Aminoff, M.J., Penn, W., "Basis of Nocturnal Polyuria in Patients with Autonomic Failure," *J. Neurol. Neurosurg. Psychiatry*, 37, No. 6 (June 1974):677-84.

(598) Nankin, H.R., Talbott, J.B., Oshima, H, Fan, D.F., Pan, S.F., Troen, P., "Down and Klinefelter Syndromes (48, XXY, G+) in a Young Man. Cytogenetic Endocrine and Testicular Steroidogenesis Studies," *Arch. Intern. Med.*, 134, No. 2 (August 1974):352-58.

(599) Casthely, S., Maheswaran, C., Levy, J., "Laparoscopy: An Important Tool in the Diagnosis of Rokitansky-Kuster-Hauser Syndrome," *Am. J. Obstet. Gynecol.*, 119, No. 4 (15 June 1974):571-72.

(600) Reddy, P.R., "Proceedings: Reversible Contraceptive Action of Testosterone in Males," *J. Reprod. Fertil.*, 38, No. 1 (May 1974):232.

(601) Uematsu, K., Morimura, Y., Matsumoto, K., Koto, K., Tsujino, G., Minagawa, J., Miyaji, T., "Leprechaunism (Donohue's Syndrome)—Two Autopsy Cases," *Acta Pathol. Jap.*, 24, No. 2 (March 1974):309-24.

(602) Beckett, Arnold, *Personal Communication*, August, 1978 with E.C. Percy.

(603) Glendhill, N., Buick, F.G., Froese, A.B., Spriet, L., and Myers, E.C., "An Optimal Method of Storing Blood for Blood Doping," *Med. Science in Sports*, 10, (1978):40.

(604) McCollum, E.V., *A History of Nutrition*. Boston: Houghton, Mifflin Co., 1957.

(605) Goldblith, S.A. and Joslyn, M.A., *Milestones in Nutrition*. Westport, Conn.: Avi Publishing Co., 1964.

(606) Hopkins, F.G., *The Analyst*, 31 (1906):385; Hopkins, F.G., *J. Physiol.* (London), 44 (1912):425.

(607) Funk, C.J., *State Medicine*, 20 (1912):341.

(608) Drummond, J.C., *Biochem. J.*, 14 (1920):660.

(609) Gyorgy, P. and Eckardt, R.E., *Nature*, 144 (1939):512.

(610) Axelrod, A.E. and Traketellis, A.C., *Vitamins and Hormones*, 22 (1964):581.

(611) Watt, B.K. and Merrill, A.L., *Composition of Foods: Raw, Processed, Prepared*, U.S.D.A. Handbook No. 8, Washington, D.C., 1963.

(612) Orr, M.L., "Pantothenic Acid, Vitamin B-6 and Vitamin B-12 in Foods," U.S.D.A., Washington, D.C., *Home Economics Res. Rep.*, 36, 1969.

(613) Hardinge, M.G. and Crooks, H., *Journal American Dietet. Assoc.*, 38 (1961):240.

(614) Underwood, E.J., *Trace Elements in Human and Animal Nutriton*, 3rd ed. New York: Academic Press, 1971.

(615) Holmberg, C.G. and Laurell, C.B., *Acta Chem. Scan.*, 1 (1947):944; Bates, G.W. and Wernicke, J., *J. Biol. Chem.*, 246 (1971):3679.

(616) Multani, J.S., Cepurneek, C.P., Davis, P.S., and Saltman, P., *Biochem.*, 9 (1970):3970.

(617) Holmberg, C.G. and Laurell, C.B., *Acta Chem. Scand.*, 2 (1948):550; Frieden, E., *Nutr. Rev.*, 28 (1970):87; Osaki, S., Johnson, D.A., and Frieden, E., *J. Biol. Chem.*, 246 (1971):3018.

(618) Dyment, P.G., "Drug Misuse by Adolescent Athletes," *Pediatr. Clin. North Am.*, No. 6 (29 December 1982):1363-69.

(619) Solberg, S., "Anabolic Steroids and Norwegian Weightlifters," *Br. J. Sports Med.*, 16, No. 3 (1982):169-71.

(620) Sledhill, N., "Blood Doping and Related Issues: A Brief Review," *Med. Sci. Sports Exerc.*, 14, No. 3 (1982):183-89.

(621) Lucking, M.T., "Steroid Hormones in Sports. Special Reference: Sex Hormones and Their Derivatives," *Int. J. Sports Med.*, Suppl. 1, (February 1982):65-67.

(622) Horwitz, D.L., "Drugs and the Athlete, (editorial),*Compr. Ther.*, (8 March 1982):3-4.

(623) Beckett, A.H., "Use and Abuse of Drugs in Sport," *J. Biosoc Sci.* (suppl.), 7 (1981):163-78.

(624) Mangi, R.J. and Jokl, P., "Drugs and Sport," *Conn. Med.*, 45, No. 10 (October 1981):637-41.

(625) Laties, V.G. and Weiss, B., "The Amphetamine Margin in Sports," *Fed. Proc.*, 40, No. 12 (October 1981):2689-92.

(626) Burks, T.F., "Drug Use in Athletics: Introduction," *Fed. Proc.*, 40, No. 12 (October 1981):2690-91.

(627) Lucking, M.T., "Experimental Random Spot Testing for Drugs in Sportsmen," *Br. J. Sports Med.*, 15, No. 1 (March 1981):33.

(628) Arblaster, C.I. and Blackman, G.L., "Drugs in Sport: The Extent of the Problem, Toxic Effects, and Control," *Aust. Fam. Physician.*, 10, No. 3 (March 1981):145-46, 148.

(629) Massey, P.M., "General Practitioner at the Olympic Games," *Br. Med. J. Clin. Res.*, 282, No. 6277 (23 May 1981):1675-76.

(630) Wright, James, *Anabolic Steroids and Sports*, volume II.

(631) Todd, Terry, "The Steroid Predicament," *Sports Illustrated* (1 August 1983):63-78.

(632) Annitto, W.J. and Layman, W.A., "Anabolic Steroids and Acute Schizophrenic Episode," *J. Clin. Psych.*, 41, No. 4 (April 1980).

(633) Mandell, A.J. and Stewart, K.D., "The Sunday Syndrome: From Kinetics to Altered Consciousness," *Fed. Proc.*, 40, No. 12 (October 1981):2693-98.

INDEX

About the Author

ROBERT M. GOLDMAN HAS BEEN A COMPETITIVE ATHLETE SINCE THE AGE OF TWELVE. COMPETING IN SIX SPORTS IN HIGH SCHOOL AND FOUR IN COLLEGE, HE WAS THE NEW YORK ALL-CITY WRESTLING CHAMPION, MIDDLE LINEBACKER ON THREE ALL-CITY FOOTBALL TEAMS, ALL-CITY TRACK AND FIELD SHOT-PUTTER, AND THE UNDEFEATED ALL-COLLEGE PHYSICAL FITNESS CHAMPION, 1973-76. BOB STILL HOLDS NUMEROUS COLLEGE AND NEW YORK PHYSICAL FITNESS MARKS.

THE THREE-TIME WINNER OF THE J.F.K. PHYSICAL FITNESS AWARD, HE WAS ALSO A YMCA POWERLIFTING CHAMPION AND IS A BLACK BELT IN KARATE. HE WAS VOTED ATHLETE OF THE YEAR IN 1981 AND 1982 BY KING OF FITNESS CORPORATION AND WAS THE RECIPIENT OF THE 1983 CHAMPIONS AWARD. HE HAS BEEN SETTING WORLD RECORDS FOR OVER A DECADE AND HOLDS SEVERAL RECORDS RECOGNIZED BY *THE GUINNESS BOOK OF WORLD RECORDS.*

HE GRADUATED FROM BROOKLYN COLLEGE IN 1977, AFTER WHICH HE DID THREE YEARS OF POSTGRADUATE RESEARCH IN ANABOLIC STEROIDS. AT PRESENT, HE IS A FELLOW IN SPORTS MEDICINE AT THE CHICAGO COLLEGE OF OSTEOPATHIC MEDICINE.

HE HAS AUTHORED MORE THAN FIFTY ARTICLES IN PHYSICAL CULTURE MAGAZINES AND A NUMBER OF SCIENTIFIC PAPERS IN MEDICAL JOURNALS, MOST RECENTLY BEING THE FIRST CLINICAL RESEARCH STUDY EVER PUBLISHED EVALUATING THE PHSYIOLOGICAL EFFECTS OF GRAVITY INVERSION BOOTS.

IN 1980, HE WAS INDUCTED INTO THE WORLD HALL OF FAME FOR BODY BUILDING AND PHYSICAL FITNESS FOR HIS RESEARCH IN COMBATING STEROID ABUSE. HE IS INTENT ON SPECIALIZING IN SPORTS INJURY PREVENTION AND REHABILITATION

HIS CLOSE WORKING RELATIONSHIP WITH THE LATE JOHN B. ZIEGLER, M.D., HAS RESULTED IN DR. ZIEGLER BESTOWING ON HIS DISCIPLE ALL HIS RESEARCH AND WORK. DR. ZIEGLER, THE "FATHER OF SPORTS MEDICINE," WAS U.S. NATIONAL TEAM PHYSICIAN DURING THE 1950S AND WAS THE FIRST TO REFINE ANABOLIC STEROIDS (WITH CIBA PHARMACEUTICAL), CREATING THE FORMULA FOR DIANABOL. HE WAS THE FIRST MAN TO NOTE THE SOVIETS USING THESE DRUGS IN THE OLYMPICS AND WAS THE MAN WHO BROUGHT THEM BACK TO THIS COUNTRY, ONLY TO SEE THEM ABUSED. HIS SUBSEQUENT REJECTION AND FIGHT AGAINST ANABOLIC STEROIDS WAS EVEN MORE EMPHATIC THAN HIS ORIGINAL ADVOCACY OF THEM.

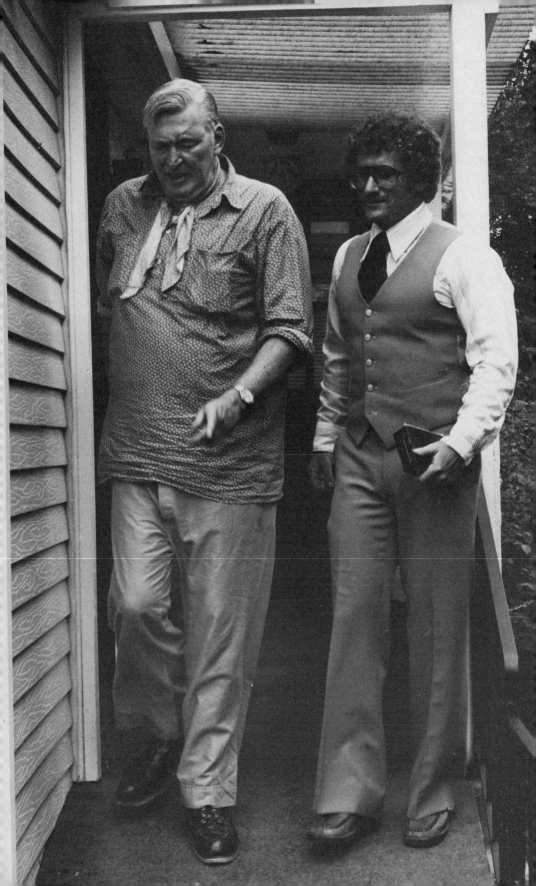